Endoscopic Skull Base Surgery

Endoscopic Skull Base Surgery

A Comprehensive Guide with Illustrative Cases

Hrayr K. Shahinian, MD, FACS

Co-Authors

M. S. Kabil, MD
R. Jarrahy, MD
M.-P. Thill, MD

Humana Press

Author
Hrayr K. Shahinian
Skull Base Institute
Los Angeles, CA 90048, USA
Shahinian@skullbaseinstitute.com

ISBN 978-1-61737-790-7 e-ISBN 978-1-59745-340-0

DOI: 10.1007/978-1-59745-340-0

Cover Design by Jadi Communications

Front Cover Image:

Skull Base and Brain Anatomy including Facial Nerves and Internal Carotid Artery. 0 Degree 4mm Neuroendoscope.

Back Cover Images:

Left Foreground Image: Endoscopic Supraorbital Approach.
Right Foreground Image: Endoscopic Retromastoid Approach.
Right Mid Image: Pituitary Resection.
Right Background Image: Endoscopic Endonasal Approach.

Printed on acid-free paper.

9 8 7 6 5 4 3 2 1

springer.com

Author

Hrayr K. Shahinian, MD, FACS
Director, Skull Base Institute
Los Angeles, California

Co-Authors

Mohamed S. Kabil, MD
Lecturer of Neurosurgery
Department of Neurosurgery, Faculty of Medicine,
Ain Shams University, Cairo, Egypt
Research Associate,
Skull Base Institute, Los Angeles, California

Reza Jarrahy, MD
Assistant Professor
Division of Plastic and Reconstructive Surgery,
UCLA School of Medicine,
Skull Base Surgery Fellow,
Skull Base Institute, Los Angeles, California

Marie-Paule Thill, MD
Associate Chief of Service,
Otolaryngology and Head and Neck Surgery,
St. Peter University Medical Center, Brussels, Belgium

Contributors

René Chapot, MD
Professor of Neuroradiology
Head of Department of Interventional Neuroradiology
Krupp Krankenhaus
Essen, Germany

Theodore C. Friedman, MD, PhD
Chief, Division of Endocrinology, Metabolism and Molecular Medicine
Charles R. Drew University of Medicine and Science, Associate Professor of Medicine,
UCLA School of Medicine, Los Angeles, California
Director
Endocrinology Fellowship Program, Charles R. Drew University of Medicine and Science

Richard J. Tamman, MD
Attending Anesthesiologist,
Cedars-Sinai Medical Center, Los Angeles, California

Ahmed B. ElSerwi, MD
Consultant of Interventional Neuroradiology,
Ain Shams University Specialized Hospital,
Cairo, Egypt

— *To my wife Leslie and children Alexander and Karina for their patience with my long hours and for giving me the joys of fatherhood every single day.*

— *To my parents Karnig and Maro, my grandmother Makrouhi, and my sisters Houry and Lara for my education and making me who I am.*

— *To my surgical teachers, mentors, true masters—Block, Shehadeh, Sawyers, Herrington, Edwards, Abumrad, McCarthy, Baker, Beasley, Thorne, Tabbal, Siebert, Kassabian, Fisch, Sanna, Magnan, and many others—for inspiring me and guiding my professional career.*

— *To my critics ... for strengthening my resolve.*

Foreword

I am honored to be asked to write a foreword to this comprehensive and fascinating book on skull base surgery (SBS) by Dr. Shahinian, who I consider among the pioneers in the field. I should start by writing a disclaimer. I first met Dr. Shahinian when he was a brilliant surgical resident at Vanderbilt University Medical Center in 1986. Over the next several years, I had the pleasure of following his career through different training rotations in the United States and abroad. I remember well when he told me that skull base surgery was his career choice. I thought it was a high-risk career move considering that the discipline was still in its early development. As a result, I was quite gratified to follow Dr. Shahinian's professional success as he developed the Skull Base Institute, initially in New York, and later in Los Angeles.

I would like to first define SBS from my perspective as a general surgeon. SBS denotes a group of operations involving the base of the skull or its contents. The skull base is divided into an anterior (attached to the facial skeleton), middle, and posterior areas. Vital arteries, veins, as well as cranial nerves pass through the skull base. Consequently, this part of the skull has historically been the most difficult to access, and lesions of the skull base were often associated with a poor prognosis.

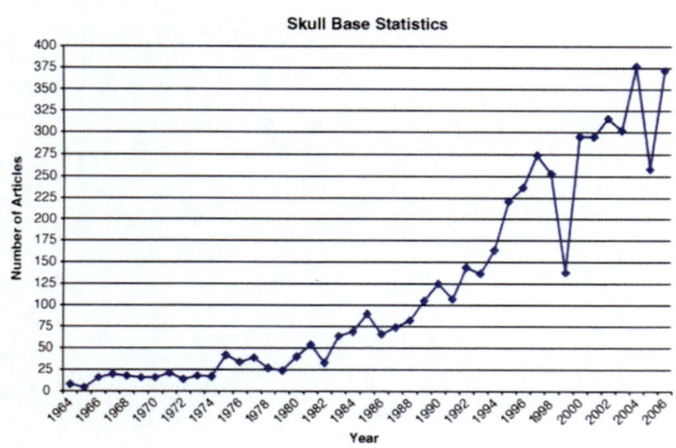

A recent search of PubMed and Google databases for "Skull Base Surgery" revealed the significant recent progress in the field. As shown in the graph, the number of published scientific articles related to SBS experienced an exponential rise beginning in the mid-1980s. This reflected major advances in technology and technical expertise that pushed firmly the field forward. Advances in imaging (computed tomography; magnetic resonance imaging [MRI], including intraoperative MRI, ultrasound); instrumentation (frameless stereotaxy, ultrasonic aspirators, etc.); microscopy; endoscopy; and anesthetic techniques played a major role. A major benefit of this progress has been the significant improvements in the diagnosis and management of skull base tumors with improved mortality and morbidity.

This book, with its comprehensive illustration of surgical cases and techniques, should serve as a valuable reference to physicians and health practitioners in many medical specialties. Although skull base surgery is a discipline that for some would be classified as a branch of one specific specialty, canvassing the related literature makes it clear that such a classification is too narrow. Possibly this is best reflected by the decision of the only journal dedicated to the field *Skull Base* to drop the word *Surgery* from its title. It is also supported by the realization that advances to SBS have come from various surgical and nonsurgical specialties. A quick survey of the articles in *Skull Base* indicates that they are largely interdisciplinary in nature. A partial and nonexhaustive list of contributors would include those in surgical disciplines such as head and neck surgery, neurosurgery, plastic and reconstructive surgery, general surgery, otolaryngology, and neuro-ophthalmology and nonsurgical clinical disciplines such as radiology (particularly neuroradiology), intensive care medicine, optics, and basic sciences such as physics, biochemistry, and so on. The gamut of these disciplines now usually forms what has become known as "skull base centers."

Like all surgical disciplines, the advances in the field of SBS have favored less-invasive surgical approaches. The first and clever use of an endonasal transseptal, transsphenoidal approach to resect a pituitary tumor was performed by a Viennese otolaryngologist, Dr. Oskar Hirsch, in 1910. Since then, the procedure has been refined and become widely practiced. SBS has also developed a battery of minimally invasive techniques or adapted those developed by other disciplines. A survey of PubMed and Google reveals 104 publications in that field for the same time period shown in the graph, again published by a multitude of investigators in various subspecialties. Based on our experience of the technical progress in the fields of general surgery and obstetrics and gynecology, it is reasonable to expect that the trend toward less-invasive procedures will continue and even accelerate. Conceivably, the majority of procedures currently carried out by skull base surgeons (and for that matter, neurosurgeons, otolaryngologists, head and neck surgeons, neuro-otologists, and others) will be performed in the not too distant future using minimally invasive approaches. If anything, this will continue to make SBS even more multidisciplinary, increasing the potential contribution of this unique book.

Naji N. Abumrad, *MD, FACS*
John L. Sawyers, Professor and Chairman,
Department of Surgery,
Vanderbilt University School of Medicine,
Nashville, Tennessee

Preface

At every crossing on the road that leads to the future, each progressive spirit is opposed by a thousand appointed to guard the past.

Maurice Maeterlinck

As a medical student, I was confounded by the skull base and its insurmountable portrayal as "no man's land." During my 9 years of postgraduate training, I had the inspiring privilege of learning from master surgeons from different subspecialties around the world in my quest to find solutions, studying general surgery, plastic and reconstructive surgery, neurosurgery, otolaryngology, and vascular surgery in cities such as Chicago, Nashville, New York, Zurich, Marseilles, and Piacenza. It is this expansive, hybrid training, along with rigorous fellowships in craniofacial surgery and skull base microsurgery, that has allowed me to exclusively devote the last 15 years of my practice to demystifying the art and science of skull base surgery.

To date, more than 3,000 brain and skull base tumors, along with various vascular problems, have been treated using advanced, fully endoscopic, minimally invasive techniques that were first introduced in 1996. These techniques have been continually refined and progressively evolving at the Skull Base Institute since that time.

This book is the product of my journey and is dedicated to future generations of skull base surgeons whose pursuit of medical excellence will inevitably advance this challenging field down the road that leads to the future. In doing so, they shall continue our mission as physicians to fulfill our duty and destiny in alleviating suffering and proudly honoring the gift of healing.

Hrayr K. Shahinian, MD, FACS
Director
Skull Base Institute
Los Angeles, California

Contents

AUTHOR v

CO-AUTHORS vii

CONTRIBUTORS ix

DEDICATION xi

FOREWORD xiii

PREFACE xv

1. Introduction 1

1. The Evolution from the Open Craniotomy to Fully Endoscopic Skull Base Surgery 1
2. Endoscopic Skull Base Surgery in Practice 2

2. Anesthetic Considerations in Endoscopic Skull Base Surgery 5

1. Introduction 5
2. Preoperative Assessment 5
3. General Considerations 6
4. Special Considerations 6
5. Future Challenges 9

3. Neuroendocrine Aspects of Skull Base Surgery 11

1. Introduction 11
2. Pituitary Tumors 12
3. Hormonal Deficiencies Caused by Pituitary Tumors 16
4. Long-term Follow-up of Patients with a Pituitary Tumor 18

4. Interventional Neuroradiology Aspects of Skull Base Surgery 21

1. Introduction 21
2. Embolization of Skull Base Tumors 21
3. Test and Permanent Occlusion of the Internal Carotid Artery 25
4. Inferior Petrosal Sinus Sampling 26

5. Instrumentation in Endoscopic Skull Base Surgery 29

1. Introduction 29
2. Rigid Endoscopes 29
3. Irrigation Sheaths and Pumps 29
4. Pneumatic Holding Arms 30
5. Xenon Light Sources 31
6. High-Definition Digital Cameras 31
7. Digital Monitors 31
8. DVD Recorders 31
9. Polaroid Digital Printers 31
10. Cranial Nerve Monitors 31
11. Microdrill Handpieces, Attachments, and Burrs 32
12. Micro-Cavitron Ultrasonic Surgical Aspirator (MicroCUSA) Handpieces and Tips 32
13. Specialized Endoscopic Microinstruments 33

6. The Fully Endoscopic Endonasal Approach 43

1. Introduction 43
2. Indications 43
3. Instrumentation 43
4. Operating Room Setup 43
5. Patient Positioning 44
6. Operative Technique 45
7. Illustrative Cases 48
8. Potential Complications 60
9. Avoiding Complications in Author's Experience 65

7. The Fully Endoscopic Transglabellar Approach 73

1. Introduction 73
2. Indications 73
3. Instrumentation 73
4. Operating Room Setup 73
5. Patient Positioning 74
6. Operative Technique 74
7. Illustrative Cases 76
8. Potential Complications 80
9. Avoiding Complications in Author's Experience 82

8. The Fully Endoscopic Supraorbital Approach 89

1. Introduction 89
2. Indications 89
3. Instrumentation 90
4. Operating Room Setup 90
5. Patient Positioning 90
6. Operative Technique 90
7. Illustrative Cases 93
8. Potential Complications 101
9. Avoiding Complications in Author's Experience 107

9. The Fully Endoscopic Retrosigmoid Approach 109

1. Introduction 109
2. Indications 109
3. Instrumentation 109
4. Operating Room Setup 109
5. Patient Positioning 110
6. Operative Technique 110
7. Illustrative Cases 113
8. Potential Complications 130
9. Avoiding Complications in Author's Experience 171

10. The Fully Endoscopic Subtemporal Approach 173

1. Introduction 173
2. Indications 173
3. Instrumentation 173
4. Operating Room Setup 174
5. Patient Positioning 174
6. Operative Technique 174
7. Illustrative Cases 178
8. Potential Complications 179
9. Avoiding Complications in Author's Experience 183

Index 189

1 Introduction

This chapter discusses the evolution from traditional surgical approaches to the anterior, middle, and posterior skull base to fully endoscopic skull base surgery. The field of skull base surgery is currently being transformed into an endoscopy-based specialty that is distinguished by excellent outcomes, shorter operating times, faster recoveries, fewer complications, and overall decreased patient morbidity. The chapter provides insight into the practice of fully endoscopic skull base surgery at the Skull Base Institute in Los Angeles, California. These techniques are routinely used in the surgical management of anterior, middle, and posterior skull base tumors, both primary and recurrent, as well as for various neurovascular compression syndromes, such as trigeminal neuralgia, hemifacial spasm, and others. In our experience, these endoscopic techniques have provided superior access and resulted in better surgical results and an unsurpassed intraoperative definition of neurovascular conflicts and tumor morphologies. More than 90% of all patients undergoing endoscopic skull base surgery are discharged from the hospital within 48 h of their operation.

Keywords: Brain; Endonasal; Endoscope; Endoscopic; Keyhole; Minimally invasive; Pituitary; Retrosigmoid; Skull base; Subtemporal; Supraorbital; Surgery; Surgical; Transglabellar.

1. THE EVOLUTION FROM THE OPEN CRANIOTOMY TO FULLY ENDOSCOPIC SKULL BASE SURGERY

For decades, surgeons interested in the field of skull base surgery have debated which techniques provide the best access to the skull base with the least amount of associated risk. Traditional approaches to the anterior, middle, and posterior skull base have included complex transcranial or transfacial operations. These procedures, facilitated by progress in the designs of surgical instruments and advances in perioperative intensive care, have afforded excellent exposure, allowing for complete removal of massive tumors. However, these open procedures have also been associated with significant morbidity and long-term convalescence; the burden on the patient has been great. As a result, the evolution of skull base surgery over the past decade has been characterized by an emphasis on the development of minimally invasive techniques that do not compromise surgical outcomes but do significantly diminish the perioperative burden on the patient.

Innovations in medical technology have again provided the raw materials needed for this progress. Advances in fiber-optic technology, including improved design of endoscopes, light sources, video cameras, and special microinstruments, have culminated in the development of safe and effective alternatives to traditional neurosurgical, neuro-otologic, and craniofacial techniques. From its original reliance on microsurgical techniques, the field of skull base surgery is currently being transformed into an endoscopy-based specialty that is distinguished by excellent outcomes, shorter operating times, faster recoveries, fewer complications, and overall decreased patient morbidity (Fig. 1A, B).

Progress is continuing, changing many scenarios in daily clinical life. The expectation of achieving the greatest therapeutic effect with the least iatrogenic injury is higher now than ever. In addition, because of excellent diagnostic modalities such as computed tomography and magnetic resonance imaging, smaller lesions are being encountered, resulting in the increased use of early surgery. The best way to preserve collateral structures is not to touch them and, even better, not to expose them. Wide exposure of the brain, skull, and soft tissues under nonphysiological circumstances for several hours is certainly undesirable.

The main purpose of the keyhole approach is to use a more targeted approach that eliminates many of the steps necessary with conventional approaches. Although the radical cranial base approaches are well established and their features are widely

From: *Endoscopic Skull Base Surgery: A Comprehensive Guide with Illustrative Cases.*
Edited by H. K. Shahinian © Humana Press, Totowa, NJ.

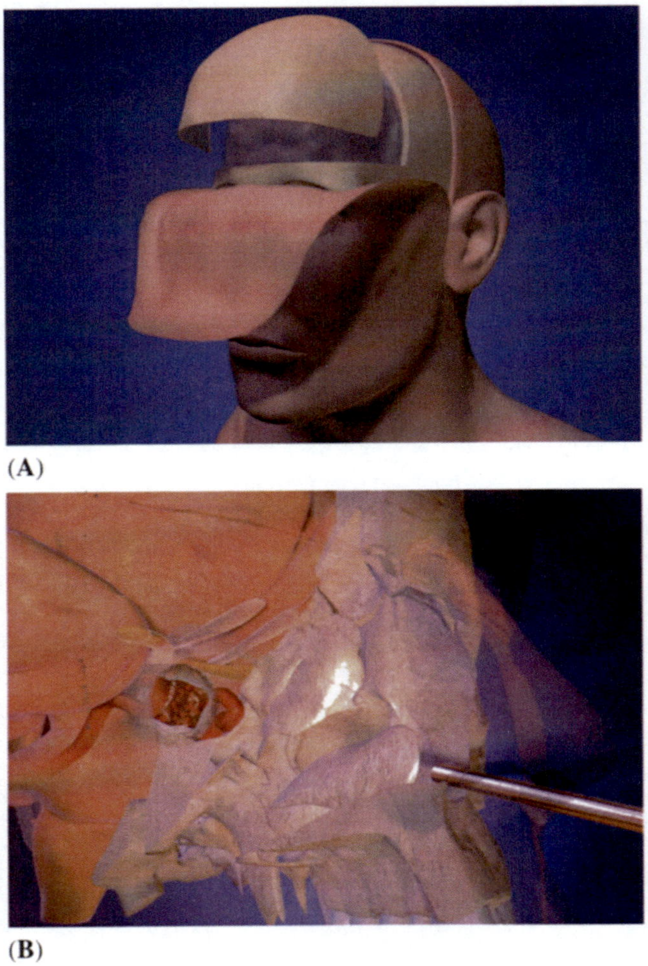

Fig. 1 **A** Traditional bifrontal. **B** Endoscopic endonasal.

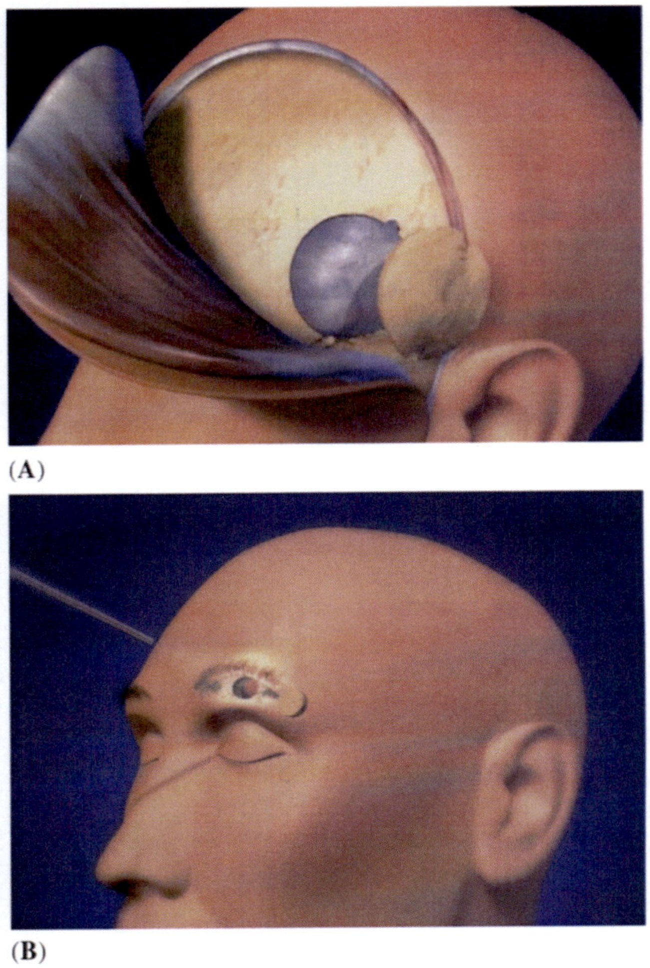

Fig. 2 **A** Traditional pterional. **B** Endoscopic supraorbital.

recognized, it is not always necessary to resect or expose wide extracranial or intracranial compartments. The more the cranial base techniques become established, the more they can be refined and limited to the essential compartment. As this process is accelerated, lesions will be diagnosed when they are smaller, and the extent of the craniotomy will be reduced as a result (Fig. 2A, B).

Selecting short, direct, and precise routes to brain and skull base lesions without manipulating and exposing unaffected areas is essential for keyhole surgery. Because the surgeon does not have the flexibility to correct the angle of approach during the procedure, the surgeon must be familiar with the anatomic features of keyhole craniotomy to determine its adequate location and size in each case. Precise knowledge about three-dimensional space characteristics of the target region with its corresponding windows is indispensable. Furthermore, affected structures are commonly displaced, so the individual anatomy and concomitantly the individual approach need to be evaluated in detail for each patient preoperatively.

The parallel use of rigid lens scopes during open microsurgical procedures offers an enormously increased panoramic overview with excellent visual quality in deep and narrow fields. Furthermore, this not only helps to inspect vessels and nerves around corners but also assists in manipulating and resecting residual lesions beyond the direct view of the microscope. With the endoscope attached to the holding arm, two-hand manipulation with regular microsurgical instruments beside the endoscope is feasible. This endoscope-assisted microsurgical technique is an important transitional step between traditional open techniques and fully endoscopic techniques and may provide the surgeon a gradual learning opportunity (Fig. 3A, B).

2. ENDOSCOPIC SKULL BASE SURGERY IN PRACTICE

For the past decade at the Skull Base Institute in Los Angeles, California, we have been performing endoscope-assisted and fully endoscopic surgery of the anterior, middle, and posterior skull base. Applications of endoscopy at our institution have included treatment of primary and recurrent pituitary tumors (both with and without suprasellar extension); treatment of the various neurovascular compression syndromes (trigeminal neuralgia, hemifacial spasm, glossopharyngeal neuralgia, spasmodic torticollis) at the cerebellopontine angle (CPA); removal of vestibular schwannomas and other CPA tumors; as well as resection of various other skull base lesions, both malignant and benign. More than 90% of all patients undergoing endoscopic procedures of the skull base are discharged from the hospital within 48 h.

For many indications, we now use only fully endoscopic techniques via keyhole craniotomy access points; the need for extensive craniotomies for intracranial exposure and retraction

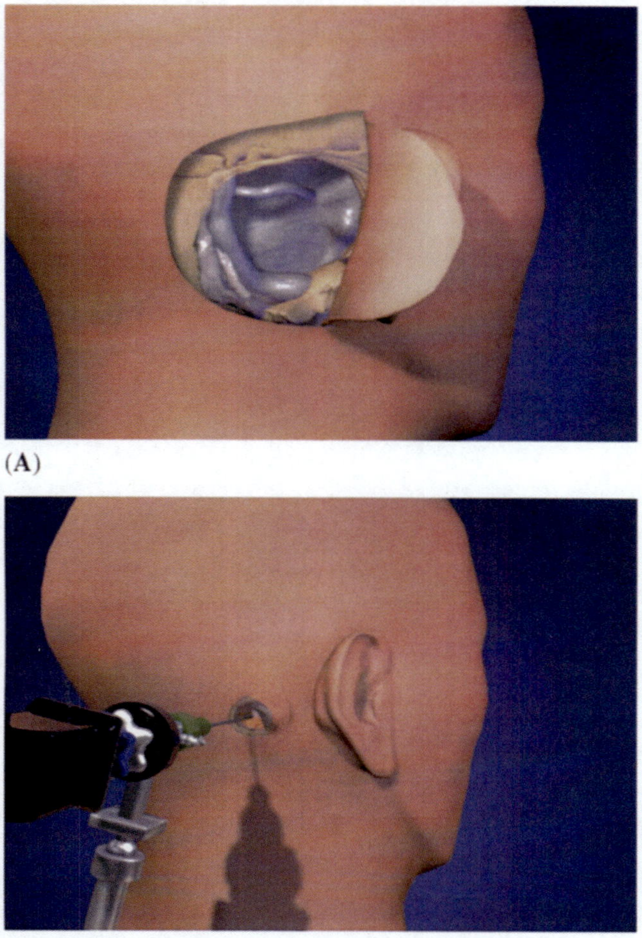
(A)
(B)

Fig. 3 **A** Traditional translabyrinthine. **B** Endoscopic retrosigmoid.

has been all but obviated. Visualization of the relevant anatomy has proven to be improved over microscopic imaging. Endonasal, supraorbital, transglabellar, retrosigmoid, subtemporal, and other tailored keyhole approaches have made virtually all skull base tumors amenable to endoscopic resection. Rigid endoscopes of varying lengths and angles of view have broadened the available surgical exposure without the need for additional dissection or retraction; the resulting panoramic perspectives of the surgical field have allowed for thorough evaluations of the extent of intracranial disease. The maneuverability of the endoscope has allowed the surgeon to position it directly at the level of dissection, effectively reducing the viewing and operating distances.

In pituitary surgery, this has meant abandoning the transseptal–transsphenoidal microscopic technique in favor of a completely endoscopic endonasal approach. For larger tumors with significant suprasellar extension, endoscopic transcranial approaches—whether transglabellar or supraorbital—in conjunction with the endoscopic endonasal approach have been effective adjuncts that provide significantly less-invasive alternatives to traditional transcranial approaches to the floor of the anterior fossa. Surgical outcomes and complication rates of endoscopic pituitary surgery have compared favorably to those that have been reported in large series of patients who have undergone microscopic transseptal pituitary surgery. At the CPA, the use of endoscopy, particularly implementing rigid endoscopes of varying angles of view, has vastly improved visualization around the contour of the petrous portion of the temporal bone, one of the most significant impediments to exposure using traditional microscopic techniques. In our experience this superior access has resulted in better surgical results due to better intraoperative definition of neurovascular conflicts and tumor morphology.

We offer this atlas as a resource for current practitioners of skull base surgery as well as students of the discipline. It contains detailed intraoperative photos demonstrating the endoscopic surgical anatomy encountered in a variety of approaches to the skull base, as well as rendered schematic images that assist in presurgical planning. It is our hope that this work will contribute to the ongoing evolution of minimally invasive skull base surgery.

2 Anesthetic Considerations in Endoscopic Skull Base Surgery

This chapter discusses the unique challenges that endoscopic skull base surgery present to the neuroanesthesiologist. The neuroanesthesiology team plays a vital role in ensuring a safe outcome to this delicate surgery. Highly specialized endoscopic techniques and equipment, together with the use of sophisticated intraoperative monitoring, all mandate skillful anesthesia management that is tailored to the needs of minimally invasive, fully endoscopic skull base surgery. The specific neuroanesthetic considerations for fully endoscopic endonasal, supraorbital, and retrosigmoid approaches as well as future challenges are discussed.

Keywords: Anesthesia; Endonasal; Endoscopic; Minimally invasive; Neuroanesthesiologist; Neuroanesthesiology; Neuroanesthetic; Retrosigmoid; Skull base; Supraorbital; Surgery; Surgical.

1. INTRODUCTION

Endoscopic skull base surgery represents a major advance in patient outcome and recovery. It also presents a unique challenge to the neuroanesthesiologist. Highly specialized endoscopic techniques and equipment, together with the use of sophisticated intraoperative monitoring, all mandate skillful anesthetic management that is tailored to the needs of minimally invasive, fully endoscopic skull base surgery. The neuroanesthesiology team plays a vital role in ensuring a safe outcome to this delicate surgery.

2. PREOPERATIVE ASSESSMENT

Patients undergoing skull base surgery commonly present with coexisting manifestations of their operative disease. Perioperative management of patients with endocrine and other neurological disorders has been well covered in the literature; however, patients with pituitary neoplasms present frequently enough for endoscopic skull base surgery to warrant a review of anesthesia management for these patients.

Pituitary adenomas cause a spectrum of presenting symptoms. They are the most common cause of hypopituitarism in patients presenting for pituitary resection. Less common causes of hypopituitarism include Rathke's cleft cysts and childhood craniopharyngiomas. Patients with pituitary hypofunction are usually receiving hormone replacement therapy that must be continued perioperatively. They also typically require "stress" doses of corticosteroids on the day of surgery.

All patients undergoing pituitary surgery are at risk for perioperative antidiuretic hormone (ADH) deficiency, which presents clinically as diabetes insipidus (DI). The production of large volumes of dilute urine can result in dangerously high serum osmolality, and both urine output and serum osmolality should be monitored closely, with replacement of vasopressin/ADH as indicated.

Pituitary hyperfunction may also be present in patients presenting for skull base surgery. Most common are prolactin-secreting adenomas, but of more concern are the adenomas responsible for Cushing's disease and acromegaly. Patients with a pituitary adenoma secreting ACTH (corticotropin) present with classic symptoms of Cushing's disease. Adrenocorticoid excess leads to obesity with centripetal fat accumulation, hypertension, osteopenia, fluid retention, and hyperglycemia. Perioperative testing should include careful monitoring of serum glucose and serum electrolytes, which may be deranged as a result of mineralocorticoid-induced effects. The neuroanesthesiologist should take into account the obesity and possible delayed gastric emptying that may be present, as well as the risk of pathologic fractures during positioning at the time of surgery.

Growth hormone-secreting pituitary adenomas cause acromegaly. Of particular concern to the neuroanesthesiologist is the thickened, enlarged tongue, which may complicate laryngoscopy and endotracheal intubation. In addition, cartilaginous hypertrophy of the arytenoids and tracheal rings may actually narrow the patient's functioning airway, necessitating smaller-caliber

From: *Endoscopic Skull Base Surgery: A Comprehensive Guide with Illustrative Cases.*
Edited by H. K. Shahinian © Humana Press, Totowa, NJ.

endotracheal tubes. Both airway abnormalities may also contribute to postoperative airway obstruction, especially if deep extubation is attempted.

3. GENERAL CONSIDERATIONS

Fully endoscopic skull base surgery presents a unique operating room environment for the neuroanesthesiologist. The skull base surgeon uses highly advanced technology to perform the surgery, including complex robotic equipment to fix the endoscopes and other instruments in place, thus freeing both hands for bimanual dexterity. The patient's head is typically fixed in a Mayfield three-pin head clamp in a position that affords good surgical access. However, for the neuroanesthesiologist, this position provides poor access to the patient's face and airway. All hoses, intravenous lines, arterial lines, and the like must be of sufficient length to provide secure "long-distance" anesthesia, and special care must be given to securing the patient's airway. For emergency vascular access, it is a good idea to have the patient's foot exposed and easily accessible.

Large-bore intravenous and arterial lines are usually indicated in intracranial procedures, and central venous access may be considered if the potential for venous air embolism is high. Armored endotracheal tubes are used to prevent the tube from becoming kinked or obstructed; this is especially important in retrosigmoid approaches, for which repeated jaw clenching may result from cranial nerve stimulation. Of paramount importance during endoscopic skull base surgery is a stationary field; any patient movement carries the risk of intracranial injury by the endoscope or endoscopic instruments and the risk of possible spine injury from the head being fixed in the Mayfield frame.

4. SPECIAL CONSIDERATIONS

4.1. NEUROANESTHESIA FOR THE FULLY ENDOSCOPIC ENDONASAL APPROACH (FIG. 1) The fully endoscopic endonasal approach to the pituitary gland and its surrounding structures involves some intranasal dissection and dilation, turbinate manipulation, or out-fracture and approaching the sella turcica through the posterior nasopharynx. These structures are very vascular, and surgical visualization can be severely compromised by bleeding. Therefore, the neuroanesthesiologist should maintain blood pressure in the low-normal range throughout the whole surgery. This can be quite challenging as endonasal surgery elicits a strong sympathetic response; thus, a combination of deep anesthesia and antihypertensive medications is usually necessary. A balanced narcotic/inhalational anesthetic technique may be supplemented by propofol infusion. Intermittent or continuous infusion of antihypertensive drugs such as labetalol and sodium nitroprusside constitutes the next line of therapy. It is advisable, of course, to perform continuous intra-arterial blood pressure monitoring.

Endoscopic endonasal surgery, unlike the posterior cranial fossa approaches, typically does not require monitoring of cranial nerves or the brain stem. Therefore, the patient may be kept on muscle relaxants, fully sedated, and "deep." Toward the end of the operation and as the surgeon assesses the field for bleeding, the patient may be "lightened," and the blood pressure may be allowed to increase up to 110 to 130 mmHg systolic. It is important that the patient does not become too "light" at this point because periods of intense stimulation may still occur. Before closure, the surgeon will typically request one or more Valsalva maneuvers, to intrathoracic pressures of 30 to 40 cm H_2O; this permits the surgeon to visualize the surgical cavity and to check for cerebrospinal fluid (CSF) leaks. It is wise to

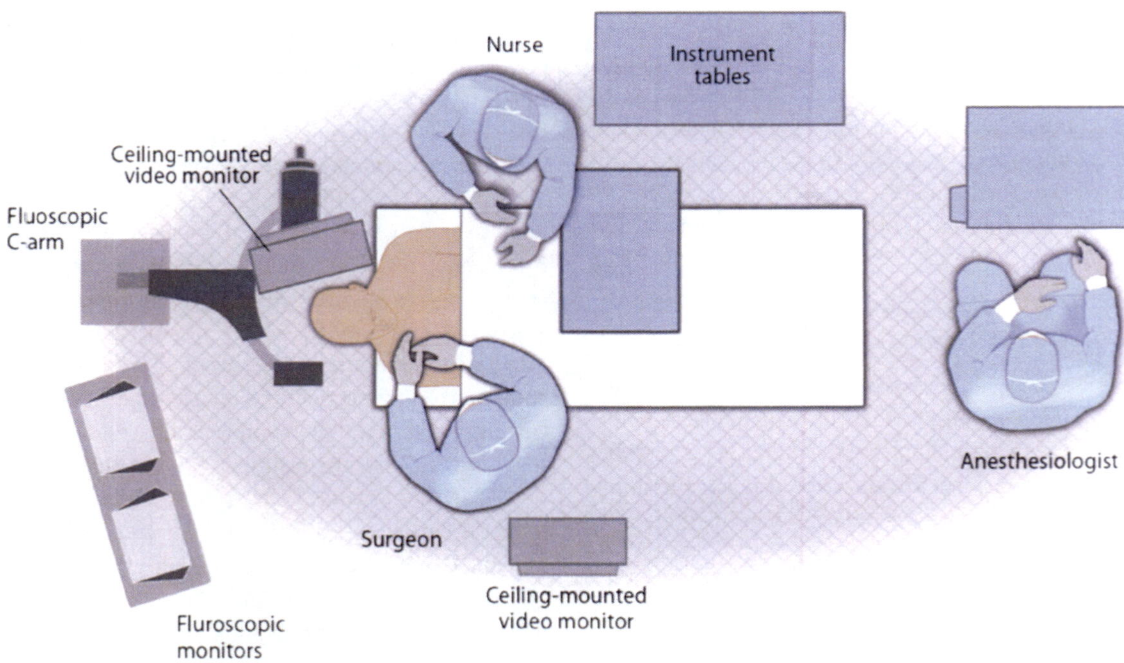

Fig. 1 Operating room setup for the endoscopic endonasal approach.

maintain paralysis for as long as possible, reversing it only after the Mayfield head clamp has been removed.

Smooth emergence from anesthesia is particularly important because violent "bucking" while intubated and coughing after extubation may cause bleeding in the surgical bed or dislodgement of the fat graft. This may predispose the patient to further complications, such as postoperative infection and persistent CSF leak. One approach to ensure a smooth emergence from anesthesia is to establish adequate spontaneous ventilation while the patient is still intubated under deep inhalational anesthesia. After good gastric and pharyngeal suctioning, an oral airway is placed, and the endotracheal tube cuff is slowly deflated (known as "taming the trachea"). If breathing remains regular—a sign that the patient is still deep—the patient is extubated, and supplemental oxygen is administered. The patient can thus emerge from anesthesia without the need for endotracheal stimulation. The oral airway is kept in to prevent airway obstruction until the patient is more awake.

4.2. NEUROANESTHESIA FOR THE FULLY ENDOSCOPIC SUPRAORBITAL APPROACH (FIG. 2) The fully endoscopic supraorbital approach is used to access and resect different tumors of the anterior and middle cranial base, such as meningiomas, craniopharyngiomas, supra- or parasellar extensions of pituitary tumors, esthesioneuroblastomas, and others. Conventional open craniotomies entail creating large bicoronal scalp flaps and retracting one or both frontal lobes to gain access to the anterior or middle cranial base. In contrast, the fully endoscopic approach uses a small incision, which is hidden in the hair of the eyebrow, and a 1.5-cm keyhole craniotomy to accesses these same areas. The patient may be positioned semisitting facing the surgeon or supine with the neck extended and the surgeon operating from a location cephalad to the patient's head. The latter approach allows the brain to "retract" away from the skull base and helps the surgeon to drain CSF from the surrounding cisterns, thus assisting the neuroanesthesiologist in maintaining a lax brain and eliminating the need for any brain retraction.

The neuroanesthetic management for the supraorbital approach to the skull base is similar to that used in surgical clipping of brain aneurysms. The area of the skull base near the optic chiasm is crossed by major vascular structures, and there is the potential for rapid blood loss if these vessels are injured. As in aneurysm surgery, it may be necessary to induce hypotension for short periods of time in case the surgeon needs to identify and control the source of hemorrhage. The patient must have good venous access, and blood must be readily available should rapid transfusion be necessary.

Intraoperative cranial nerve or brainstem monitoring is not usually performed with the supraorbital approach, so muscle relaxation is generally permissible. This approach to the skull base does not disrupt major sensory nerves, so surgical stimulation remains low throughout the procedure (with the exception of the Valsalva maneuver, used occasionally to help the surgeon drain CSF from the operative field and further improve the exposure). After adequate brain relaxation is achieved, a balanced anesthetic using shorter-acting agents provides for quicker emergence as postoperative pain is minimal with this surgery and patients may remain asleep for a long time if longer-acting agents are used.

A smooth emergence from anesthesia is vital. The skin over the eyebrow is fairly loose, and violent bucking and coughing can cause a CSF collection to form subcutaneously around the eye. It may help to maintain gentle pressure over the surgical site during extubation to avoid this complication. Unlike the endonasal and retrosigmoid approaches, the supraorbital approach requires loading and maintaining phenytoin for about 6 months.

4.3. NEUROANESTHESIA FOR THE FULLY ENDOSCOPIC RETROSIGMOID APPROACH (FIG. 3) The fully endoscopic retrosigmoid approach is used to access tumors and the cranial nerves of the posterior cranial fossa. The approach

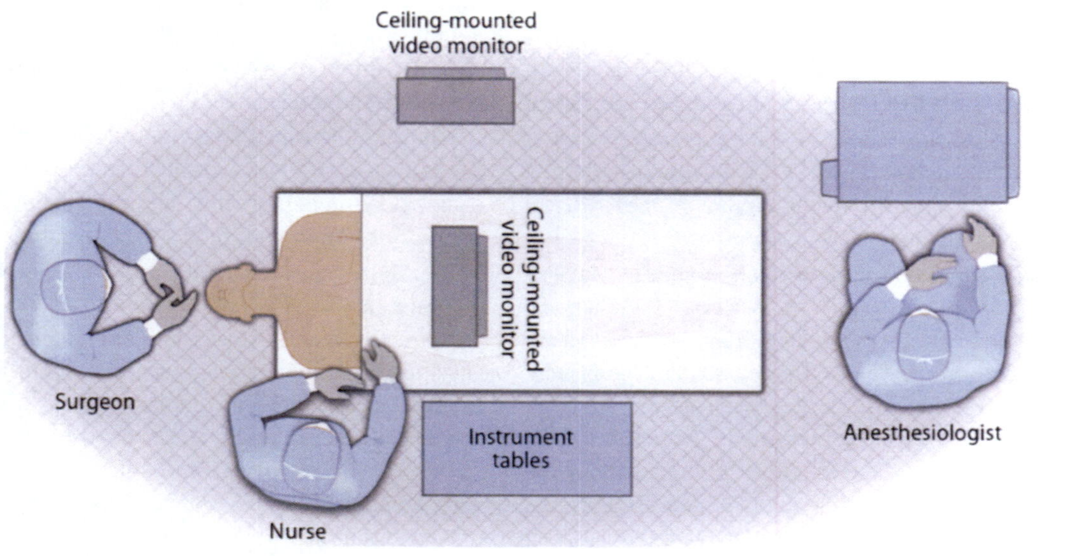

Fig. 2 Operating room setup for the endoscopic supraorbital approach.

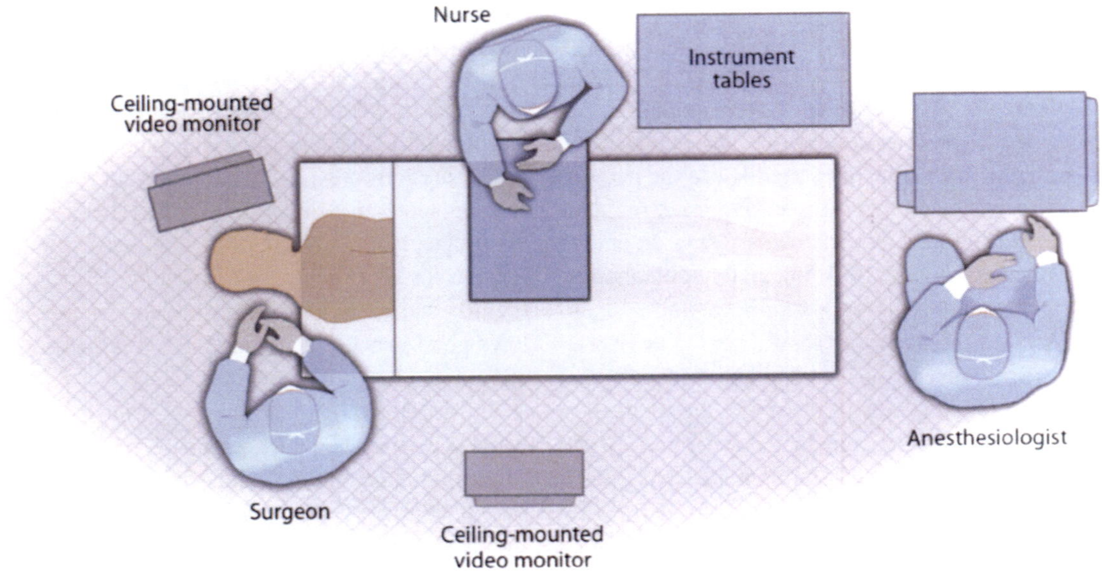

Fig. 3 Operating room setup for the endoscopic retrosigmoid approach.

is mainly used for resection of cerebellopontine angle tumors, such as vestibular (acoustic) schwannomas and meningiomas. It is also used for microvascular decompression of cranial nerve V (trigeminal) for trigeminal neuralgia or, less commonly, cranial nerve VII (facial) for hemifacial spasm or cranial nerve IX (glossopharyngeal) for glossopharyngeal neuralgia.

Similar to other approaches used in endoscopic skull base surgery, after induction of anesthesia, the patient's head is placed in a Mayfield clamp. Precautions related to the remoteness of the surgical field and the need for complete stillness should be taken by the neuroanesthesiologist as previously described. The lateral oblique (park-bench) position, with the patient facing away from the surgeon, is preferred for this approach. This position, however, makes it more difficult for the neuroanesthesiologist to gain access to the patient's face; therefore, strict measures must be taken to protect the airway.

Intravenous access and intra-arterial blood pressure monitoring must be established, and dehydrating measures with mannitol and hyperventilation must be initiated. Effective brain relaxation obviates the need for brain retraction, thus reducing unnecessary trauma to the brain tissue. Relaxation is typically achieved with 1 g/kg mannitol, hyperventilation to an arterial pco_2 of 25 to 30 mmHg, and infusion of propofol.

After anesthesia is induced, intraoperative monitoring devices are connected to the patient. For most posterior fossa surgeries, cranial nerve electromyograms (EMGs) and brainstem auditory and somatosensory evoked potentials are monitored. The EMGs assess the integrity of the facial nerve (VII) and motor function of the trigeminal nerve (V). Brainstem auditory-evoked responses assess the function of the acoustic nerve (VIII). Brainstem somatosensory-evoked responses asses the function of the upper and lower extremities; therefore, after the patient is put in the appropriate position for surgery, neuromuscular blockade must be allowed to wear off, and the patient should remain unparalyzed throughout the procedure. This presents a particular challenge to the neuroanesthesiologist as inadvertent patient movement during surgery can be very dangerous. Furthermore, the use of an armored endotracheal tube, or at least an oral airway, is advisable to prevent the patient from biting and occluding the tube during facial or trigeminal nerve stimulation.

In addition to the contraindication of neuromuscular blockade, use of intraoperative cranial nerve and brainstem monitoring dictates that only moderate doses of inhalational anesthetic be used; higher doses are damaging to motor potentials and to evoked cortical responses. Fortunately, endoscopic retrosigmoid surgery is, for the most part, minimally stimulating to the patient. After the surgeon infiltrates the scalp and periosteum with local anesthetic, the only stimulation comes from the Mayfield pins and the endotracheal tube. At certain times during the procedure, however, stimulation may increase dramatically. Common sources of intense stimulation are the Valsalva maneuver and direct trigeminal nerve irritation.

The anesthetic technique must accomplish the necessary depth of anesthesia to avoid patient movement during periods of intense stimulation while permitting sensitive cranial nerve monitoring. This is particularly challenging for the neuroanesthesiologist. However, an effective approach to solve the dilemma (anesthesia light enough to monitor, deep enough to prevent movement) is to combine elements of total intravenous anesthesia with inhalational techniques. On a baseline of low-to-moderate levels of inhalational agent, infusion of propofol and a short-acting opioid such as remifentanil can provide a stable level of anesthesia and still permit good neurophysiologic monitoring. To have a reasonable margin of safety against movement during cranial nerve stimulation, it may be necessary to increase the intravenous agents to fairly high doses, doses that may cause hypotension during quieter periods.

In this situation, during periods of little stimulation, infusion of vasopressors such as phenylephrine may be necessary.

After closure, emergence from anesthesia following this approach may sometimes be prolonged. This is due to the lingering effects of intravenous anesthetics and the absence of postoperative pain. This delay can frustrate the surgeon's postoperative neurologic assessment. Again, tailored anesthetic management can help by reinstating short-acting neuromuscular blockade during surgical closure and cranioplasty (cranial nerve and brainstem monitoring is no longer needed). The patient may be safely lightened while immobilized in the Mayfield head clamp. The patient's position also permits the use of bispectral index (BIS) monitoring, a useful technological tool that is used to assess anesthetic depth and speed of emergence. The patient is then ready for extubation and neurological assessment fairly soon after the Mayfield head clamp is removed.

5. FUTURE CHALLENGES

As endoscopic skull base surgery progresses, new and novel approaches will be used to access deeper areas at the base of the skull. Just as these operations will be custom tailored to a particular patient's pathology, neuroanesthetic management will have to be customized for the surgical approach. Specialized neurologic monitoring equipment and three-dimensional imaging will provide further challenges to the neuroanesthesiologist. With special care and a tailored approach analogous to that of skull base surgeons, neuroanesthesiologists can continue to make major contributions to fully endoscopic skull base surgery.

3 Neuroendocrine Aspects of Skull Base Surgery

In this chapter, the neuroendocrine aspects of skull base surgery are discussed, with special emphasis on the pituitary gland and the various tumors or disorders that may affect it. The different pathological conditions that may result from pituitary tumors, such as Cushing's syndrome, acromegaly, and others, are also reviewed. The chapter explains the clinical effects of pituitary hormonal deficiencies and overproduction and the methods used in the neuroendocrine evaluation of patients with pituitary tumors, such as blood tests and bilateral inferior petrosal sinus sampling in Cushing's syndrome. In addition, the chapter provides insight into perioperative neuroendocrine management of patients with a pituitary tumor, including the various drugs and drug categories that are used, hormonal supplementation therapy for pituitary failure, and long-term management and outpatient care of pituitary tumor patients.

Keywords: Acromegaly; Cushing's disease; Cushing's syndrome; Diabetes insipidus; Gigantism; Hypopituitarism; Neuroendocrine; Petrosal sinus sampling; Pituitary gland; Prolactinoma.

1. INTRODUCTION

1.1. THE PITUITARY GLAND The pituitary gland is considered the master gland of the body, and it lays at the base of the skull in the sella turcica. It secretes several hormones that regulate other endocrine organs throughout the body, and its proper function is vital for the well-being of an individual. The hormones that the pituitary gland secretes include corticotropin (ACTH), thyroid-stimulating hormone (TSH), luteinizing hormone (LH), follicle-stimulating hormone (FSH), growth hormone (GH), and prolactin (PRL). These hormones are made in the anterior pituitary gland. In addition, the posterior pituitary gland makes arginine vasopressin (AVP), which is also known as antidiuretic hormone (ADH), and oxytocin.

From: *Endoscopic Skull Base Surgery: A Comprehensive Guide with Illustrative Cases.*
Edited by H. K. Shahinian © Humana Press, Totowa, NJ.

The pituitary hormones are all regulated by hypothalamic hormones. ACTH secretion is regulated by corticotropin-releasing hormone (CRH) and AVP. Growth hormone secretion is regulated by growth hormone-releasing hormone (GHRH). LH and FSH secretions are regulated by gonadotropin-releasing hormone (GnRH). TSH and prolactin secretions are positively regulated by thyrotropin-releasing hormone (TRH); prolactin secretion also is inhibited by dopamine. In addition, somatostatin (SMS) inhibits secretion of growth hormone and TSH.

There are distinct cells in the pituitary gland that secrete each of the pituitary hormones. ACTH is secreted by corticotroph cells, LH and FSH are secreted by gonadotroph cells, growth hormone is secreted by somatotroph cells, prolactin is secreted by lactotroph cells, and TSH is secreted by thyrotroph cells. These pituitary hormones go to peripheral end organs to stimulate hormone release. For example, TSH stimulates the thyroid gland to secrete thyroxine (T_4) and triiodothyronine (T_3). Prolactin acts on the breast to allow for milk release. Growth hormone acts on the liver to secret insulin-like growth factor-1 (IGF-1). LH acts on the ovaries and the testes to stimulate the secretion of estrogen and testosterone. FSH also acts on the ovaries and the testes and is involved in follicle stimulation and spermatogenesis as well as increasing the secretion of the hormone inhibin. ACTH acts on the adrenal glands to stimulate the stress hormone, cortisol, and to a lesser extent the salt-regulating hormone aldosterone. In addition, the posterior hormones also affect peripheral target tissues. Vasopressin has three receptors: in the kidney to regulate free water uptake, in the pituitary to regulate ACTH secretion, and in the smooth vessels to regulate vasoconstriction. Oxytocin acts in the uterus and the breast (Fig. 1).

1.2. SKULL BASE TUMORS AND OTHER DISORDERS THAT AFFECT THE PITUITARY GLAND Disorders of the pituitary gland can be caused by pituitary tumors that produce excessive hormones or by tumors that cause decreased hormone production, leading to hormonal deficiencies. Larger tumors can have a mass effect and may affect peripheral vision or cause headaches and elevated intracranial pressure (ICP).

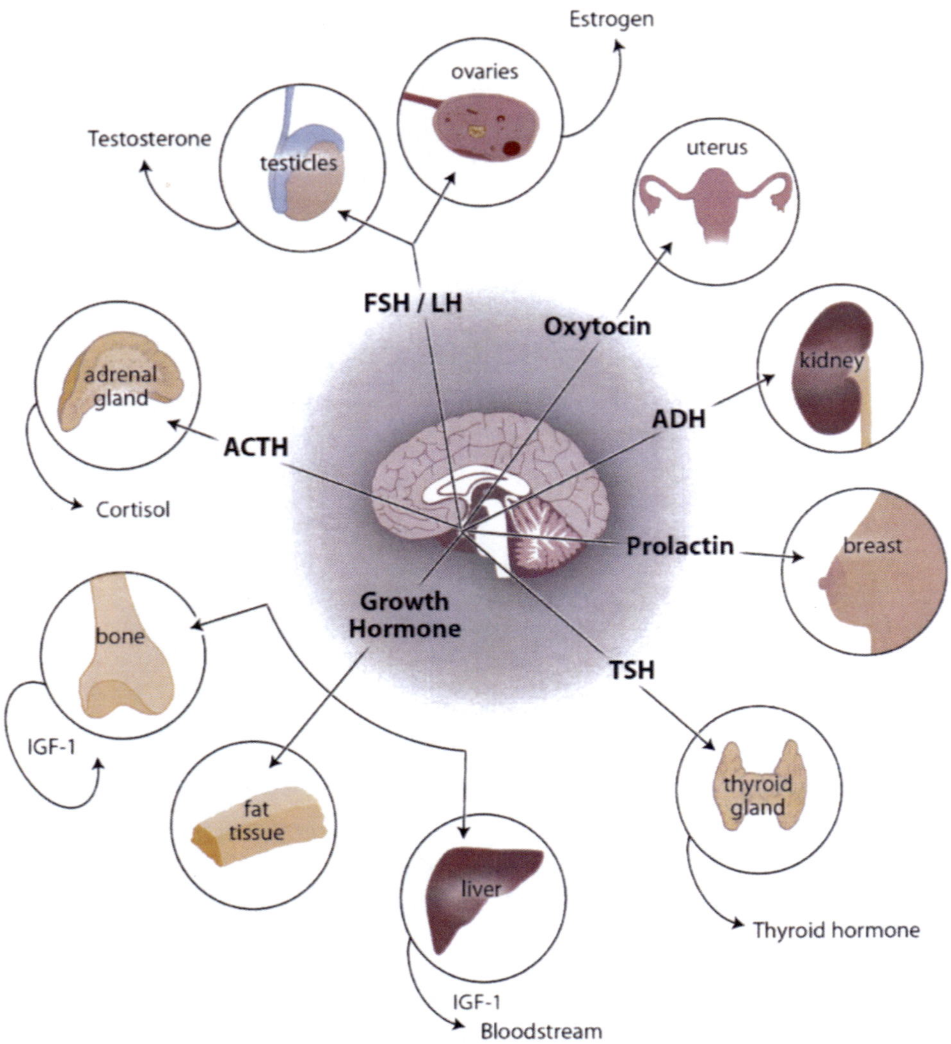

Fig. 1 The pituitary as a master gland.

Rarely, pituitary tumors can become malignant, invading surrounding tissues and leading to metastases.

Tumors and disorders that affect the pituitary gland include the following:

Prolactin-producing pituitary tumors
ACTH-producing pituitary tumors
Growth hormone-producing pituitary tumors
Thyroid hormone-producing pituitary tumors
Nonfunctioning pituitary tumors
Pituitary carcinomas

Other pathologies that may affect the pituitary gland are as follows:

- Meningiomas: tuberculum sellae, planum sphenoidale, olfactory groove
- Craniopharyngiomas
- Rathke's cleft cysts
- Chordomas
- Epidermoid tumors (epidermoid cysts)
- Inflammatory and other rare conditions: hypophysitis, sarcoidosis, histiocytosis, pituitary abscess, hypothalamic gliomas, tuberculomas, germinomas, and others

2. PITUITARY TUMORS

2.1. PROLACTINOMAS Prolactin-secreting tumors are the most common pituitary tumors. Most prolactinomas are relatively small in females, although they can be quite large in males. The clinical effects of prolactinomas in females include galactorrhea (breast milk discharge) and irregular (oligomenorrhea) or absent (amenorrhea) periods. Prolactinomas inhibit the GnRH–LH–estradiol axis, which leads to estrogen deficiency. Estrogen deficiency, if untreated, can lead to osteoporosis. Prolactinomas are very responsive to medical treatment with dopamine agonists.

Besides prolactinomas, there are other causes of elevated prolactin; these include other large lesions that affect the hypothalamic–pituitary axis. This is called *stalk effect*. In addition, stimulation of the breasts, pregnancy, and primary hypothyroidism (by the stimulation of TRH, which increases prolactin secretion) lead to elevated prolactin. Psychiatric medicines that have dopamine antagonist activity also raise prolactin. These medicines classically include the psychotropic medicines such as Haldol used for schizophrenia, but also include the newer selective serotonin reuptake inhibitors (SSRIs) and some antidepressants.

In female patients presenting with galactorrhea or oligomenorrhea or amenorrhea, a prolactin level should be measured; if elevated, the other causes of elevated prolactin besides prolactinoma need to be excluded. This includes a careful review of all medications. Magnetic resonance imaging (MRI) should be performed to exclude a large pituitary lesion. If the patient has a microadenoma or a macroadenoma that is not compressing the optic nerves, the patient should be treated medically with dopamine agonists. Although classically bromocriptine has been the agent used to treat prolactinomas, the use of this drug has been largely replaced by the use of cabergoline (Dostinex), which is a specific D_2 agonist. This medicine has much fewer side effects compared to bromocriptine and is usually given once or twice a week. Cabergoline and other dopamine agonists are also effective at reducing the size of the tumor, so in most patients with a prolactinoma, medical treatment should be initiated. Surgical treatment is indicated for patients who fail to have a response to dopamine agonists or cannot tolerate the side effects (Fig. 2).

2.2. CUSHING'S DISEASE The second most common hormone-secreting pituitary tumor is an ACTH-secreting tumor. This condition is called Cushing's disease. Cushing's disease results in elevated cortisol levels and a wide range of clinical symptoms and signs. These manifestations include rapid and unexplained weight gain, central obesity, stretch marks (striae), bruising, round plethoric face, a buffalo hump, thinning of extremities, acne, and hirsutism. Decreased libido and severe fatigue are also noted. Muscle weakness and psychiatric problems, including mania, anxiety, and depression, are common. Diabetes or high blood pressure usually occur in patients with more severe disease.

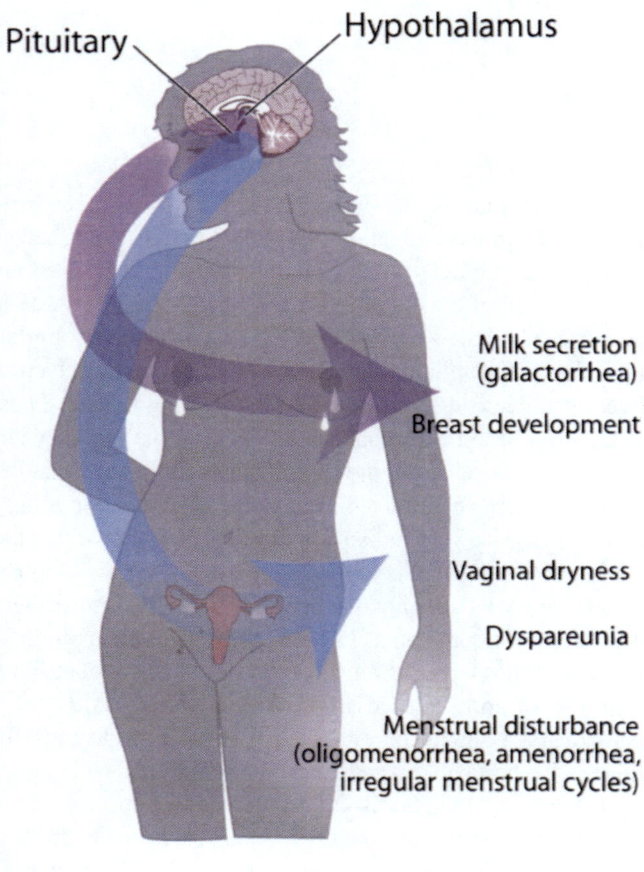

Fig. 2 Clinical effects of prolactinomas.

The causes of hypercortisolism can be divided into endogenous and exogenous. Exogenous hypercortisolism occurs when patients are given steroids, and this is quite common. Of the endogenous causes of hypercortisolism, Cushing's disease is the most common; it occurs in between 80% and 90% of patients with Cushing's syndrome and is much more common in females than males. Other causes of endogenous hypercortisolism are adrenal tumors that secrete cortisol and ectopic tumors, most likely bronchial or lung tumors that secrete ACTH. In addition, an entity called pseudo-Cushing's exists in which disorders such as depression, alcoholism, and alcohol withdrawal lead to elevated cortisol secretion without the stigmata of Cushing's syndrome. However, pseudo-Cushing's appears to be decreasing in frequency, possibly due to more sensitive urinary free cortisol (UFC) assays that only detect cortisol and not cortisol metabolites. Nevertheless, it is important to distinguish among exogenous Cushing's syndrome due to steroid use or abuse, endogenous Cushing's syndrome due to Cushing's disease, and pseudo-Cushing's syndrome.

Cushing's syndrome is now more recognized by both patients and endocrinologists and is diagnosed much earlier, with patients having milder signs and symptoms. With the recognition of mild cases, the occurrence of Cushing's syndrome is probably much more frequent than previously thought. Because of this, a high degree of suspicion for Cushing's syndrome is needed, and multiple testing needs to be performed. Plus, some patients with Cushing's syndrome have what is described as an episodic or periodic type in that they have higher cortisol secretion rates at some times than at other times. Again, multiple testing is needed, and a single normal test cannot be used to exclude Cushing's syndrome (Fig. 3).

The most common tests used for the diagnosis of Cushing's syndrome are 24-h urinary free cortisol measurements, nighttime blood cortisol measurements, dexamethasone suppression tests, and nighttime salivary cortisol measurements. A 24-h urinary cortisol collection involves collecting all urine for 24 h; a creatinine should also be measured to determine that collection was complete. A 24-h urinary collection should have both a urinary free cortisol and a 17-hydroxysteroid collection as the latter may be positive in some patients with normal urinary free cortisol collection. Because patients with Cushing's syndrome can have the periodic type, it is important that the collection be done at the time when they have signs and symptoms of high cortisol production.

Nighttime blood cortisol levels are usually done between 11:00 p.m. and 1:00 a.m. A value greater than 7 μg/dL is consistent with Cushing's syndrome. This test has been somewhat replaced by salivary cortisols, which reflect free cortisol in the blood. Salivary cortisols are convenient to measure, and specimens can be mailed. Sampling should be done between 11:00 p.m. and midnight. Each laboratory has a different normal range.

Dexamethasone suppression tests have been widely used to screen and diagnose patients with Cushing's syndrome. The most common test to screen for Cushing's syndrome is an

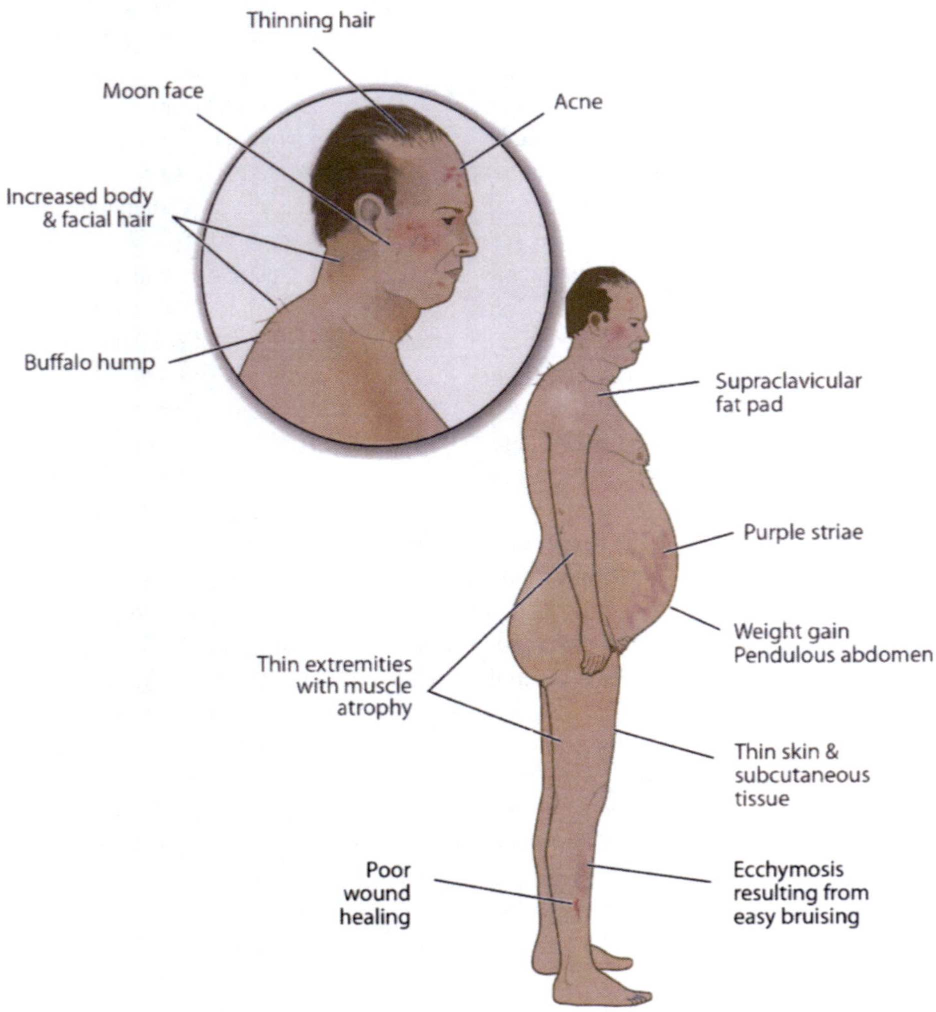

Fig. 3 Clinical effects of Cushing's syndrome.

overnight dexamethasone test in which the patient takes 1 mg dexamethasone at midnight, and an 8:00 a.m. blood specimen for cortisol measurement is drawn. The recommended cutoff for the cortisol has been decreasing, and it is now recommended to use a value between 1.8 and 3 µg/dL. This lower cutoff not only may detect more patients with Cushing's syndrome but also will detect more patients without it. In addition, many patients do suppress in response to the overnight dexamethasone test, so this test is no longer recommended to exclude patients as having Cushing's syndrome. Plus, there is a low-dose dexamethasone suppression test in which the patient takes 0.5 mg dexamethasone every 6 h for 2 days. This dose of dexamethasone should suppress cortisol levels in normal patients but not in patients with Cushing's syndrome of any type. However, patients with Cushing's disease have been found to quite readily suppress cortisol in response to this 2-day dexamethasone suppression test, so this test is also unlikely to be of much use. Therefore, the recommended tests for the diagnosis of Cushing's syndrome include multiple measurements of 24-h urine for urinary free cortisol and 17-hydroxysteroids, nighttime salivary cortisol, and nighttime blood cortisol.

Although traditionally imaging tests have not been performed at the initial evaluation of a patient with Cushing's syndrome, the high quality of new pituitary MRIs has allowed the early detection of most tumors. Also, dynamic pituitary MRIs have focused on the slow infusion and diffusion of gadolinium into and out of the pituitary gland, further refining the detection of very small lesions typical of ACTH-secreting tumors. Thus, the MRI has become a valuable technique for the initial evaluation of the disease and could be performed at the time that the diagnosis is being entertained. A negative MRI makes pituitary Cushing's disease very unlikely, although it is possible that the patient could still have ectopic or adrenal Cushing's. A positive pituitary MRI does not diagnose Cushing's disease as there are pituitary incidentalomas in which the patient has a pituitary tumor that is not secreting any hormone. Thus, all patients with symptoms of cortisol excess that have a positive MRI for a microadenoma should be evaluated with 24-h urine tests for urinary free cortisol and 17-hydroxysteroids and with nighttime salivary or blood cortisols.

Once the diagnosis of Cushing's syndrome is made, the next step is determining whether the patient has ACTH-dependent (pituitary Cushing's disease or ectopic ACTH syndrome) or ACTH-independent (adrenal) Cushing's syndrome. The distinction is made by measuring a morning plasma ACTH level. If this value is low (<10 pg/mL), the patient likely has adrenal Cushing's syndrome, and the patient should have adrenal computed tomography (CT) or MRI. If the ACTH level is above 100 pg/mL, the patient most likely has ectopic Cushing's syndrome; if the patient has an ACTH between 10 and 100 pg/mL, then pituitary Cushing's is more likely. However, the ACTH levels indicative of ectopic and pituitary Cushing's do overlap, so further investigation is needed. In most patients, ectopic Cushing's syndrome is more severe than pituitary Cushing's syndrome, and these patients can usually be detected by their failure to suppress in response to an overnight or low-dose dexamethasone suppression test. In addition, a high-dose dexamethasone suppression test can be done; patients with pituitary Cushing's disease suppress in response to high-dose dexamethasone, while patients with ectopic Cushing's do not.

Once the diagnosis of pituitary Cushing's disease is obtained, surgical intervention should be recommended. Most patients can be cured of their disease with selective pituitary surgery, either thru traditional transphenoidal techniques or more recently thru a minimally invasive endoscopic endonasal approach. Postoperatively, many patients become hypocortisolemic due to the fact that before surgery the normal pituitary corticotrophs were suppressed by the elevated cortisol levels. However, some patients have episodic and mild Cushing's disease, and they do not have suppression of the normal pituitary corticotrophs; therefore, they do not have low cortisol values postoperatively. Although this is the case, most patients do become mildly hypocortisolemic after surgery and do require cortisol replacement for a period between 3 months and 1 year. The cortisol replacement should be tapered off, and within a year the patient is usually off cortisol supplementation. Also, during surgery the pituitary may be damaged, and postoperatively it is quite common for patients to require growth hormone replacement. Patients may also require thyroid hormone, estrogen, or testosterone replacement and occasionally develop diabetes insipidus and require DDAVP® (desmopressin acetate).

In those patients who fail initial pituitary surgery, another MRI should be performed. Our approach is that patients who have a visible lesion on MRI should undergo a second pituitary surgery. If no lesion is seen, we usually recommend bilateral adrenalectomy to cure the hypercortisolism. Although pituitary radiation can also be done at this stage, the effects are quite delayed. In addition, most patients who receive pituitary radiation develop hypopituitarism and require pituitary hormone replacement.

2.2.1. Bilateral Inferior Petrosal Sinus Sampling in Cushing's Disease If the patient has biochemical evidence of pituitary Cushing's disease and a pituitary tumor, the patient should have pituitary surgery. However, if the patient has biochemical evidence supporting ectopic Cushing's syndrome and has a pituitary microadenoma or the patient does not have a pituitary tumor yet has biochemical evidence of pituitary Cushing's disease, petrosal sinus samplings should be performed. In this procedure, also called bilateral inferior petrosal sinus sampling (BIPSS), blood in the petrosal sinuses that drain each side of the pituitary is sampled for ACTH. This is usually done before and after CRH is given, and this is customarily measured at 0, 2, 5, and 10 min afterward. In pituitary Cushing's disease, the ACTH level is much higher in the petrosal blood than in a simultaneously drawn peripheral sample. In contrast, in ectopic ACTH the values between petrosal and peripheral blood are similar. A rise in ACTH with CRH is also indicative of Cushing's disease, and the lateralization may help determine on which side of the pituitary the tumor is. In tumors that are large, the blood drainage is often compromised; therefore, the ACTH levels between the two petrosal sinuses may not be valid for lateralization. However, in patients with small microadenomas the petrosal sinus sampling is most useful, and the lateralization is often effective.

Petrosal sinus sampling cannot be used to distinguish individuals with pituitary Cushing's disease from normal individuals as normal individuals and patients with pituitary Cushing's disease have similar petrosal ACTH values. Both normal individuals and patients with pituitary Cushing's disease respond to CRH, and both have lateralization of ACTH. However, it is reassuring when petrosal sinus sampling shows lateralization that is on the same side as the pituitary tumor seen on MRI. This helps confirm that the pituitary tumor seen on MRI is indeed secreting ACTH. Most important, petrosal sinus sampling is good at distinguishing between pituitary and ectopic Cushing's (Fig. 4).

2.3. ACROMEGALY Excess growth hormone in adults is called *acromegaly*, and growth hormone-secreting pituitary tumors are the third most common types of hormone-secreting pituitary tumors. Patients with acromegaly have traditionally

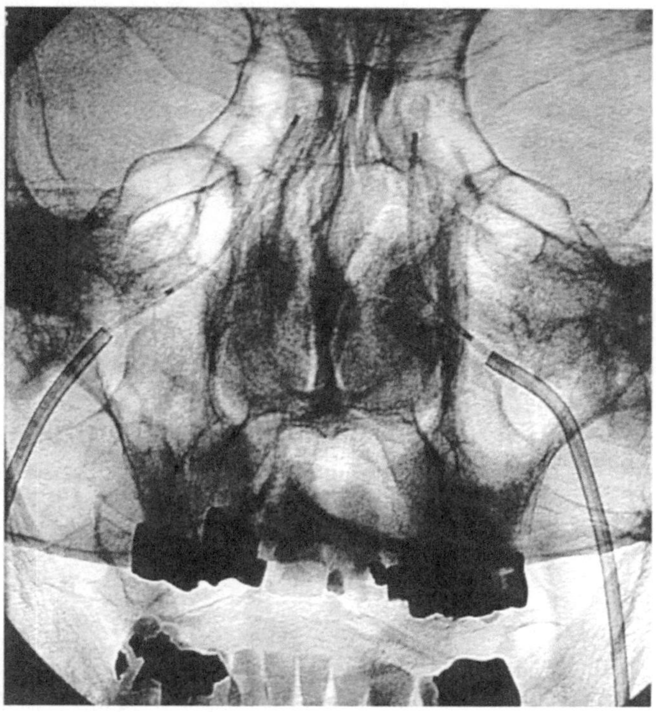

Fig. 4 Anteroposterior fluoroscopy view showing BIPSS.

had large pituitary tumors as the signs and symptoms of acromegaly are relatively nonspecific, and there has often been delay in seeking treatment and diagnosis. More recently, acromegaly has been recognized earlier as a condition, and now many of the tumors are smaller. Women usually seek medical attention before men, and this is often the case with acromegaly.

Patients with acromegaly usually have multiple slow changes in the body habitus. These include increase in ring and foot size, increase in tongue size, a wide forehead, widening of the nose, enlarged and sweaty hands, and gaps between the teeth. They also have arthritis; cardiac problems, including congestive heart failure; and increased instance of polyps in the gastrointestinal tract.

The initial workup for acromegaly usually involves measuring a serum IGF-1 level, which is almost always elevated in patients with acromegaly. In patients with an elevated IGF-1, an oral glucose tolerance test is obtained. In the normal population, glucose should suppress plasma growth hormone levels. In patients with acromegaly, the suppression is blunted, and patients usually have a growth hormone value following glucose of >1 ng/mL. In general, measuring random growth hormone is not helpful for the diagnosis of acromegaly due to pulsatility of growth hormone.

Once the diagnosis of acromegaly is made, pituitary imaging should be obtained. If the patient can be cured with pituitary surgery, surgery should be done, and no other treatment is needed. If the patient cannot be cured with surgery because the tumor is invading the cavernous sinus or other brain regions, the usual approach is to undergo pituitary surgery for reduction of the tumor mass and to decrease growth hormone.

Following this, medical treatment is initiated with one or two drugs. One family of drugs are somatostatin analogs, which act to both decrease the IGF-1 level caused by the excess growth hormone as well as control the tumor size. The somatostatin analogs are based on the structure of an octreotide and are modified to be long lasting. The side effects of octreotide-based drugs include nausea, vomiting, gallstones, or gallbladder sludge formation. A newer drug is pegvisomant, also called Somavert, which acts as a growth hormone antagonist. This drug prevents endogenous growth hormone from binding at the growth hormone receptor and stimulating IGF-1 and is very effective at decreasing IGF-1 levels. However, it does not have any effect on tumor size. In some patients, the combined use of pegvisomant plus octreotide analogs is effective. Radiation therapy can be used but is only a third-line approach (Fig. 5).

2.4. TSH-SECRETING TUMORS TSH-secreting tumors are extremely rare and manifest with symptoms of hyperthyroidism with an elevated TSH and free T_4 levels. Patients usually have a goiter. This can be distinguished from thyroid hormone resistance by a positive pituitary MRI if there is also an elevated TSH and T_4 level. Patients with TSH-secreting pituitary tumors should be aggressively treated with surgery.

2.5. LH- AND FSH-SECRETING TUMORS Patients with LH- and FSH-secreting tumors are also rarely identified clinically. Although many nonsecreting pituitary tumors, when examined by immunohistochemistry, do secrete small amounts of LH and FSH, patients with true LH- and FSH-secreting tumors are usually males who present with either mass effect or low testosterone levels. They may have erectile dysfunction and decreased libido. Females would have irregular or no periods, and in postmenopausal women the diagnosis is extremely difficult to make. Sometimes, these tumors secrete high levels of alpha subunits of LH and FSH, and these can be measured.

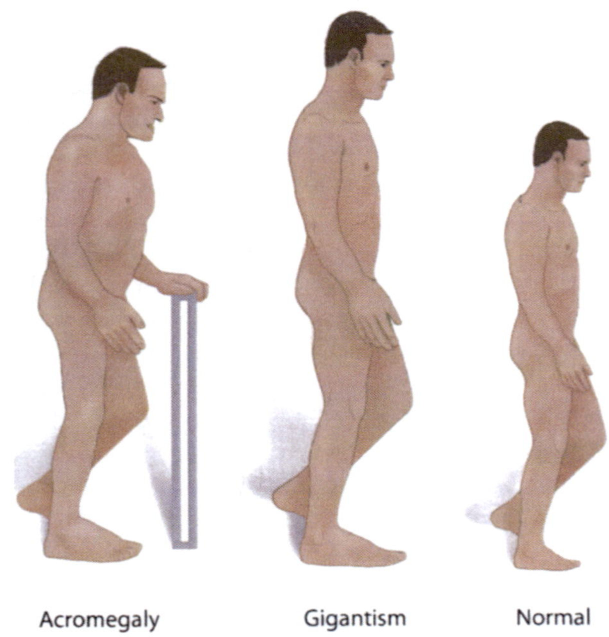

Fig. 5 Clinical effects of acromegaly and gigantism.

2.6. NONFUNCTIONING PITUITARY TUMORS Another very frequent type of tumor that secretes no hormones is known as a silent or nonfunctioning pituitary tumor. These tumors affect the pituitary because of their mass effect. Tumors usually larger than 1.5–2.0 cm; those that cause visual field cuts are surgically resected.

3. HORMONAL DEFICIENCIES CAUSED BY PITUITARY TUMORS

Any tumor that is large enough to compress the pituitary gland can give rise to pituitary hormonal deficiencies. However, it is increasingly recognized that small pituitary tumors such as microadenomas, which are defined as tumors <10 mm in size, can also cause pituitary dysfunction. The pituitary hormone that is most easily affected by pituitary damage, and therefore by relatively small pituitary tumors, is growth hormone. This hormone susceptibility is followed by susceptibility of LH, FSH, and TSH. ACTH is the last hormone affected. Therefore, in all patients with pituitary damage (tumors or prior surgery or radiation), growth hormone deficiency should be tested. In addition, testosterone in females is due to secretion of ACTH and gonadotropins. Thus, testosterone deficiency may be an early sign of decreased pituitary function in patients with relatively small pituitary tumors or other pituitary damage. All patients with large pituitary tumors deserve a complete hormonal workup. To test for hyperfunction, we recommend measuring an IGF-1 for growth hormone, thyroid function tests, and a 24-h urine for urinary free cortisol.

3.1. GROWTH HORMONE DEFICIENCY Diagnosing growth hormone deficiency is becoming more important as it is realized that growth hormone deficiency plays a crucial role in adults. Patients with growth hormone deficiency have relatively nonspecific complaints, but these symptoms have been shown to be due to decreased growth hormone and improve with growth hormone therapy. These symptoms include severe fatigue, trouble sleeping, joint and muscle pains, depression, and other mood disturbances. Patients with growth hormone deficiency also have decreased lean muscle mass, increased body fat, and osteopenia or osteoporosis.

A screening test for growth hormone deficiency is an IGF-1 level. However, IGF-1 levels can be normal in patients with growth hormone deficiency and can be low in patients without growth hormone deficiency. An IGF-1 level also needs to be adjusted for age and gender. IGF-1 levels that are within one standard deviation of the median for age argue against growth hormone deficiency. Patients who have very low IGF-1 levels and have other pituitary deficiencies are very likely to have growth hormone deficiency. Patients with a low-normal or mildly low IGF-1 level should be tested with growth hormone stimulation testing to determine the ability of the pituitary to secrete growth hormone. The most common of these is called an arginine–GHRH test in which arginine and GH are given, and response to growth hormone is measured. We use a growth hormone measured by radioimmunoassay of 9 ng/dL as a cutoff any time following arginine–GHRH stimulation.

3.2. CENTRAL HYPOTHYROIDISM To assess central hypothyroidism, which is hypothyroidism caused by pituitary problems, we measure free T_4 and TSH. A free T_4 measurement below or at the lower limit of normal coupled with a low TSH level in a patient with a pituitary problem is consistent with central hypothyroidism, and that patient should be treated with thyroid hormone replacement.

3.3. GONADOTROPIN DEFICIENCY Female patients with irregular or no periods are likely to be estrogen deficient. Thus, for those patients a physician should measure estradiol, LH, and FSH levels; if consistent with low LH, FSH, and estradiol, a pituitary cause of hypogonadism is likely. The patient should be treated with an estrogen replacement, especially if the patient is premenopausal. Female patients can also have androgen deficiency, and testosterone levels should be measured, with the caveat that many commercially available assays for testosterone lack precision and sensitivity in the range of female testosterone levels. However, in a patient with low testosterone levels and signs of testosterone deficiency, such as decreased libido and decreased muscle mass, testosterone replacement may be indicated. There is no form of testosterone replacement approved by the Food and Drug Administration (FDA) for women. One option is to give over-the-counter DHEA (dihydroepiandrosterone), which is converted to testosterone. Alternatively, compounding pharmacies can compound testosterone in doses suitable for females.

Hypogonadism in men is manifested as erectile dysfunction and decreased libido. In these patients, total and free testosterone levels should be measured, as should LH and FSH levels, to determine if the cause is pituitary in nature. Patients with a low testosterone level benefit from testosterone replacement. The forms of testosterone replacement include AndroGel, which is testosterone cream; Androderm, which is a testosterone patch; buccal testosterone preparation (Striant); and testosterone injections. Also, human chorionic gonadotrophin injections, which stimulate the testes to make testosterone, are also an option.

3.4. ACTH DEFICIENCY ACTH is the last hormone to be affected in the case of pituitary damage, and most patients have an intact ACTH–cortisol axis. Chronic ACTH deficiency leads to cortisol deficiency. Our approach in patients suspected of ACTH and cortisol deficiency is to measure a morning cortisol level. If this level is < 4 μg/dL, then it is pretty certain that the patient has cortisol deficiency and needs to be placed on cortisol. If the cortisol value is > 12 μg/dL, then it is unlikely that the patient has cortisol insufficiency. If the cortisol level is between 4 and 12 μg/dL, then a cosyntropin test should be done. Cosyntropin is $ACTH_{1-24}$ and it is given by intramuscular or subcutaneous injection, and cortisol is drawn at 0, 30, and 60 min. We recommend a 1-μg cosyntropin test as this is more sensitive in revealing pituitary insufficiency. A cortisol at 30 min of > 18 μg/dL is considered normal. If the value is between 12 and 18 μg/dL, then the patient should have cortisol replacement in when facing such stresses as surgery or an accident. If the cortisol value is < 12 μg/dL, then the patient most likely needs daily cortisol replacement.

3.5. DIABETES INSIPIDUS Another complication of pituitary surgery or radiation that patients can develop in terms of hypopituitarism is diabetes insipidus. Diabetes insipidus is due to a deficiency of antidiuretic hormone (ADH), also called arginine vasopressin (AVP). AVP is made in the posterior pituitary, so only when this portion of the pituitary is damaged does diabetes insipidus occur. Manifestations of diabetes insipidus are polyuria, polydipsia, and hypernatremia. Immediately following pituitary surgery, there is occasionally a transient diabetes insipidus. This can be followed by episodes of hyponatremia due to excess ADH secretion at around day 7 postoperatively. This can resolve, or it can lead to permanent diabetes insipidus.

The diagnosis of diabetes insipidus is usually made by noticing increased urinary volume. Our cutoff is that a 24-h urinary volume of > 3 L is abnormal, and diabetes insipidus should be considered. We also perform a modified water deprivation test and have the patient fast for 12 h, including no liquids. A normal individual should have an elevated urine osmolality. However, patients with diabetes insipidus fail to have concentrated urine and have a urine with low osmolality. Usually after a 12-h fast, their spot urine osmolality is < 500 mosm/kg, with normal values greater than this cutoff. With an increased 24-h urine volume and dilute urine following a 12-h fast, a formal water deprivation test is usually not needed.

The treatment for diabetes insipidus is to give the AVP analog DDAVP® either orally or intranasally The goal would be to eliminate nighttime awakenings due to the need to urinate and still have the patient retain a normal fluid balance. The urine volume, urine and serum osmolality, and serum sodium should be monitored after initiation of DDAVP® treatment (Fig. 6).

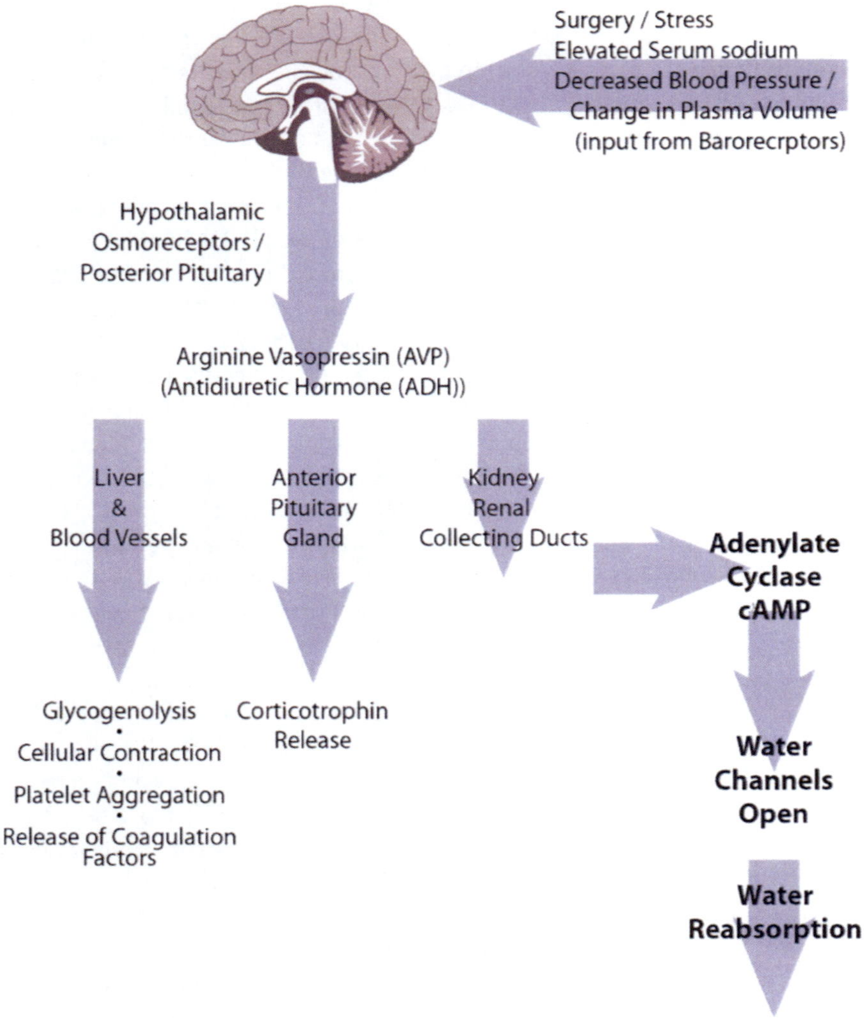

Fig. 6 Physiology and effects of antidiuretic hormone.

3.6. OTHER CAUSES OF HYPOPITUITARISM Any lesion around the hypothalamic stalk or pituitary can give hypopituitarism. These lesions include craniopharyngiomas, meningiomas, chordomas, and Rathkes' cysts. In addition, other lesions in the hypothalamus, including sarcoidosis, hemochromatosis, tuberculosis, and histiocytosis X can lead to hypopituitarism. Head trauma can lead to hypopituitarism, as can other lesions in the pituitary, including lymphomas and other space-occupying lesions. All of these patients should be evaluated for each pituitary hormone as discussed above.

4. LONG-TERM FOLLOW-UP OF PATIENTS WITH A PITUITARY TUMOR

Following pituitary surgery, patients are seen within a few days for clinical evaluation. The postoperative evaluation of pituitary function is carried out weeks after surgery.

Endocrinologically active adenomas are followed by regular testing of marker hormones. As long as the endocrine data are within the normal limits, no imaging studies are required. In acromegaly, the easiest parameter to follow is IGF-1; prolactinomas are followed by serum prolactin level, and so forth. In our practice, the initial examination is performed 8–12 weeks after surgery and repeated annually for the next 5 years.

Medications are given based on hormonal abnormalities. For instance, dopaminergic agents are used for hyperprolactinemia, and somatostatin analogs are used for acromegaly. Patient education, including diet, daily activity, and awareness of the symptoms of recurrence, are all part of a long-term follow-up plan. Of note, in patients who received radiotherapy or radiosurgery for their pituitary tumors, pituitary dysfunction may occur years following therapy. These patients are monitored for development of hypopituitarism, and long-term evaluation of pituitary hormones is necessary. In the case of those with endocrine-inactive adenomas, the follow-up depends essentially on serial MRI and visual studies (Table 1).

Table 1
Pituitary: target organ hormone axis

Hypothalamic hormone	*Pituitary target cell*	*Pituitary hormone affected*	*Peripheral target gland*	*Peripheral hormone affected*
Anterior lobe of pituitary gland				
Corticotropin-releasing hormone (CRH)/vasopressin	Corticotroph	Corticotropin (ACTH)	Adrenal gland	Cortisol, aldosterone
Thyrotropin-releasing hormone (TRH)	Thyrotroph Lactotroph	Thyroid-stimulating hormone (TSH) Prolactin	Thyroid gland Breast	Thyroxine (T_4) Triiodothyronine (T_3)
Growth hormone-releasing hormone (GHRH)	Somatotroph	Growth hormone (GH)	Liver	Insulin-like growth factor-1 (IGF-1)
Gonadotropin-releasing hormone (GnRH)	Gonadotroph		Ovary	Progesterone
		Luteinizing hormone (LH)	Testis	Testosterone
			Ovary Testis	Estradiol Inhibin
		Follicle-stimulating hormone (FSH)		
Somatostatin (inhibitory)	Somatotroph	GH		
Dopamine (inhibitory)	Lactotroph	Prolactin		
Posterior lobe of pituitary gland				
Vasopressin			Kidney Smooth vessels Pituitary	
Oxytocin			Uterus Breast	

4 Interventional Neuroradiology Aspects of Skull Base Surgery

Interventional neuroradiology procedures have evolved and now have an established role in the treatment and diagnosis of various skull base pathological conditions. In this chapter, the most common aspects of interventional neuroradiologic procedures related to skull base surgery are discussed, namely, embolization of skull base tumors, test and permanent occlusion of the internal carotid artery, and inferior petrosal sinus sampling, with emphasis on indications, techniques, and potential complications of each procedure.

Keywords: Angiofibromas; Inferior petrosal sinus sampling; INR; IPSS; Interventional neuroradiology; Meningiomas carotid artery occlusion; Paragangliomas; Preoperative embolization; Skull base; Skull base tumor.

1. INTRODUCTION

In interventional neuroradiology, *embolization* refers to occlusion or obliteration of a vascular channel or obliteration of a vascular bed. Numerous factors determine the technique and material to be used for any embolization procedure. Differences in the location and structure of the target mandate the use of different techniques and materials. The goal of the embolization procedure is mostly preoperative devascularization shortly before surgery. In rare cases, it may be a palliative or permanent treatment.

2. EMBOLIZATION OF SKULL BASE TUMORS

2.1. PARAGANGLIOMAS Paragangliomas are vascular, locally aggressive tumors with a low metastatic potential; they arise from paraganglionic chemoreceptor cells of neural crest origin. They may be multicentric in about 10% of cases, which requires looking for familial tumor syndromes such as multiple endocrine neoplasia type 2 (MEN 2), von Hippel–Lindau (VHL), and neurofibromatosis type 1 (NF-1).

From: *Endoscopic Skull Base Surgery: A Comprehensive Guide with Illustrative Cases.*
Edited by H. K. Shahinian © Humana Press, Totowa, NJ.

These tumors may secrete vasoactive substances such as catecholamines and serotonin. Release of these substances may be triggered by selective catheterization and injection of iodine contrast agent, leading to increased heart rate and blood pressure. Secretory activity and multicentricity are associated with an increased incidence of malignancy. These lesions have an intense hypervascularization made of numerous arteries and veins interconnected via arteriovenous shunts.

Surgical removal is the treatment of choice. Preoperative embolization cannot be achieved in most cases, but it is mandatory for tumors in locations of poor surgical control such as the foramen jugulare to reduce operative bleeding and decrease the surgical morbidity.

A complete cerebral angiogram is performed as a first step to determine the precise location of the relevant vascular feeders. The ascending pharyngeal artery is a common feeder in tympanic and jugular locations. Other usual contributors are meningeal branches arising from the middle meningeal artery, the accessory meningeal artery, the occipital artery, the distal segments of the vertebral arteries (VAs), and the internal carotid artery (ICA) at the level of the carotid siphon. Selective catheterization of the feeding vessels is achieved using a microcatheter, and the embolization is performed using microparticles of various sizes. Only microparticles of less than 300 μm reach the intratumoral vessels. These small microparticles are therefore the most efficient. However, the related risk of embolization is increased when using these small size particles due to potential occlusion of the vasa vasorum, leading to cranial nerve damage or to erratic embolization due to opening and migration through collaterals. The risk of such complications, however, remains low; it is reduced by the experience of the operator, careful handling during the endovascular procedure, and application of basic rules such as avoiding injection of an embolizing agent under a blocked flow condition (Fig. 1).

In selected cases of extensive lesions fed by the ICA and the VA, the only way of achieving significant devascularization is to achieve an embolization by direct puncture and intralesional injection of a liquid adhesive embolizing agent such as acrylic

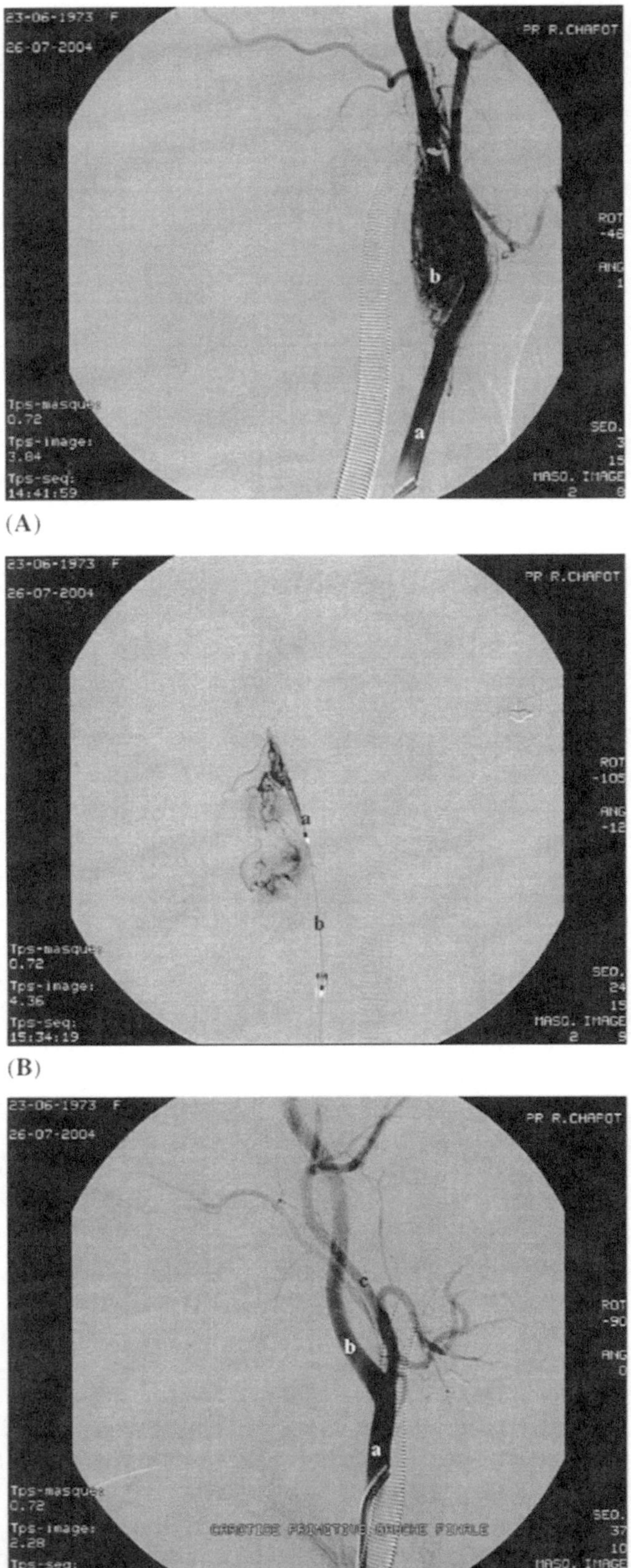

Fig. 1 (**A**)–(**C**) Carotid bifurcation paraganglioma embolized with microparticles. (**A**) Lateral view of the common carotid artery showing the hypervascular carotid bifurcation paraganglioma. *a* Common carotid artery. *b* Paraganglioma. (**B**) Selective injection of the ascending pharyngeal artery, which is the main feeder. *a* Ascending pharyngeal artery. *b*. Microcatheter. (**C**) Lateral view of the common carotid showing complete devascularization after occlusion with microparticles (calibrated 100- to 300-μm microspheres). *a* Common carotid artery. *b* Internal carotid artery. *c* External carotid artery.

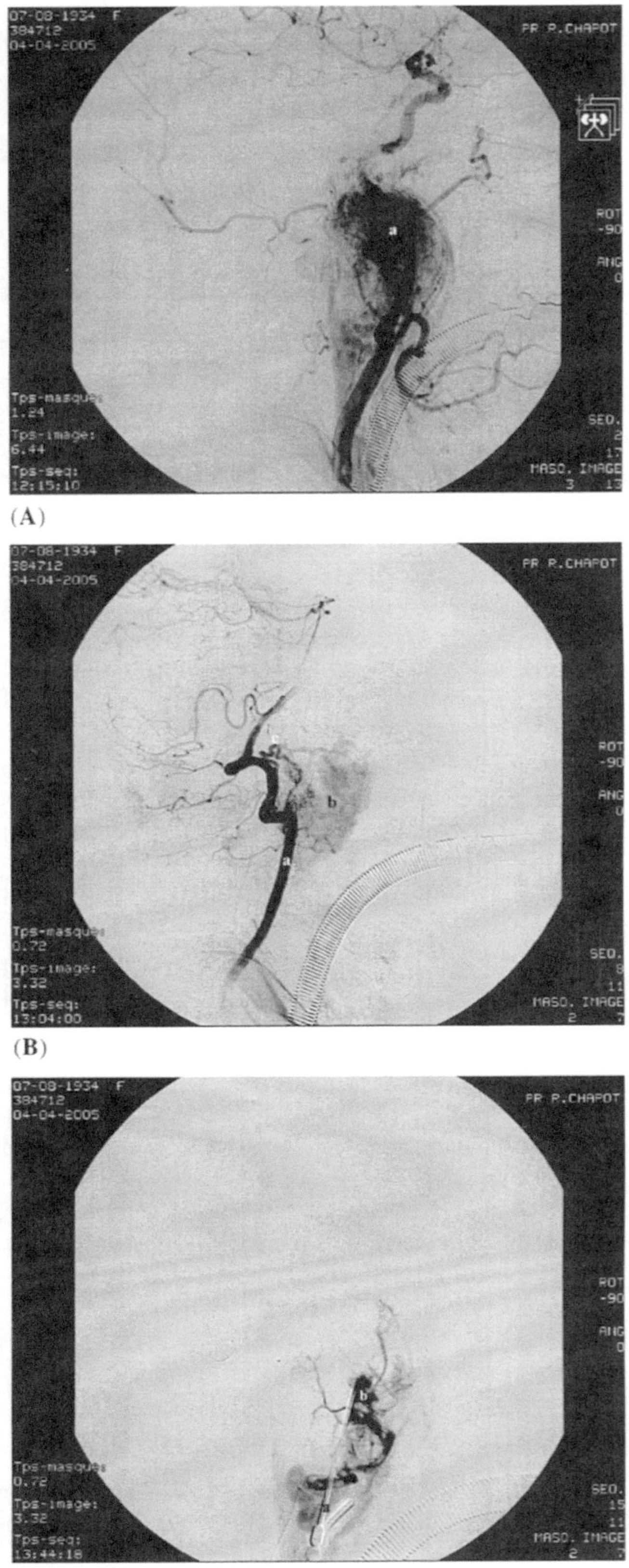

Fig. 2 Foramen jugular paraganglioma embolized with direct puncture and injection of Onyx. (**A**) Hypervascularized tumor of foramen jugular location that is fed by multiple branches from the external carotid artery. *a* Paraganglioma. (**B**) Lateral view of the vertebral artery showing refilling of the tumor. Selective catheterization and embolization of this feeder from the vertebral artery is at risk of aberrant embolization in the intracranial posterior circulation. *a* Vertebral artery. *b* Paraganglioma. *c* Feeder from vertebral artery. (**C**) Direct puncture of the tumor and injection of contrast showing opacification

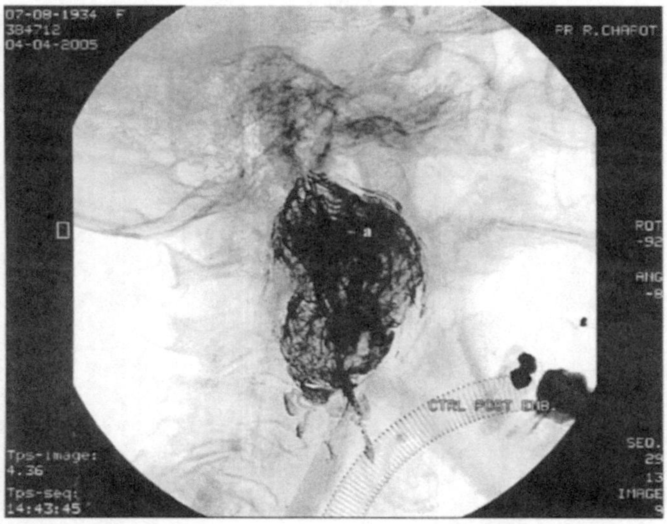

(D)

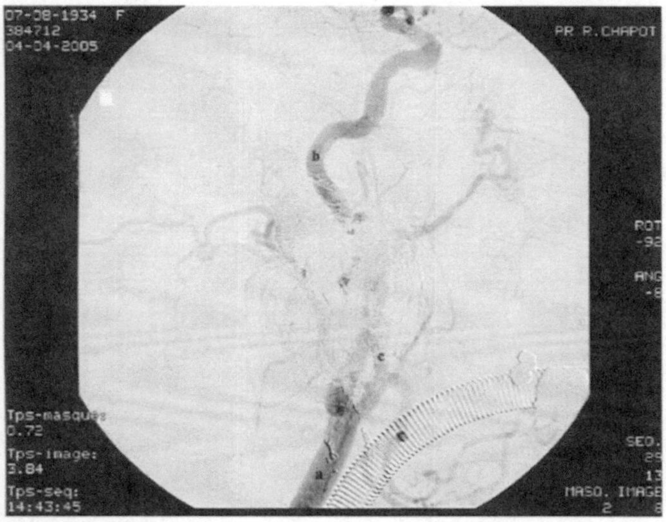

(E)

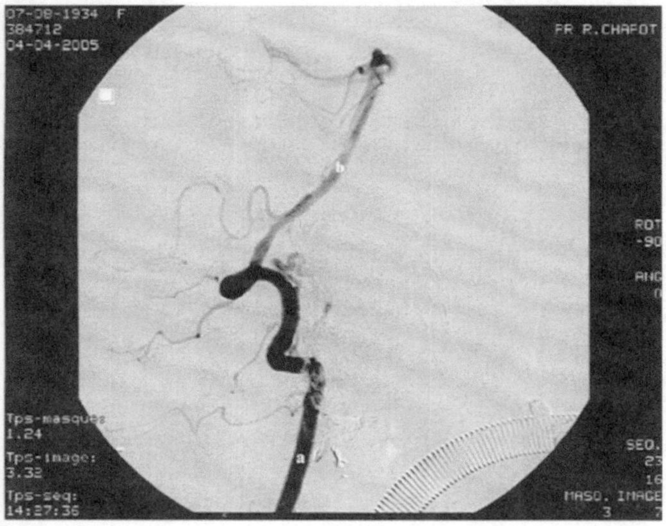

(F)

Fig. 2 (continued) of intratumoral arteries and veins. *a*. Puncture needle. *b* Contrast filling tumor vessels. (**D**) Intratumoral cast of Onyx injected by direct puncture showing widespread embolization material in all intratumoral vessels. *a* Cast of Onyx. (**E**) and (**F**) Common carotid and vertebral artery after injection of Onyx, confirming complete devascularization. (**E**) *a* Common carotid artery. *b* Internal carotid artery. *c* External carotid artery. (**F**) *a* Vertebral artery. *b*. Basilar artery.

glue or Onyx®. The high degree of vascularization of these tumors allows direct access to intratumoral vessels with a needle after direct puncture. The main advantages of this technique is to allow embolization of tumors where feeders cannot be accessed with a microcatheter and to achieve a high degree of devascularization as not only arteries but also veins are occluded by this means. The main drawback is the risk of retrograde diffusion of the embolizing agent in normal vessels by opening of anastomoses (Fig. 2).

2.2. JUVENILE NASOPHARYNGEAL ANGIOFIBROMAS Juvenile nasopharyngeal angiofibromas are benign nonencapsulated fibrovascular tumors typically occupying the nasopharynx and posterior nasal cavity of males around the age of puberty. These tumors arise from the lateral margin of the posterior nasal cavity and can show extensive local spread. The lesions are generally supplied by branches of the internal maxillary (sphenopalatine and descending palatine branches) and ascending pharyngeal arteries. In larger lesions, the vascular supply is provided by the facial and ophthalmic arteries and by branches of the internal carotid arteries.

The goal of treatment is complete surgical resection of the tumor as partial resection mostly leads to recurrence. Surgery may be technically difficult due to the high degree of vascularization. To reduce intraoperative bleeding, embolization is achieved preoperatively. Surgery should be performed 2 to 3 days after embolization to have the highest benefit of embolization and reduce the effect of subsequent recanalization.

Embolization is achieved mostly with microparticles after successive microcatheterization of all feeders. The use of small (<300 μm) microparticles increases not only the efficiency of embolization but also the risk of aberrant diffusion of these microparticles through anastomotic channels in the normal vasculature. Spherical microparticles (Embosphere®, Biosphere Medical) have better intratumoral ability to diffuse and devascularize than nonspherical microparticles. Coils should be avoided as they only achieve proximal vascular occlusion. Besides, they prevent any possible reembolization of the same feeder in case of recurrence.

In large lesions supplied by the internal carotid arteries for which an embolization with microparticles cannot be achieved, embolization by direct puncture is the only means to achieve an efficient devascularization (Fig. 3).

Craniofacial imaging should be routinely performed in the days following surgery using contrast-enhanced computed tomography (CT). This is the best way to make sure that the entire tumor has been withdrawn. If residual tumor is seen, completion surgery should be quickly implemented to avoid recurrence of a large lesion.

2.3. SKULL BASE MENINGIOMAS Meningiomas represent about 15% of all primary central nervous system neoplasms. They originate from cellular elements that form the meninges but may also arise from pial or dural fibroblasts. They typically affect adults aged 25 to 65, with a peak age of about 45 years. Multiple meningiomas are present in 1% to 2% of cases, usually associated with neurofibromatosis. Meningiomas are typically benign but can rarely be malignant. They are well-circumscribed lesions with or without lobulations. They are slow growing and do not invade, but compress local structures.

The ability for embolization mostly depends on the vessels supplying the tumor. Skull base meningiomas arising from the

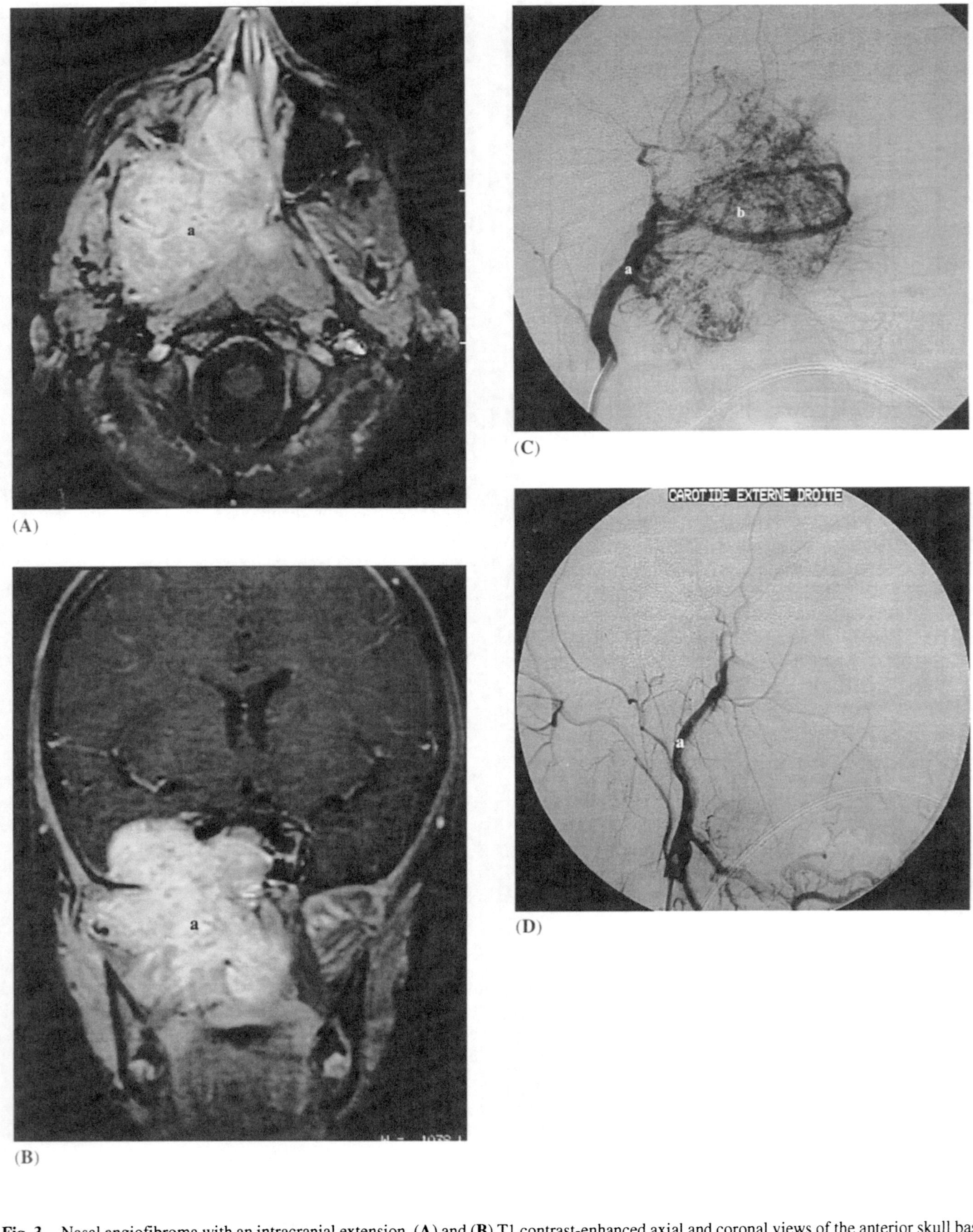

Fig. 3 Nasal angiofibroma with an intracranial extension. (**A**) and (**B**) T1 contrast-enhanced axial and coronal views of the anterior skull base showing a large nasal angiofibroma with an important intracranial extension. (**A**) and (**B**) *a* Angiofibroma. (**C**) and (**D**) Hypervascular tumoral blush provided from the external carotid artery on this lateral view, with disappearance of the blush after embolization with microparticles. (**C**) *a* External carotid artery. *b* Tumoral blush. (**D**) *a* External carotid artery. (**E**) Lateral view of the internal carotid artery showing an important recruitment that is not accessible to embolization with microparticles. *a* Internal carotid artery. *b* Tumoral blush. (**F**) Direct tumoral puncture through an anterior and lateral approach. *a* Puncture needle, anterior approach. *b* Puncture needle, lateral approach. (**G**) Postembolization intratumoral cast of glue. *a* Cast of glue. (**H**) Lateral view of the internal carotid artery after direct puncture embolization showing subtotal occlusion of the hypervascularization. *a* Internal carotid artery. *b*. Residual tumoral blush.

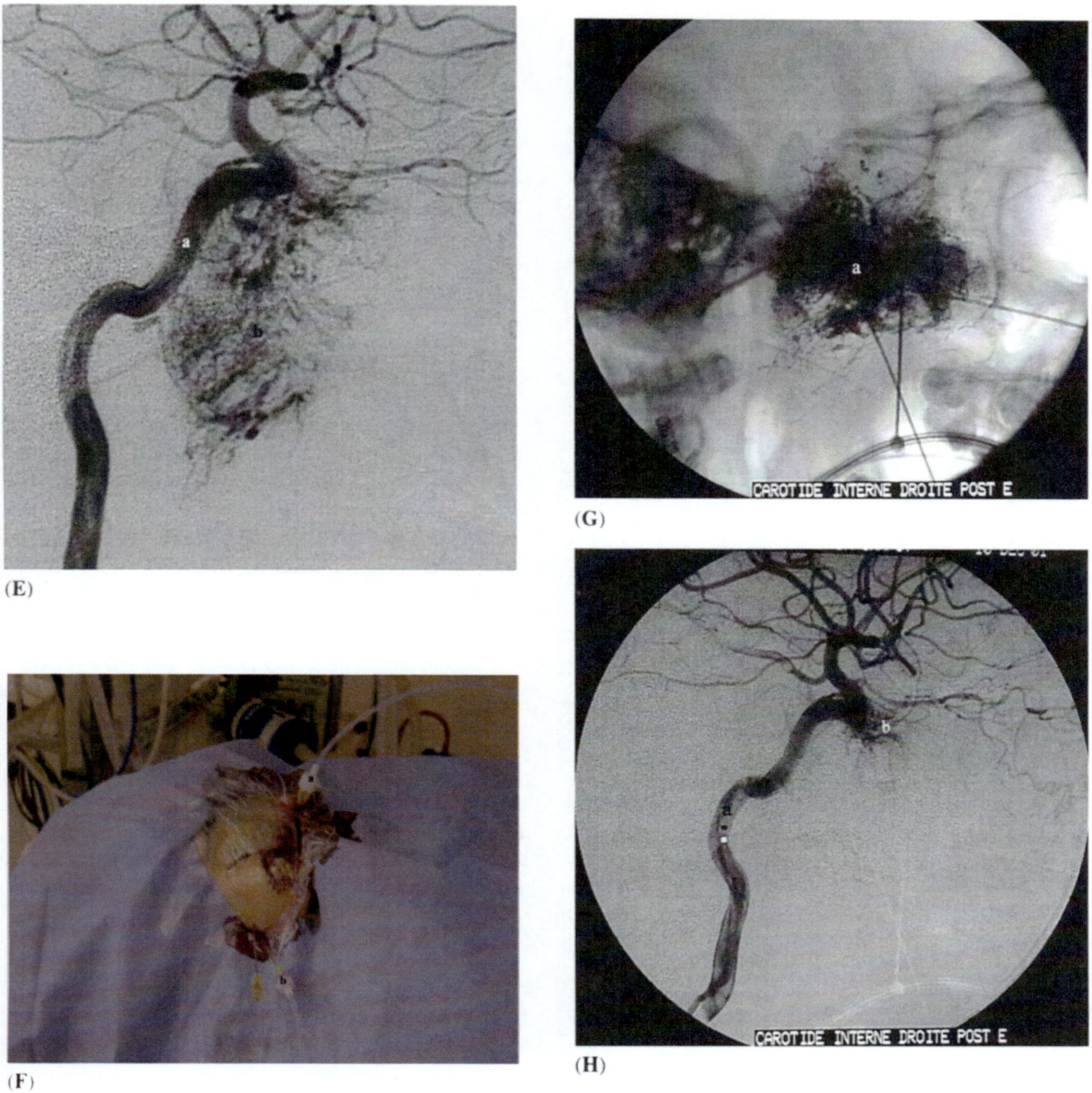

Fig. 3 (continued)

olfactory groove or the planum sphenoidale are mostly supplied from the anterior and posterior ethmoidal branches of the ophthalmic artery. Embolization cannot therefore be achieved as selective catheterization of the ethmoidal arteries is either not possible or carries a high risk of a blocked flow condition with subsequent aberrant embolization of the central retinal artery.

Cavernous sinus and parasellar meningiomas receive blood supply from the meningohypophyseal trunk and inferolateral trunk, which are branches of the cavernous ICA. These branches cannot usually be accessed selectively, and if they can, there is a significant risk of reflux from the embolizing agent into the ICA; hence, embolization is usually avoided.

The most favorable location for embolization is the convexity of the skull, at the temporal and parietal level. The vascular supply is provided by the middle meningeal artery, which is usually easily accessed selectively with a microcatheter. Embolization is then achieved with small-size microparticles. Some hemorrhagic complications have been described after embolization of meningiomas with microparticles. Such complications remain rare, but they seem to be avoided by the use of acrylic glue in the meningeal trunk at the end of the embolization with microparticles (Fig. 4).

3. TEST AND PERMANENT OCCLUSION OF THE INTERNAL CAROTID ARTERY

3.1. INDICATIONS Indications for test and permanent occlusion of an ICA include fusiform or giant wide-necked aneurysms that cannot be treated selectively by either endovascular or surgical techniques; posttraumatic lesions of the ICA; or skull base tumors when intraoperative occlusion of the ICA is contemplated.

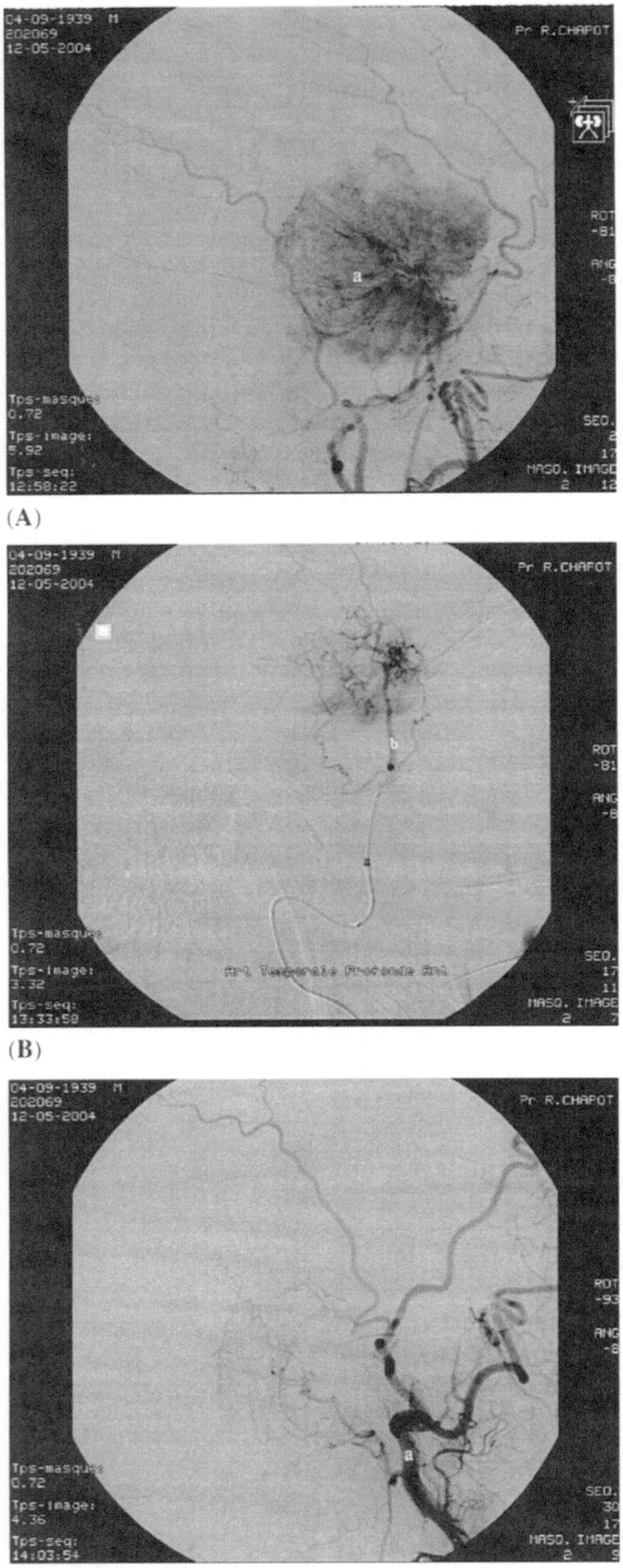

Fig. 4 Preoperative meningioma embolization. (**A**) Hypervascular blush on lateral view after injection of the external carotid artery and in relation to a meningioma located at the temporal level. *a* Tumoral blush. (**B**) Selective catheterization of the main feeder, which is the middle meningeal artery, before injection of calibrated microspheres. *a* Microcatheter. *b*. Middle meningeal artery. (**C**) Postembolization angiogram of the external carotid artery on a lateral projection. *a* External carotid artery.

3.2. TECHNICAL FEATURES The procedure is achieved under neuroleptic analgesia to enable clinical assessment of the patient during the occlusion test. Full anticoagulation with intravenous heparin is required to prevent clot formation during flow disruption.

Four-vessel cerebral angiography is achieved as a first step to evaluate the complete intracranial vasculature. A bilateral femoral approach is then required for simultaneous placement of a guiding catheter in the vessel to occlude and a diagnostic catheter in the contralateral ICA or VA. The occlusion test is then achieved with a nondetachable balloon that is inflated in the petrosal segment of the ICA. In a borderline situation, balloon inflation may last up to 30 min. The blood pressure may also be decreased by 20 mmHg during the test.

3.3 EVALUATION OF TOLERANCE Several parameters are evaluated during the test occlusion. Clinical tolerance is tested through higher, sensory, and motor functions. In case of clinical intolerance, the balloon is immediately deflated, and the test is abandoned.

Angiographic appearance with functionality of the circle of Willis is verified by injecting the contralateral ICA and the dominant VA to evaluate both anterior and posterior communicating arteries. Filling of the Middle Cerebral Artery (MCA) is mostly seen at various degrees, so that the determining aspect of the test is the venous phase; the occlusion test is well tolerated when the delay in appearance of the cortical veins between both hemispheres remains below 2 s. If this delay exceeds 4 s, the test is not tolerated. Between 2 and 4 s, further investigations may be needed, such as a hypotensive test with a decrease in blood pressure of 20 mmHg. This test shows the functional reserves as it may induce a clinical deficit due to insufficient vascular anastomoses.

In case of well-tolerated test occlusion, permanent occlusion can be performed with either a detachable balloon or coils. When using a balloon, a second safety balloon should be released just below the first one.

4. INFERIOR PETROSAL SINUS SAMPLING

4.1. RATIONALE FOR THE PROCEDURE The most important recent advance in the diagnostic evaluation of patients with Cushing's syndrome has been the use of bilateral inferior petrosal sinus sampling (BIPSS) for corticotropin (ACTH). The inferior petrosal sinuses receive drainage from the pituitary gland without mixture of blood from other sources. Therefore, if the patient has pituitary Cushing's syndrome, the ACTH levels in the inferior petrosal sinus is high compared to an ACTH drawn in the periphery. In contrast, in ectopic Cushing's, the ACTH in the inferior petrosal sinus and the periphery should be equivalent because the tumor is located elsewhere.

The inferior petrosal sinus sampling test has been shown to determine reliably whether there is a peripheral ectopic source of ACTH and has somewhat less reliably correctly predicted lateralization. The endocrinologist can then use this information to guide therapy. If a primary adenoma is determined to be present in the pituitary gland, the surgeon can use this information to decide which half of the pituitary gland contains the offending secretory tumor and thus which half to remove, rather than removing the entire gland and potentially causing panhypopituitarism.

4.2. TECHNICAL FEATURES The pituitary gland drains into the cavernous sinus and bilateral inferior petrosal sinuses, superior petrosal sinuses, and basilar venous plexus. For evaluation of the side of a possible microadenoma, simultaneous venous samples are achieved, from each inferior petrosal sinus, in addition to a concurrent peripheral sample.

Bilateral venous access is achieved by a standard transfemoral approach. Guiding catheters are placed in both internal jugular veins, allowing further catheterization of each inferior petrosal sinus. The microcatheters should be left at the inferior proximal half of the inferior petrosal sinus. Samples are then obtained from each microcatheter and from the groin, serving as the peripheral vein sample. A stimulation test with corticotropin-releasing hormone (CRH) may be added to trigger the secretion of ACTH. A significant gradient between the pituitary (central) and peripheral venous values of plasma ACTH is indicative of Cushing's disease.

5 Instrumentation in Endoscopic Skull Base Surgery

This chapter provides an in-depth description and state-of-the-art illustrations of the instrumentation utilized in endoscopic skull base surgery. Advances in technology have complemented the advances in endoscopic skull base surgery and stimulated the creation of dedicated endoscopic equipment and microinstruments specifically designed to fulfill the unique requirements of endoscopic skull base surgery. These instruments include rigid endoscopes, lens irrigation systems, pneumatically powered robotic holding arms, bipolars, light sources, high-definition digital cameras, digital processors, digital monitors, digital versatile disc (DVD) recorders, Polaroid digital photo printers, nerve monitoring devices (electroencephalographs, electromyographs, and those for somatosensory, brainstem auditory, motor, and visual evoked potentials), microdrills, micro-Cavitron ultrasonic aspirators (microCUSAs), and specialized endoscopic microinstruments.

Keywords: BAEP; Bipolar; Cavitron ultrasonic aspirators (CUSA); Digital camera; Digital monitor; Digital processor; DVD recorder; EEG; EMG; Endoscopic equipment; Endoscopic instrumentation; Endoscopic instruments; Endoscopic technologies; Endoscopic technology; Holding arm; Irrigation sheaths and pumps; Lens irrigation system; Light source; MEP; Microdrill; Microinstruments; Minimally invasive; Nerve monitoring device; Pneumatically powered robotic holding arms; Polaroid digital photo printer; Rigid endoscopes; Skull base; SSEP; Surgery; VEP.

1. INTRODUCTION

Conventional neurosurgical and microsurgical instruments are too bulky for endoscopic skull base surgery. Whereas operating microscopes require wide viewing portals for adequate illumination and visualization of the operative field, endoscopes utilize minute keyholes to precisely reach the target area. Therefore, adapting and refining regular microinstruments and equipment such as bipolars and Cavitron ultrasonic aspirators (CUSAs) to include longer, more slender shafts and smaller microtips has been essential for endoscopic skull base surgical approaches. In addition, major improvements such as the invention of sophisticated light sources, cameras, digital processors, lens irrigation systems, and robotic holding arms have all complemented the advances in endoscopic technology and stimulated the creation of dedicated endoscopic equipment and microinstruments specifically designed to fulfill the unique requirements of endoscopic skull base surgery (Fig. 1).

2. RIGID ENDOSCOPES

The design of the Hopkins rod lens system, developed by the British physicist Harold Hopkins in the late 1960s, has been revolutionized over the past several decades to yield endoscopes of variable lengths, diameters, and angles of view. The modern rigid endoscopes currently used for skull base surgery are either 2.7 or 4 mm in diameter, and their standard working length is 18 cm. The larger the diameter of the endoscope, the better the image it displays and the more light it can transmit to the operative field. Specialized endoscopic microinstruments are inserted alongside the endoscope, and the entire surgery is performed by viewing a high-definition plasma screen or liquid crystal display (LCD).

The 0° endoscopes give a "straight-on" view, while 30° endoscopes permit viewing from the side, a useful tool when looking around corners at the skull base, such as looking into the internal auditory canal (IAC) in vestibular schwannoma surgery or the cavernous sinuses during endonasal pituitary surgery. Endoscopes with a wider angle, such as 70° and 90°, are difficult and disorienting to work with and are only occasionally used (Fig. 2A,B)

3. IRRIGATION SHEATHS AND PUMPS

Imaging with an endoscope requires a clear medium and optimal illumination of the surgical field with the lowest amount of diffraction. Placement of the endoscope's lens into the surgical field exposes it to blood, fluid, and debris. To avoid the dangerous practice of frequently removing, cleaning, and repositioning

From: *Endoscopic Skull Base Surgery: A Comprehensive Guide with Illustrative Cases.*
Edited by H. K. Shahinian © Humana Press, Totowa, NJ.

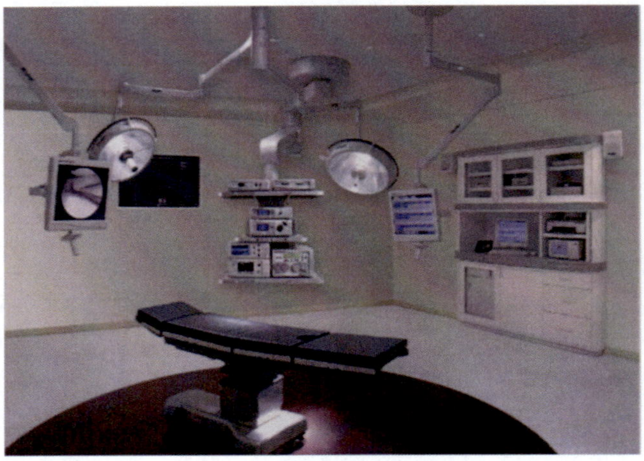

Fig. 1 Skull base surgery EndoSuite.

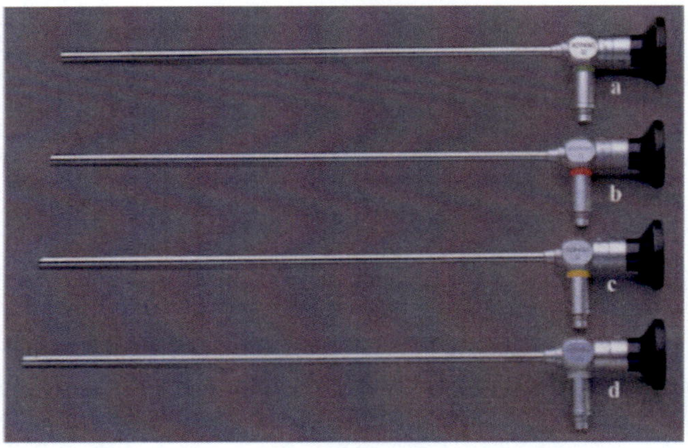

(A)

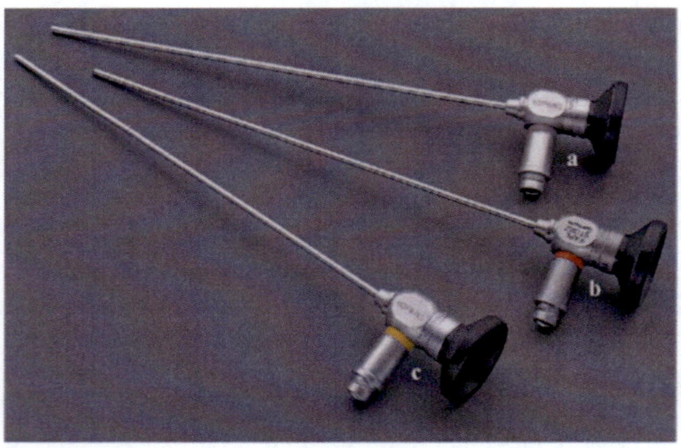

(B)

Fig. 2 Rigid endoscopes. (**A**) 4-mm endoscopes. *a* 0° endoscope. *b* 30° endoscope. *c* 70° endoscope. *d* 90° endoscope. (**B**) 2.7-mm endoscopes. *a* 0° endoscope. *b* 30° endoscope. *c* 70° endoscope.

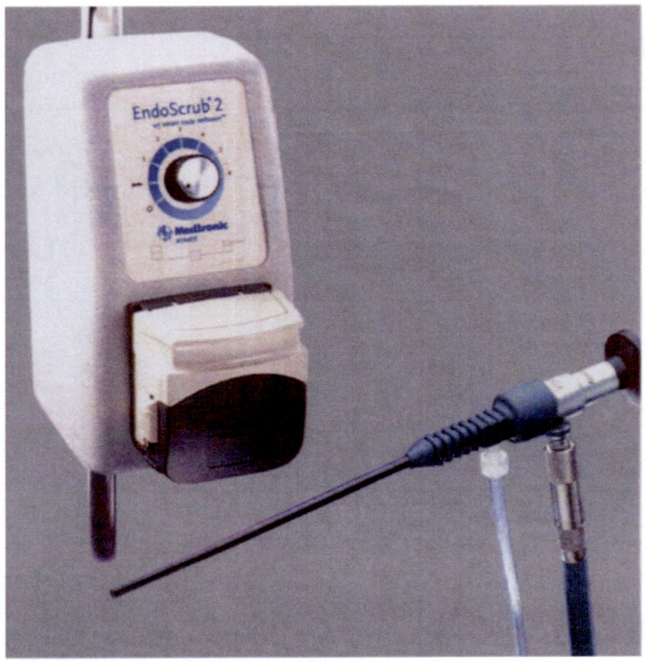

Fig. 3 Irrigation sheath and pump.

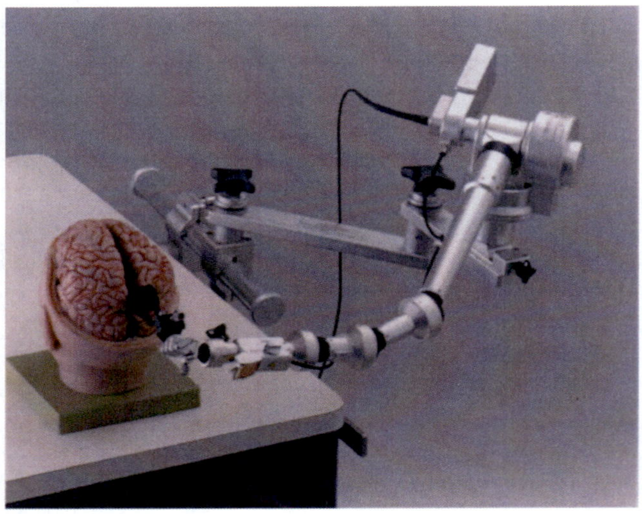

Fig. 4 Pneumatic holding arm.

the endoscope, we have fitted our endoscopes with irrigation sheaths that are attached to a pump that uses sterile saline to clear the lens while the endoscope remains in position. Irrigation sheaths are available in different diameters to fit different size endoscopes. On demand, the motorized pedal-activated pump delivers a cleansing stream of saline over the tip of the endoscope. This is immediately followed by a brief period of suction by which any remaining drops of saline that would otherwise blur the image are cleared off the lens (Fig. 3).

4. PNEUMATIC HOLDING ARMS

Bimanual dexterity is a necessity in endoscopic skull base surgery, and therefore holding arms are an essential component of the endoscopic equipment. The holding arms must be sturdy, stable, and capable of holding the endoscopes securely, yet they must be easily adjustable to allow the surgeon to manipulate them at will. Whereas earlier designs were mechanical, combining long metallic rods with movable joints, the latest generation of holding arms consists of

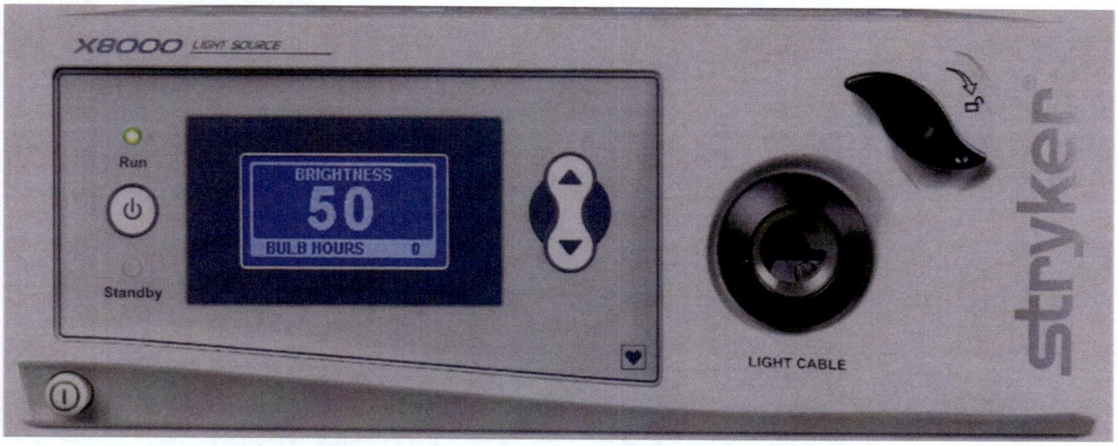

Fig. 5 Xenon light source.

ball bearing joints that are pneumatically powered. These devices are remarkably flexible and extremely reliable. Surgeons can operate them quite easily with a finger-activated mechanism that alternates between free and locked positions (Fig. 4).

5. XENON LIGHT SOURCES

Illumination is generated by a powerful cold-light source and transmitted to the endoscope via a fiber-optic cable. Light travels along the length of the endoscope to fiber-optically illuminate the operative field. The different types of light sources (tungsten, halogen, metal halide, xenon) offer light of varying brightness. Currently, the most powerful and preferred light source for endoscopic skull base surgery is a xenon system (Fig. 5).

6. HIGH-DEFINITION DIGITAL CAMERAS

Hopkins rod telescopes are manufactured with built-in standard eyepieces to which cameras are attached. The image is then projected onto one or several monitors, where it is electronically processed and recorded. Three-chip cameras contain individual chips for each of the primary colors. These produce excellent quality images and feature automatic controls over color, exposure, white balance, and digital contrast enhancement. Devices that digitally process the endoscope's image allow for optimum enhancement and image manipulation. Recently, progressive-scan, high-definition, fully digital cameras have provided further improvement in image quality (Fig. 6A,B).

7. DIGITAL MONITORS

A monitor displays the camera's image during the entire endoscopic procedure; it is the "surgeon's eye," and therefore its position is critical for the surgeon. Ceiling-mounted monitors provide maneuverability that allows the monitor to be positioned in the direct line of view of the surgeon. A second monitor is useful for viewing by the remainder of the surgical team. These color monitors should have at least 700 lines of resolution for three-chip cameras. Recently, high-definition LCD and plasma screen monitors have been coupled to high-definition cameras, resulting in superb image resolution (Fig. 7).

8. DVD RECORDERS

Digital recording devices allow single-frame or continuous imaging to be produced and stored in digital format that can then be used for presentations and publications to illustrate or document the surgery. Currently, digital versatile disc (DVD) recorders provide higher resolutions and higher data storage capacity than traditional videocassette recorders (VCRs) or digital video camera (DVCAM) recorders. They also provide direct digital formatting (Fig. 8).

9. POLAROID DIGITAL PRINTERS

Polaroid digital printers provide color prints for documentation; these prints are high quality, dry, durable, and fade resistant. They are particularly helpful for sharing information with the patient's family on completion of the surgery while the family members are in the surgical waiting room. These printers have electronic controls to manipulate brightness, contrast, orientation, image resizing, or cropping (Fig. 9).

10. CRANIAL NERVE MONITORS

Intraoperative neurophysiologic monitoring allows for real-time assessment of neurological function that helps guide the surgeon intraoperatively. In general, these devices use electrophysiological methods such as electroencephalography (EEG), electromyography (EMG), and evoked potentials to monitor the functional integrity of neural structures. Evoked potential monitoring includes somatosensory evoked potentials (SSEPs), brainstem auditory evoked potentials (BAEPs), motor evoked potentials (MEPs), and visual evoked potentials (VEPs).

Electromyography is extensively used in skull base surgery. The most common applications are in locating cranial nerves V, VII, X, XI, or XII in patients with cerebellopontine angle (CPA) and brainstem tumors and in patients undergoing microvascular decompressions. Furthermore, a selective electrical stimulation probe allows for intraoperative identification of individual cranial nerves. Depending on the specific location of the tumor, its size, and the vital structures at the skull base that might be involved, it is sometimes important to monitor other cranial nerves; for instance, occulomotor (III), trochlear (IV), and abducens (VI) nerves are monitored in

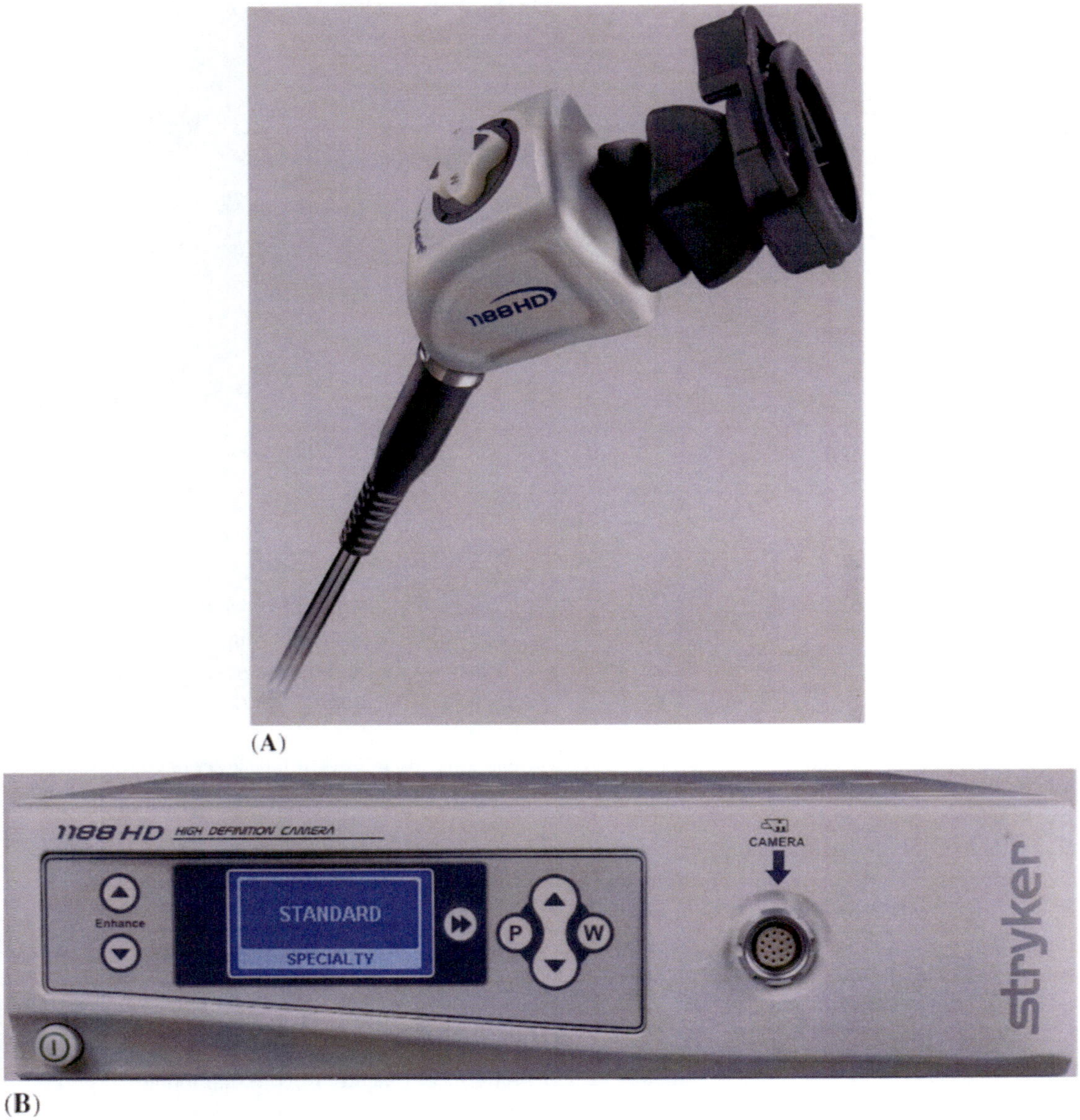

Fig. 6 (**A**) High-definition digital camera. (**B**) Camera unit.

cavernous sinus surgery. Auditory brainstem response (ABR; aka BSEP (Brainstem Evoked Potential), BSER (Brainstem Evoked Response), BAEP, etc.) is particularly important in monitoring the acoustic nerve during acoustic neuroma surgery. Recordings are obtained after stimulation with auditory clicks in the ear. This is particularly useful in small- to medium-size tumors, for which hearing preservation is important (Fig. 10).

11. MICRODRILL HANDPIECES, ATTACHMENTS, AND BURRS

Microdrills are used to create the keyhole bone flap and to drill bony structures within the skull, such as the posterior wall of the IAC in vestibular schwannoma surgery. For endoscopic skull base surgery, pen-style, compact, powerful, smooth, lightweight, high-performance microdrills provide the balance and maneuverability that enable the surgeon to work in tight spaces through keyhole access. The microdrill's attachments are tapered to provide improved visibility of the cutting or diamond burrs at its tip during surgery. They include straight or angled attachments for the creation of the keyhole craniotomy and a special extended arciform attachment for deep access and delicate bone drilling within confined surgical areas at the skull base. Craniotome attachments for both pediatric and adult cases and a range of sizes and shapes for burrs (cutting/diamond) and blades are used in combination with these attachments (Fig. 11A–E).

12. MICRO-CAVITRON ULTRASONIC SURGICAL ASPIRATOR (MICROCUSA) HANDPIECES AND TIPS

Micro-Cavitron ultrasonic surgical aspirators (microCUSAs) are used to enable ultrasonic selective fragmentation and cavitation of the inner part of a tumor. Endoscopic microCUSA

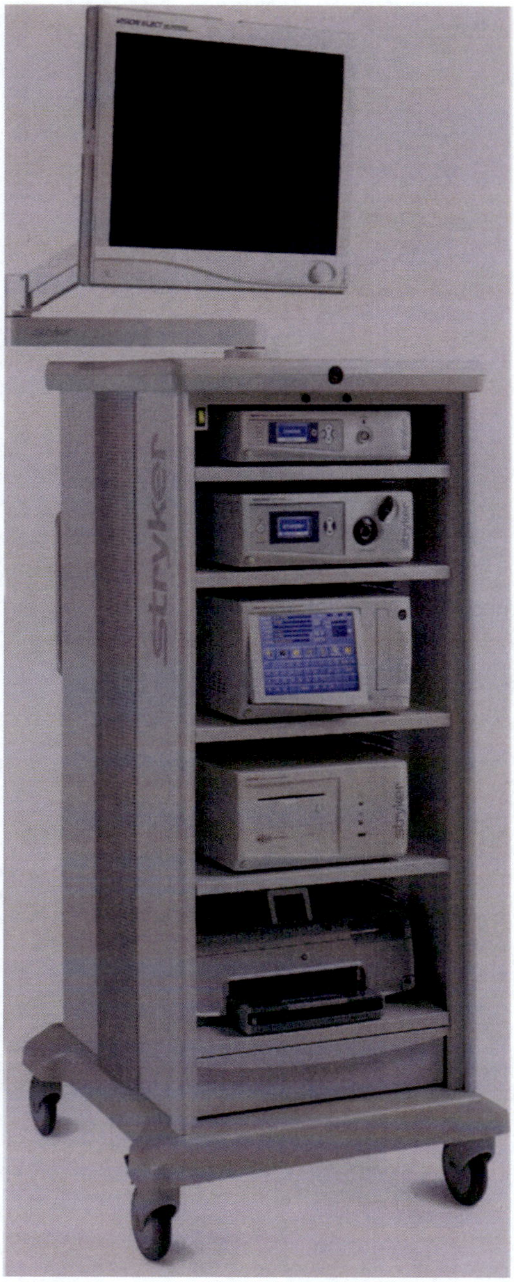

Fig. 7 Endoscopic tower and monitor.

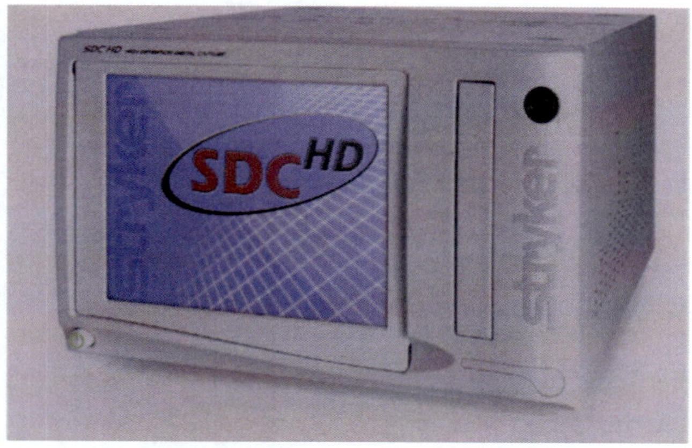

Fig. 8 DVD recorder.

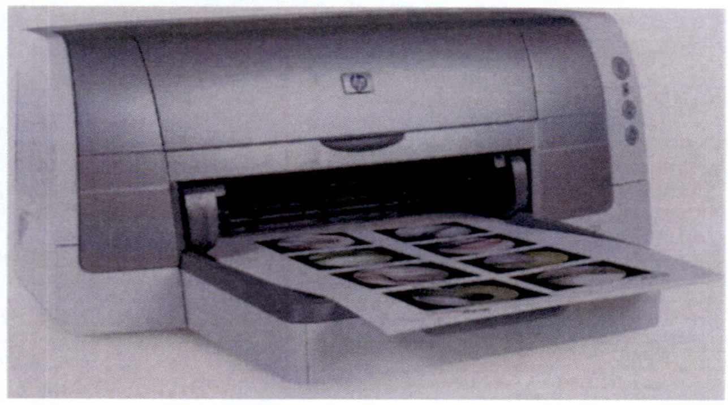

Fig. 9 Polaroid digital printer.

handpieces are more compact, lighter, lengthier, and more slender than the regular ones. They include ultrafine microtips and are angled with extended shafts that give the handpiece a better reach and allow optimal visibility during endoscopic skull base surgery. Generally, there are two different frequencies. The standard 35- or 36-kHz handpiece is ideal for soft tissue removal around critical structures, while the 23- or 24-Hz handpiece is used for harder masses. We have relied exclusively on the 36-kHz micro- and precision tips for all of our needs (Fig. 12A–E).

13. SPECIALIZED ENDOSCOPIC MICROINSTRUMENTS

A wide range of specialized microinstruments has been specifically designed for use in endoscopic skull base surgery, including microscissors, suction tubes, bipolars, microdissectors, and others. These microinstruments are generally more slender with smaller tips than those used in traditional neurosurgery. Special endoscopic bipolars with insulated sheaths and small microtips for easy introduction, 360° rotation, and maneuverability through the keyhole opening are used. Three basic sets of instruments are used exclusively at the Skull Base Institute, as illustrated in Figs. 13, 14, and 15.

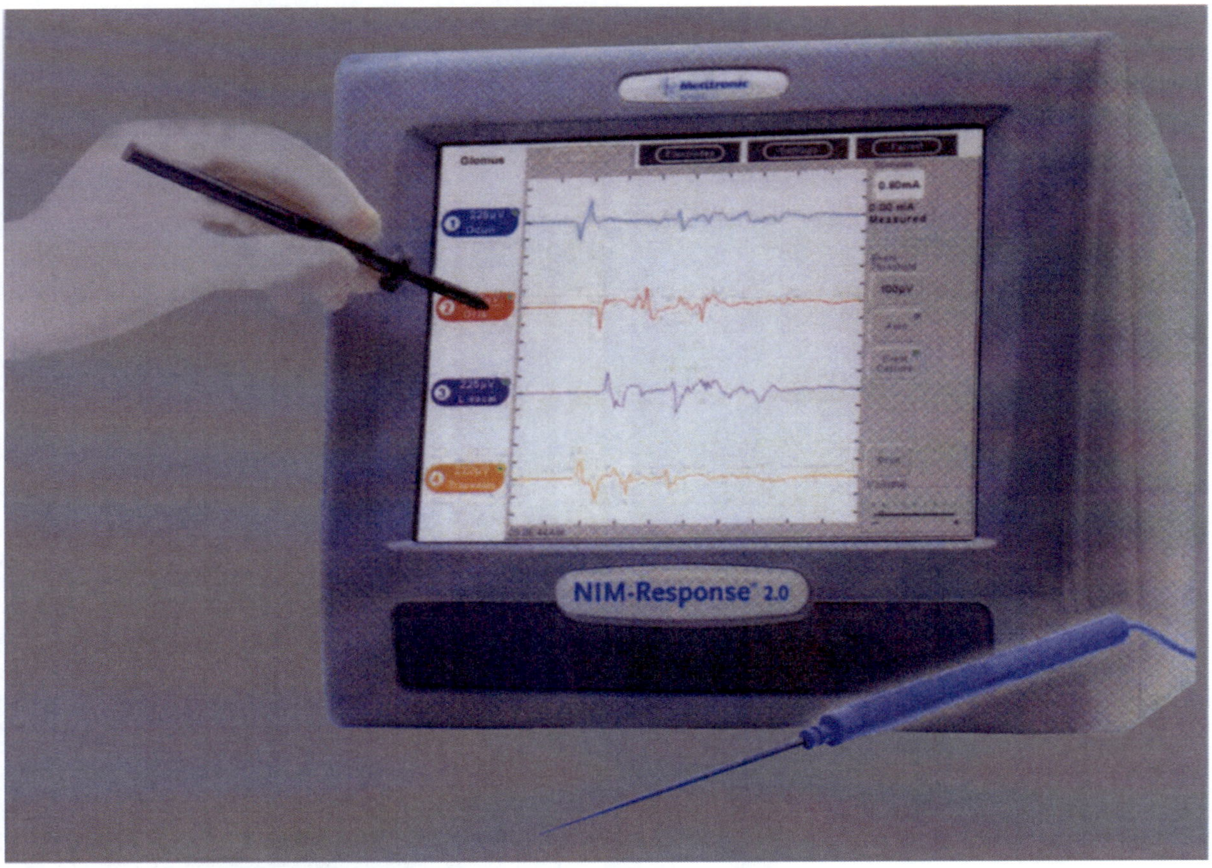

Fig. 10 Cranial nerve EMG monitor.

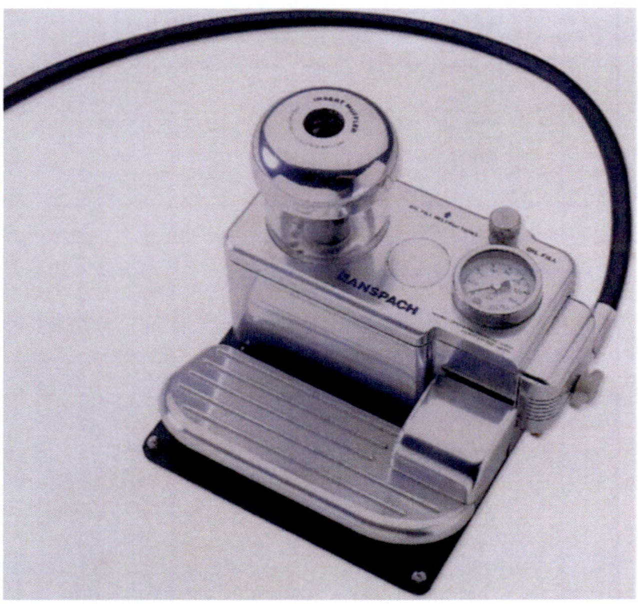

(**A**)

Fig. 11 Microdrill, handpiece, attachments, and burrs. (**A**) Foot control (**B**) Adult craniotome. (**C**) Pediatric craniotome. (**D**) Microdrill handpiece and standard attachment. (**E**) Curved extended minimal access attachments.

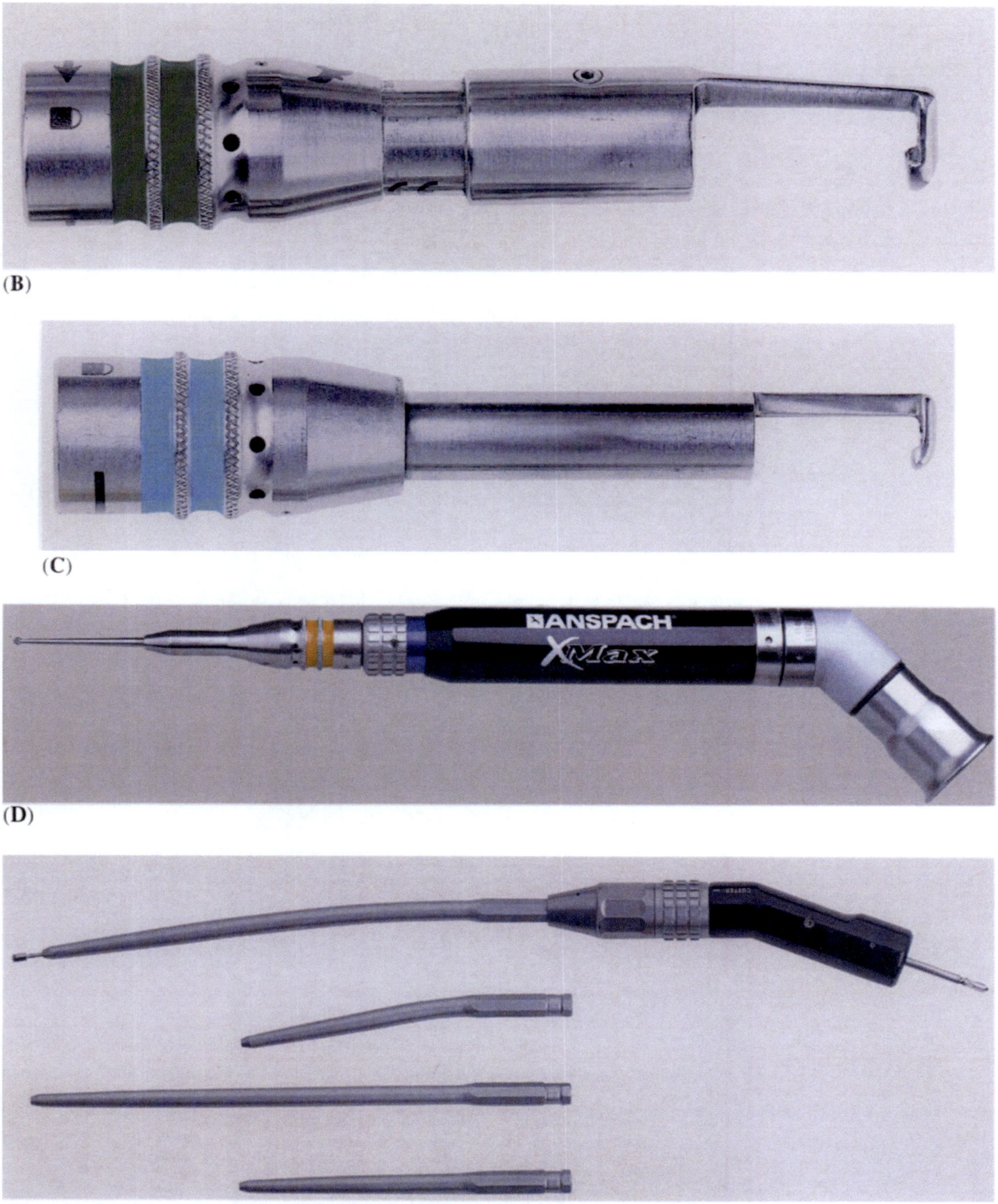

Fig. 11 (continued)

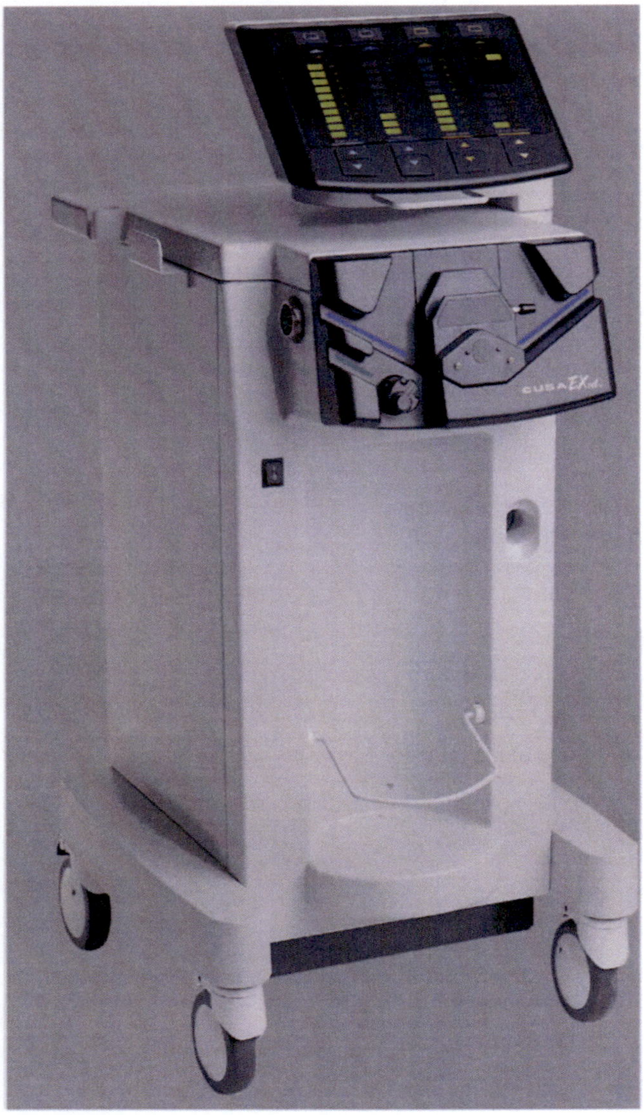

(A)

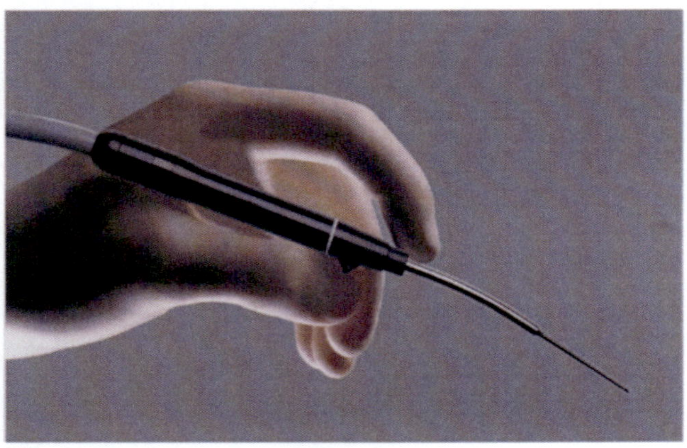

(B)

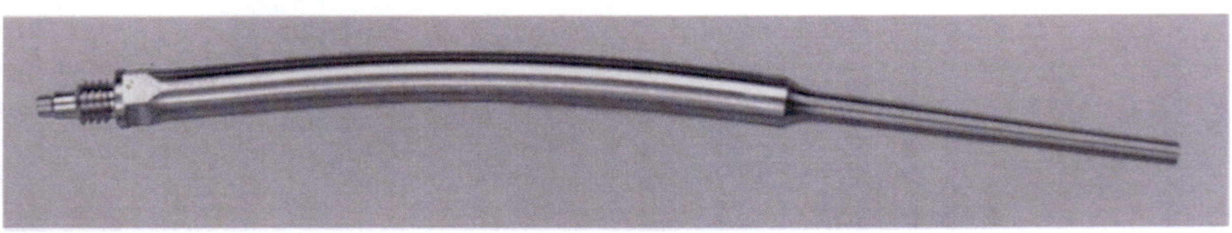

(C)

Fig. 12 MicroCUSA handpieces and tips. (**A**) MicroCUSA console. (**B**) Handpiece. (**C**) Curved extended standard tip. (**D**) Curved extended microtip. (**E**) Curved extended precision tip.

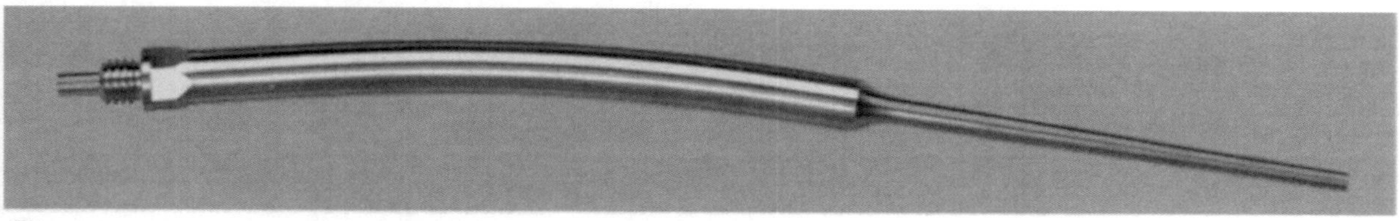

(D)

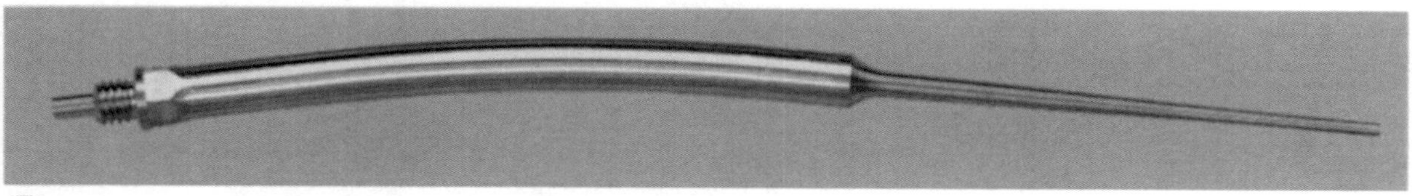

(E)

Fig. 12 (continued)

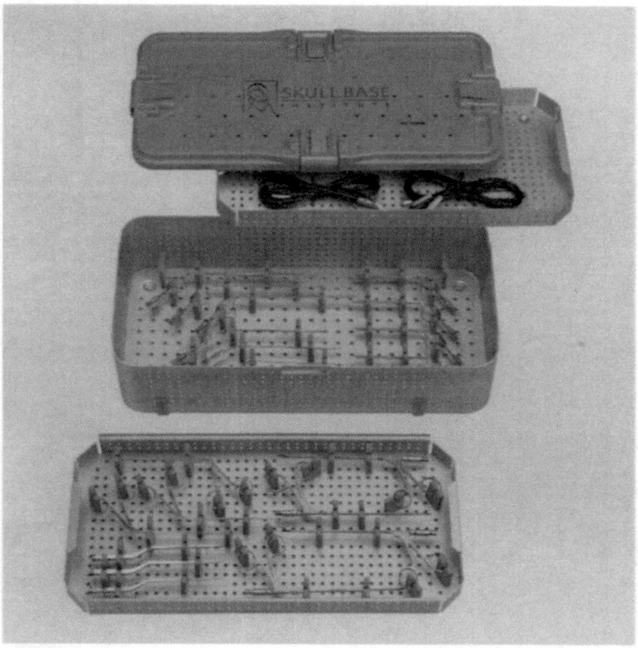

(A)

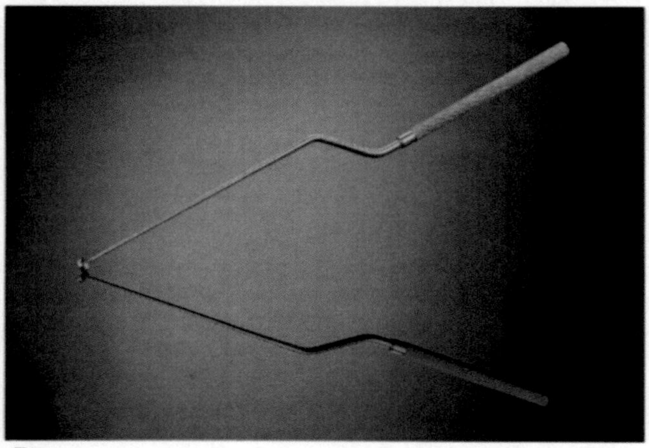

(B)

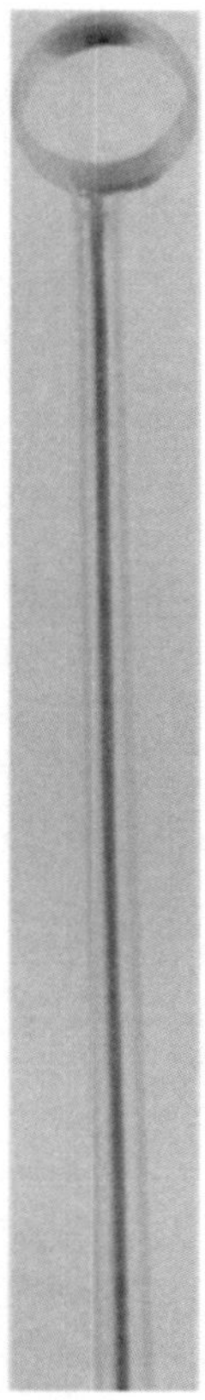

(C)

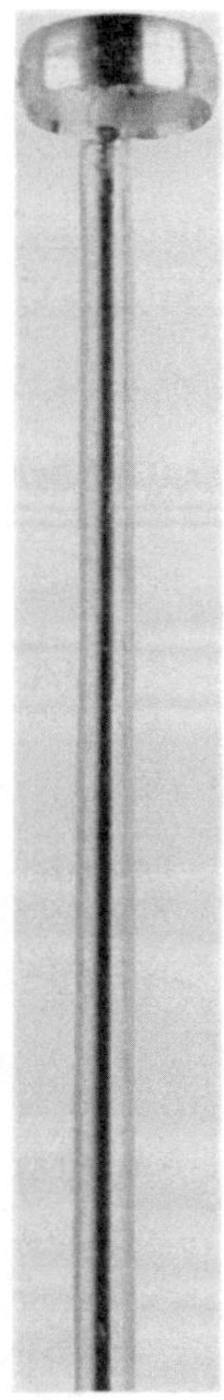

(D)

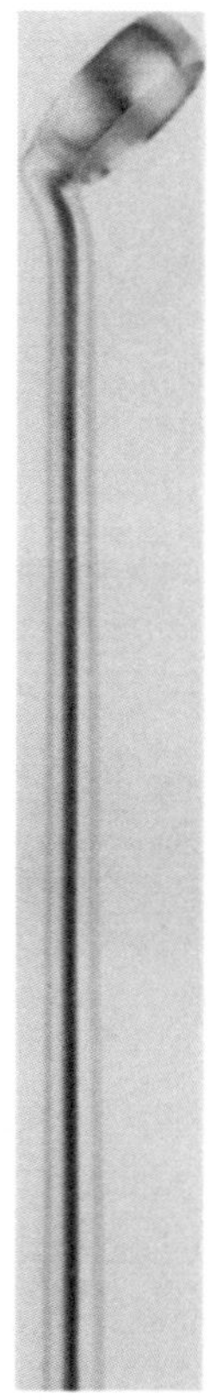

(E)

Fig. 13 (**A**) Tray 1. (**B**) Ring curette, angled 90° left. (**C**) Ring curette tip, angled 45° up. (**D**) Ring curette tip, angled 90° up. (**E**) Ring curette tip, angled 45° right. (**F**) Ring curette tip, angled 90° right. (**G**) Ring curette tip, angled 45° down. (**H**) Ring curette tip, angled 90° down. (**I**) Ring curette tip, angled 45° left. (**J**) Ring curette tip, angled 90° left.

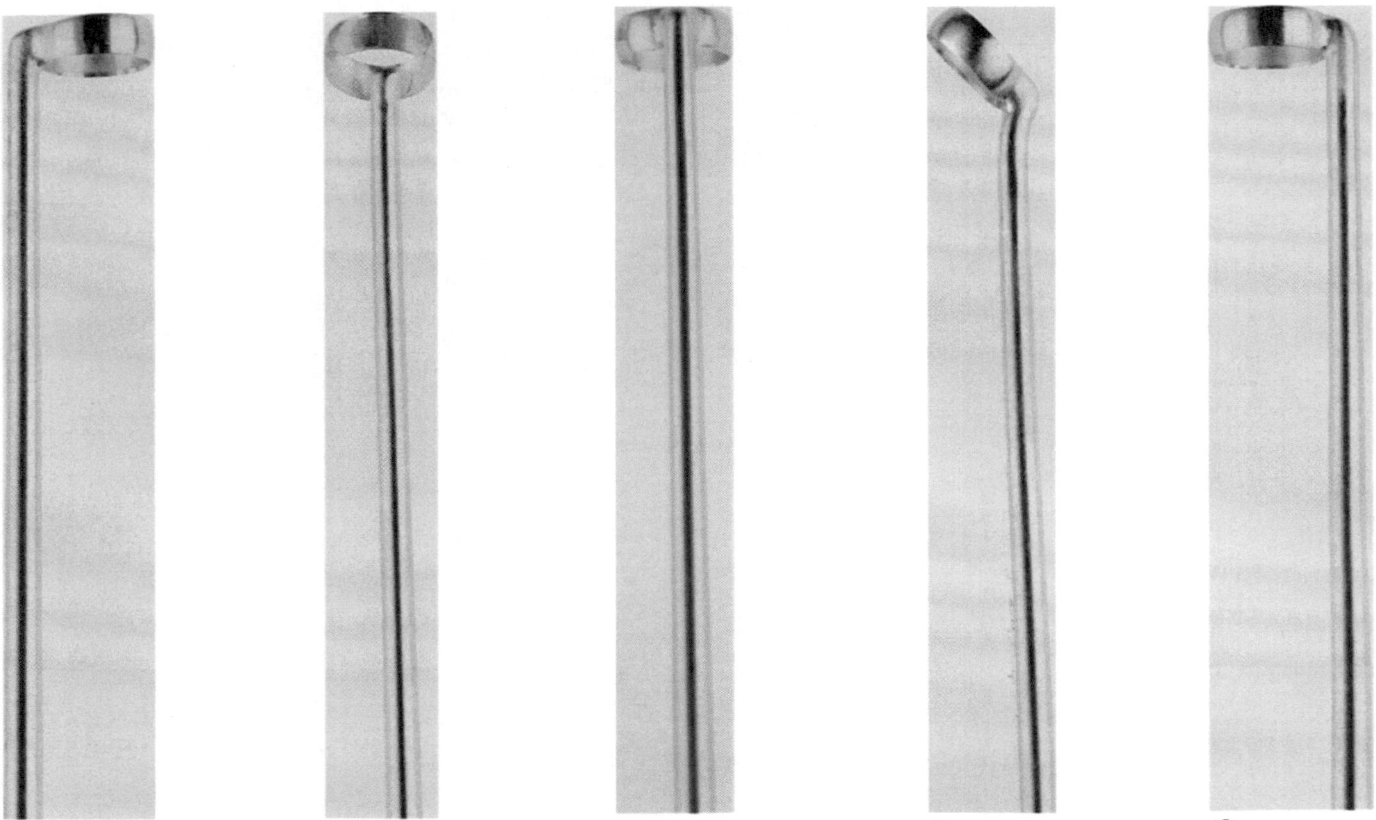

(F) (G) (H) (I) (J)

Fig. 13 (continued)

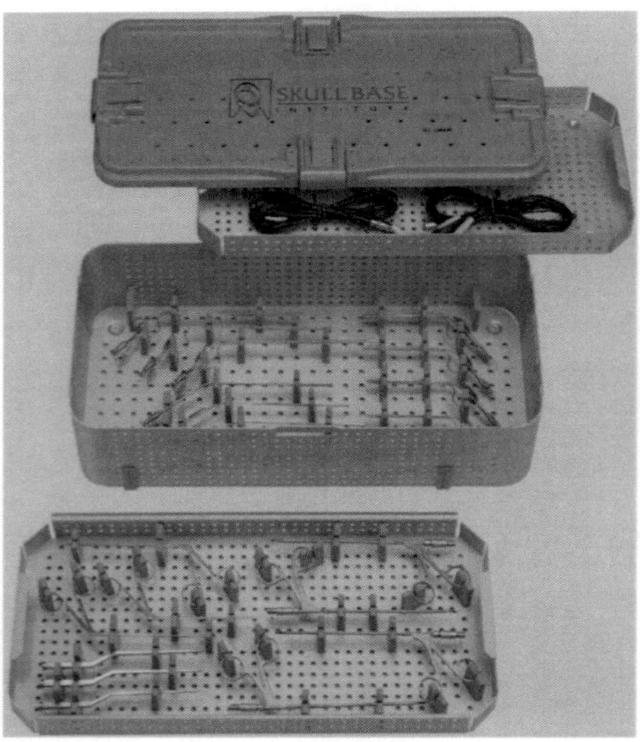

(A)

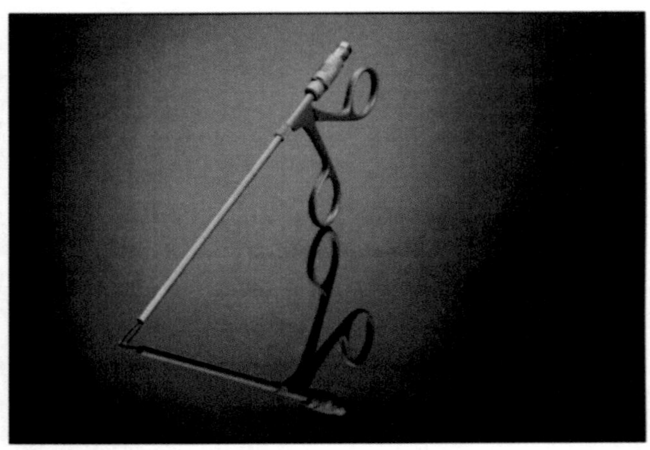

(B)

Fig. 14 (**A**) Tray 2. (**B**) Bipolar forceps. (**C**) Bipolar forceps 1.5-mm tip. (**D**) Bipolar forceps 3.0-mm tip. (**E**) Micro-osteotome medium 3.0-mm tip. (**F**) 2-mm micro-osteotome tip. (**G**) 4-mm micro-osteotome tip. (**H**) Microcupped forceps. (**I**) Microcupped forceps tip. (**J**) Atraumatic suction. (**K**) Atraumatic suction tip. (**L**) Fisch suction irrigation. (**M**) Fisch suction irrigation tip.

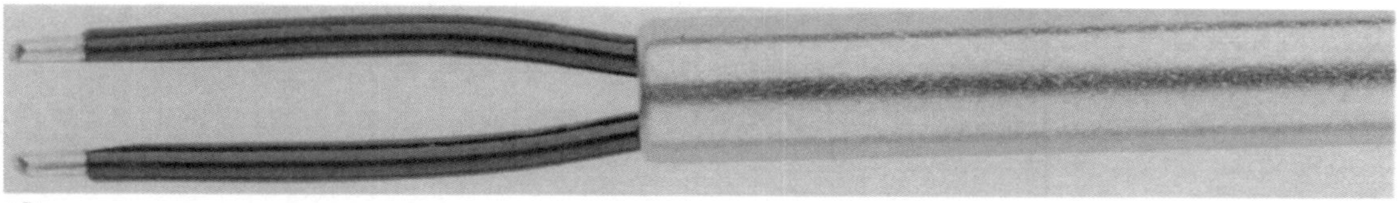

(C)

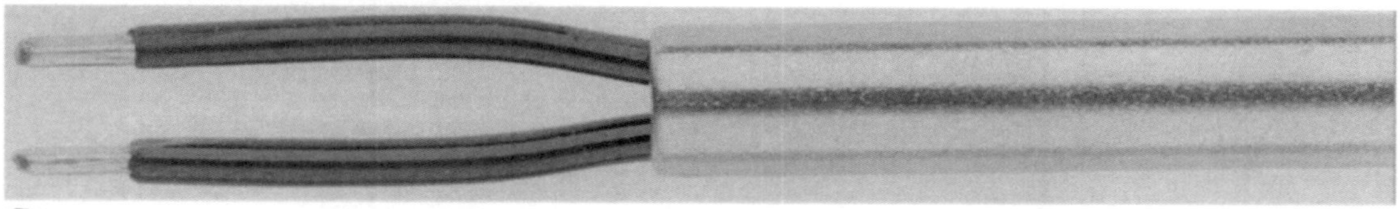

(D)

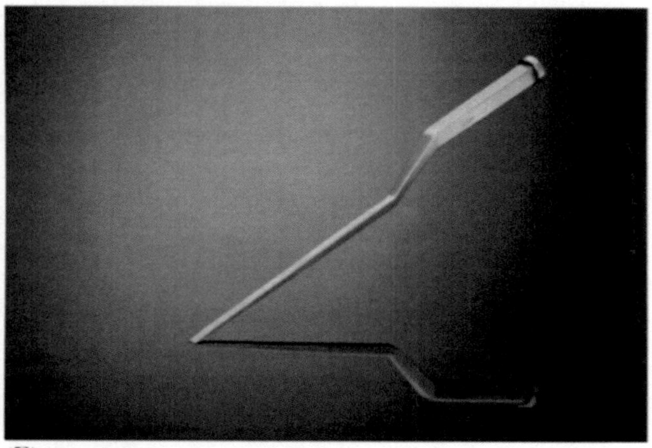

(E)

(F)

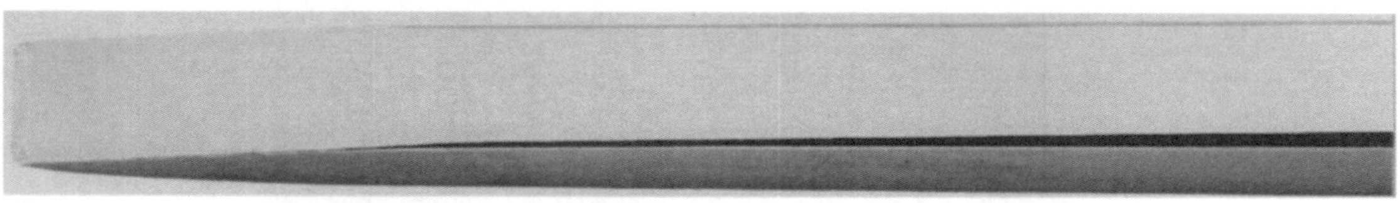

(G)

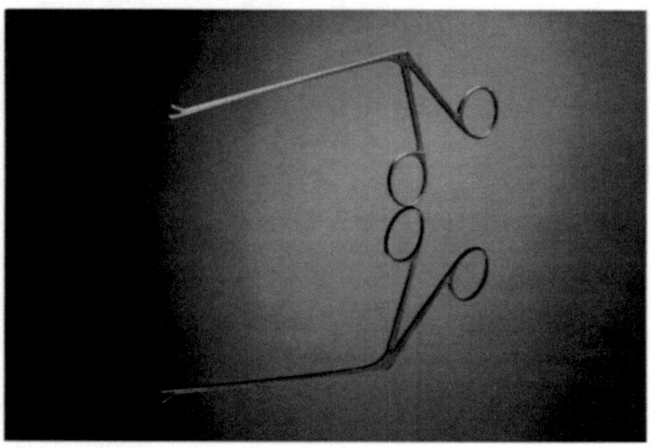

(H)

Fig. 14 (continued)

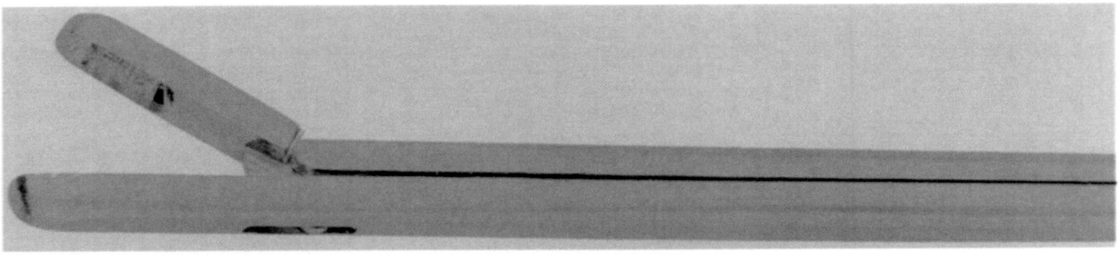

(I)

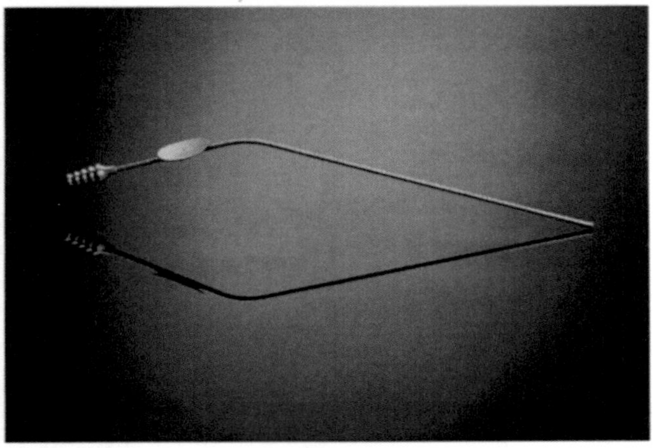

(J)

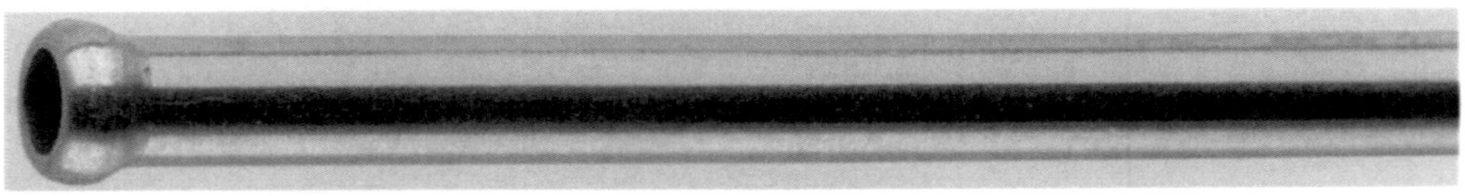

(K)

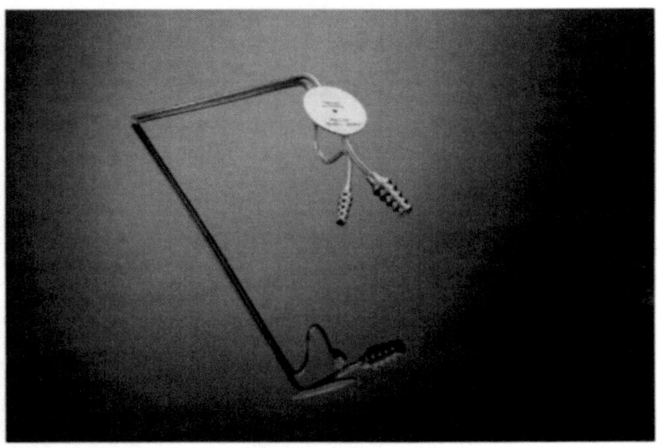

(L)

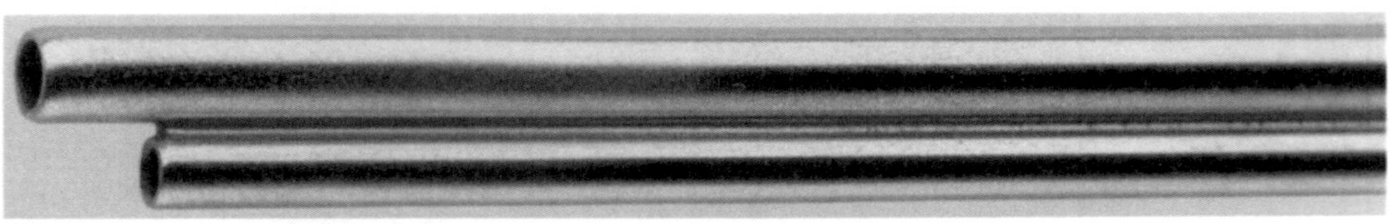

(M)

Fig. 14 (continued)

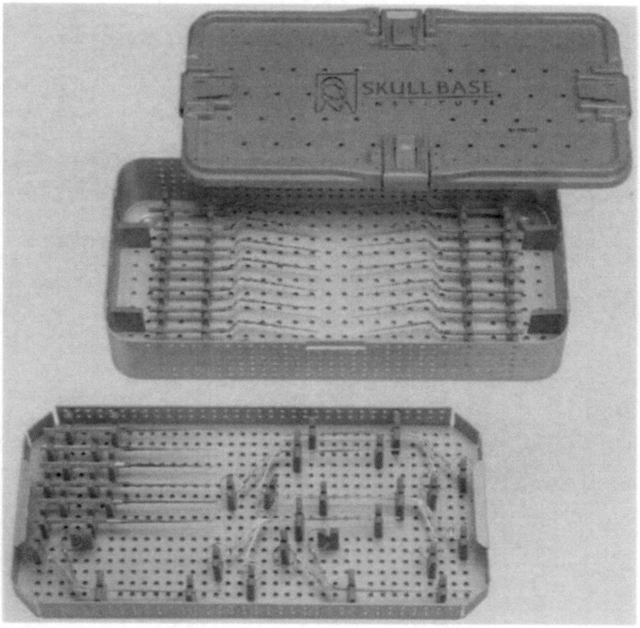

(A)

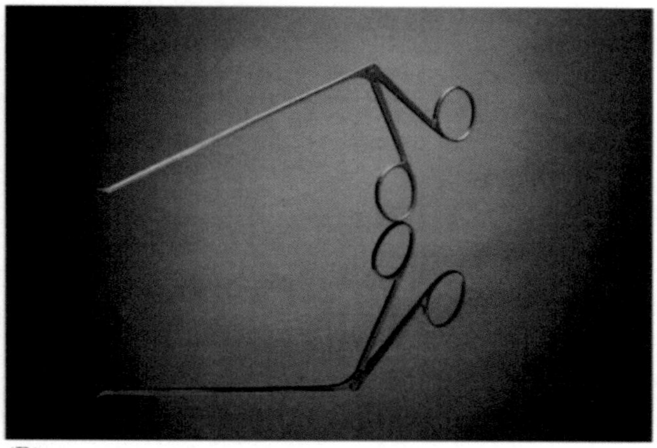

(B)

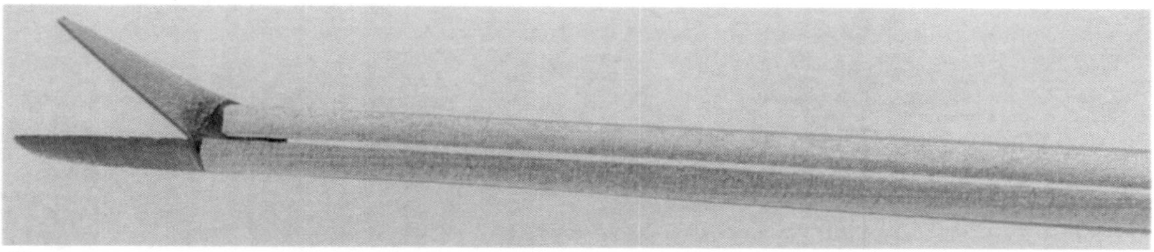

(C)

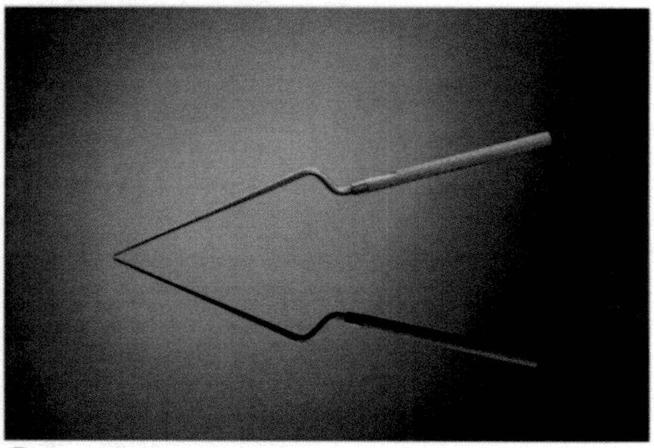

(D)

Fig. 15 (**A**) Tray 3. (**B**) Microscissors. (**C**) Straight microscissors tip. (**D**) Curved left microelevator.

6 The Fully Endoscopic Endonasal Approach

This chapter describes the fully endoscopic endonasal, also called transnasal, approach. The advantages of the endoscopic endonasal approach include more thorough tumor resection, fewer surgical complications, elimination of unnecessary steps, and reductions in operative and hospitalization times. These advantages have rendered the fully endoscopic endonasal approach the "gold standard" in pituitary surgery. In our practice, the fully endoscopic endonasal approach has improved our ability to achieve complete resection of pituitary and other sellar tumors. This chapter's description of the approach includes indications, operating room setup, patient positioning, operative technique, state-of-the-art illustrative cases (including a clinical background on the most important pathologies in this area), potential complications, and ways to avoid these complications (in the authors' experience).

Keywords: Clival chordoma; Clivus; Endonasal; Endoscopic; Macroadenoma; Microadenoma; Minimally invasive; Optic chiasm; Optic nerve; Parasellar; Pituitary; Pituitary gland; Pituitary surgery; Sella; Sellar; Skull base; Sphenoid sinus; Suprasellar; Surgery; Transnasal.

1. INTRODUCTION

Over the past few decades, surgical access to the pituitary gland and other tumors of the sellar region has, for the most part, been limited to the traditional transseptal, transsphenoidal approach. Larger tumors have often required a conventional craniotomy for optimal decompression. More recently, the introduction of the endoscopic endonasal approach has offered a less-invasive alternative to access the pituitary gland, providing superior intraoperative imaging by virtue of angled lenses that allow panoramic views of the regional anatomy. This has allowed for more thorough tumor resection and fewer surgical complications. Because the entire surgery is performed through a nostril without the need for any incisions, the need for transseptal dissection, metallic transsphenoidal retractors, and postoperative nasal packing has been eliminated, thus minimizing patient discomfort and postoperative pain.

In our practice, the fully endoscopic endonasal approach has improved our ability to achieve complete tumor resection. The elimination of unnecessary steps and reductions in complications and recovery times have rendered the fully endoscopic endonasal approach the "gold standard" in pituitary surgery. Most of our patients are able to go home the day after surgery.

2. INDICATIONS

The fully endoscopic endonasal approach provides minimally invasive access to the anterior, middle, and posterior cranial base. It is indicated for the surgical management of pituitary tumors, including secretory and nonsecretory pituitary adenomas with or without suprasellar extension, Rathke's cleft cysts, clival chordomas, craniopharyngiomas, some meningiomas and optic nerve gliomas, and it is useful in the repair of anterior cerebrospinal fluid (CSF) fistulas. These indications expand those for the traditional transseptal transsphenoidal microsurgical technique. Because this minimally invasive technique provides a distinct advantage in terms of operative time, perioperative morbidity, and faster overall recovery, the use of an endoscopic endonasal approach is particularly suited to pediatric patients, elderly patients, and patients with significant medical comorbidities.

3. INSTRUMENTATION

The instruments needed to execute this technique successfully include an endoscopic tower containing a three-chip high-definition digital camera, a xenon or halogen light source, 0° and 30° rigid endoscopes, a dedicated endoscope holding arm, an endoscope irrigation sheath, and precision microinstruments.

4. OPERATING ROOM SETUP (FIG. 1)

Once the patient is anesthetized, the operating room table is turned so that the head of the patient is rotated 180° away from the anesthesiologist. Corrugated extension tubing is used

From: *Endoscopic Skull Base Surgery: A Comprehensive Guide with Illustrative Cases.*
Edited by H. K. Shahinian © Humana Press, Totowa, NJ.

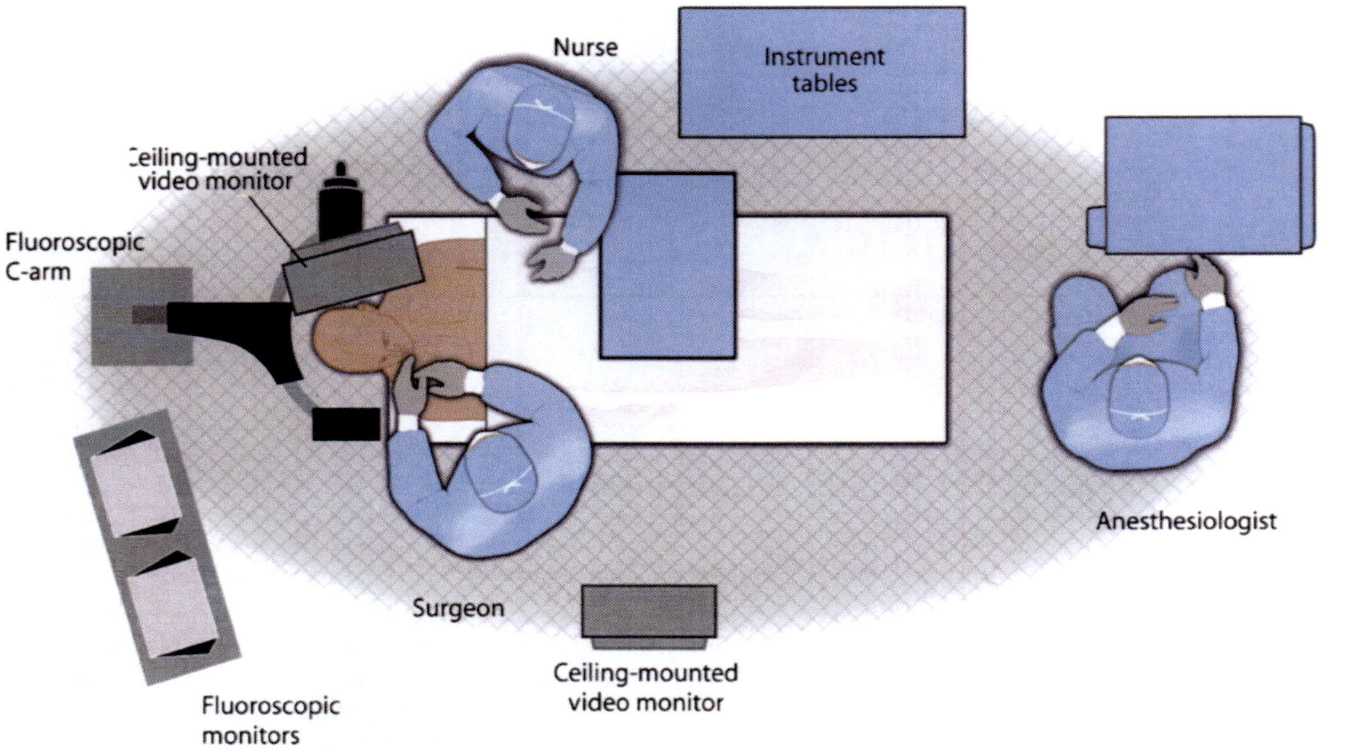

Fig. 1 Operating room setup.

to bridge the distance from airway to anesthesia machine; there are no adverse effects from adding this amount of dead space to the airway circuit. The next step is to position the imaging hardware: The C-arm fluoroscopy image intensifier is brought to the head of the table and rotated so that the trajectory of the beam yields centrally positioned sphenoid and sella contours on the fluoroscopy monitor, which is placed over the patient's right shoulder. The endoscopic tower is placed over the patient's left shoulder, directly in the line of vision of the surgeon, who stands on the patient's right side. The endoscope holding arm is affixed to the bed on the side opposite the surgeon and wrapped in a sterile drape. The arm reaches over the patient's upper body, and the grasping end rests above the patient's nose; its orientation can be adjusted to alter the position of the endoscope as necessary.

This setup provides the surgeon with an unobstructed view of the monitor displaying the endoscopic image as well as ready access to continuous and still fluoroscopic imaging. Because the surgeon is not looking down into the eyepieces of a microscope and instead is looking directly forward at the video screen, proper alignment of these components is essential to keep the surgeon oriented to a surgical plane that is perpendicular to the sphenoid rostrum.

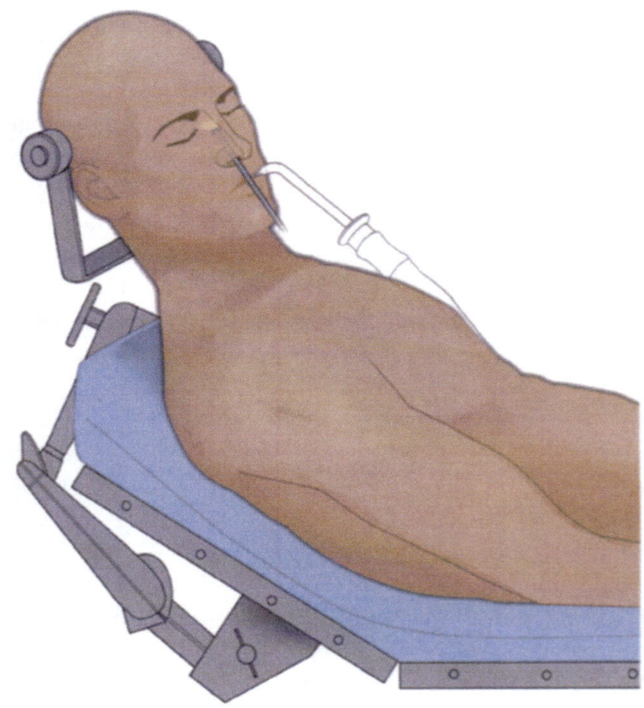

Fig. 2 Patient positioning.

5. PATIENT POSITIONING (FIG. 2)

The patient is placed supine on the operating room table with the head of the bed raised 45°. The neck is slightly extended, and the head is rotated to the right and fixed in position with a carbon horseshoe three-pin clamp. The surgeon operates through the patient's right nostril, which provides a natural axis along which the long, slender endoscopes and surgical instruments can be passed posteriorly. In patients with a significantly deviated nasal septum that effectively obliterates the working space through the right nostril, or in those with histories

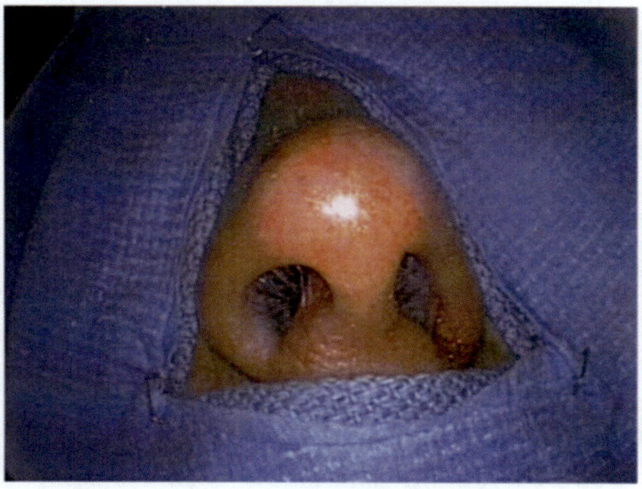

Fig. 3 Draping.

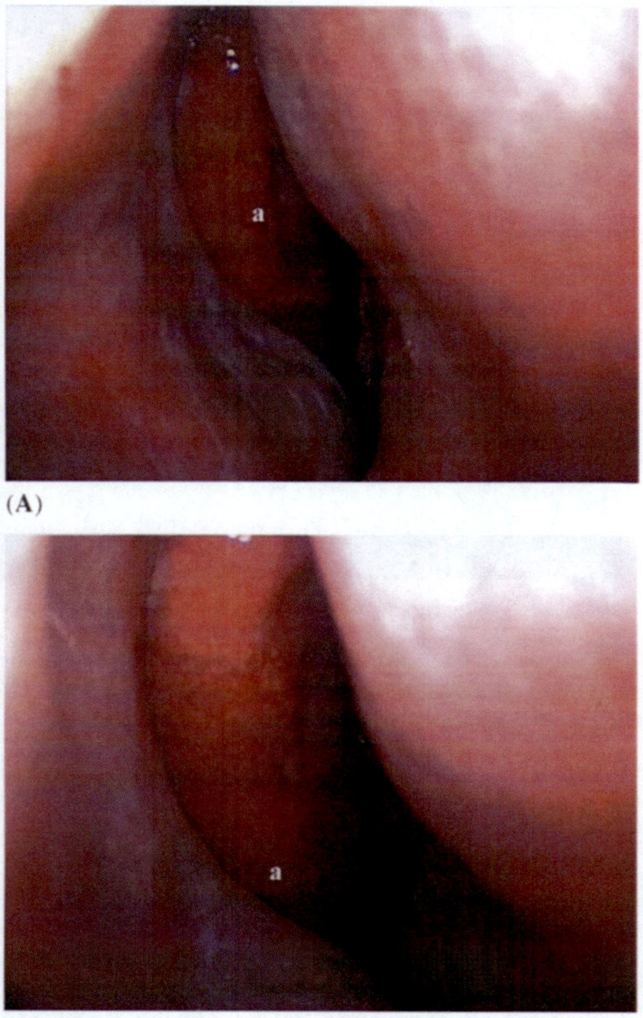

Fig. 4 (**A**) and (**B**) Endoscopic anatomy of the nose. (**A**) *a* Middle turbinate. (**B**) *a* Anterior inferior border of the middle turbinate.

of right-sided sinus surgeries or other structural abnormalities of the right nasopharynx, an approach through the left nostril should be considered.

6. OPERATIVE TECHNIQUE

The face, nares, and abdomen are prepared with antibacterial surgical scrub. Intranasal epinephrine or cocaine-soaked sponges are not used. Sterile towels are used to cover the face, leaving only the nose exposed during surgery (Fig. 3).

The first step of the operation is performed with a 0° endoscope with either 2.7- or 4-mm diameter, depending on the volume of the nasal passage. Intranasal retractors and speculums are not required during the procedure. The endoscope is attached to the grasping end of the endoscope holder, advanced into the nostril, and used to conduct a brief survey of the anterior nasal vestibule. The anteroinferior border of the middle turbinate and the architecture of the nasal septum are identified (Fig. 4A,B). An elevator is placed flatly against the surface of the nasal septum, and firm, sustained, medial pressure is applied, displacing the septal mucosa and underlying cartilage. The elevator is then intranasally rotated, and a similar force is applied laterally to displace the middle turbinate. The middle turbinate may fracture, but out-fracturing is not explicitly necessary to provide adequate exposure. Once the anterior nasal passage is widened, the holding arm is released, and the endoscope is advanced further posteriorly. The same maneuvers are then repeated along the entire face of the septum and turbinate until a passage wide enough to accommodate the endoscope and the accompanying microinstruments is created. Intranasal dissection should be performed meticulously and atraumatically as bleeding from traumatized mucosa anteriorly can obscure the vision posteriorly (Fig. 5A,B).

The posterior nasopharyngeal wall and sphenoid ostium mark the deepest extent of the intranasal dissection. Because the sphenoid ostium is often difficult to detect due to its diminutive size or mucosal inflammation, confirmation of appropriate positioning is obtained before proceeding by passing a long metallic suction cannula into the posterior nasopharynx and fluoroscopically identifying that its tip is abutting the anterior wall of the sphenoid sinus.

The mucosa overlying the anterior wall of the sphenoid sinus is cauterized using a combination suction–cautery instrument. Subperiosteal dissection with an elevator is then carried out to expose the entire anterior sphenoid; limits of dissection are the cribriform plate superiorly, the vomer inferiorly, and beyond both sphenoid ostia laterally. Fluoroscopy may again be used to confirm these anatomic limits. The perpendicular plate of the ethmoid bone, rostrum "keel" of sphenoid bone, as well as the vomer may be removed with a rongeur to more completely expose the anterior and inferior surface of the sphenoid sinus (Fig. 6A,E).

Once the sphenoid sinus is completely exposed, its mucosal lining is dissected free, grasped with a rongeur, and removed to minimize the risk of a postoperative mucocele. Any septae within the sphenoid sinus are also removed. The intersphenoidal septum is commonly bent to one or the other side and is also removed using a rongeur. The posterior wall of the sinus, which makes up the floor of the sella turcica, and the bilateral carotid prominences are immediately recognizable. The floor of the sella is usually intact; however, it may be thinned, fractured, or even completely obliterated by an expanding tumor. If the sella is intact, its floor must be removed to provide

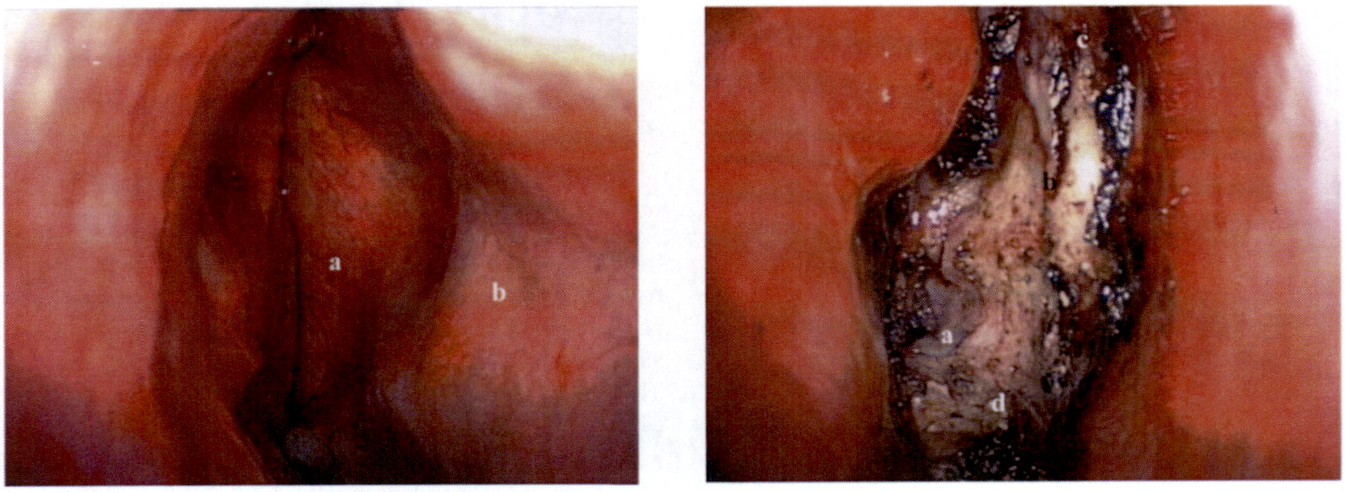

(A) (B)

Fig. 5 (**A**) and (**B**) Posterior septoplasty. (**A**) *a* Mucosa overlying face of sphenoid sinus. *b* Mucoperichondrium overlying cartilaginous nasal septum. (**B**) *a* Right sphenoid ostium. *b* Face of sphenoid sinus. *c* Ethmoidal crest (articulates with perpendicular plate of ethmoid bone). *d* Rostrum "keel" of sphenoid bone (articulates with alae of Vomer).

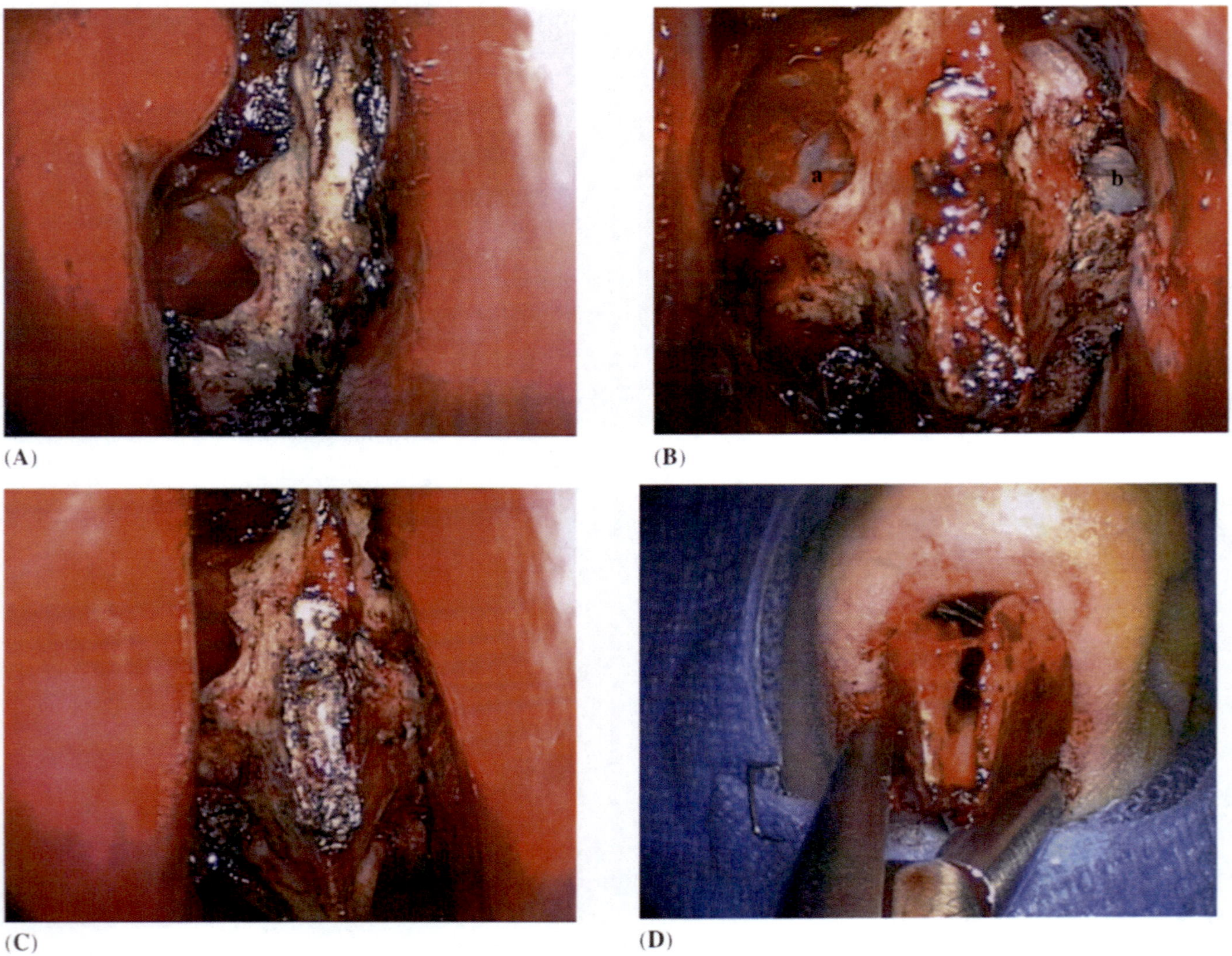

Fig. 6 (**A**)–(**E**) Opening of sphenoid sinus. (**B**) *a* Right sphenoid ostium. *b* Left sphenoid ostium. *c* Rostrum "keel" of sphenoid bone.

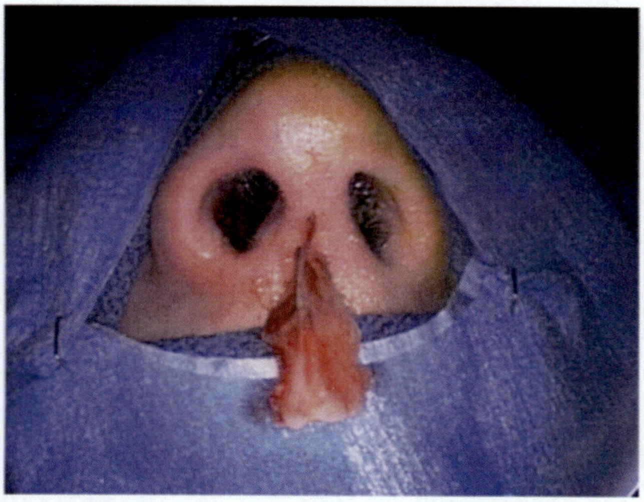

(E)

Fig. 6 (continued)

access to the tumor. As with the anterior wall of the sphenoid sinus, this is accomplished in a piecemeal fashion with the use of a fine chisel and angled rongeurs; limits of bone removal are the cavernous sinuses laterally, the planum sphenoidale superiorly, and the top of the clivus inferiorly. Maximal exposure of the tumor is achievable only with adequate removal of bone; however, serious consideration must be given to the surrounding neurovascular structures, including the carotid arteries and cavernous sinuses laterally and the optic nerves and chiasm superiorly (Fig. 7A–C).

Once the sella is adequately exposed, the overlying dura is incised in a cruciate fashion with a modified no. 11 scalpel. The ventral surface of the pituitary gland in microadenomas or the tumor in macroadenomas is exposed, and any tumor is then removed using suction and ring curettes of varying diameters and orientations. The extent of intrasellar dissection must incorporate information from preoperative imaging regarding the displacement of the normal gland by the tumor. The Valsalva maneuver, rather than saline injection through a lumbar catheter, is used to deliver suprasellar extensions of tumor into the sella (Fig. 8A–C).

Until this point of the procedure, the 0° endoscope provides all of the imaging; its optics allow near-complete exposure of the sella turcica and a partial view of the suprasellar structures, including the optic chiasm and the arachnoid membrane investing the median eminence. However, the extent of visualization under the 0° endoscope is limited by its optical capabilities. Therefore, once tumor resection under the 0° endoscope is deemed complete, it is replaced with the 30° endoscope. By advancing the 30° endoscope into the sella turcica and then rotating it in a clockwise and counterclockwise direction along its longitudinal axis, the right and left parasellar and suprasellar areas are thoroughly visualized, and any hidden tumor remnants are removed.

A fat graft is harvested from the abdomen to seal the intrasellar contents, and it is secured in place with 2 cc dural sealant or fibrin glue. Postoperative nasal packings are not used. A small gauze sponge fastened beneath the nose (a "mustache" dressing) serves to collect minimal oozing for 24 h postoperatively. Patients are monitored in a step-down unit overnight following surgery and in almost all cases are discharged home the following day (Fig. 9A,B).

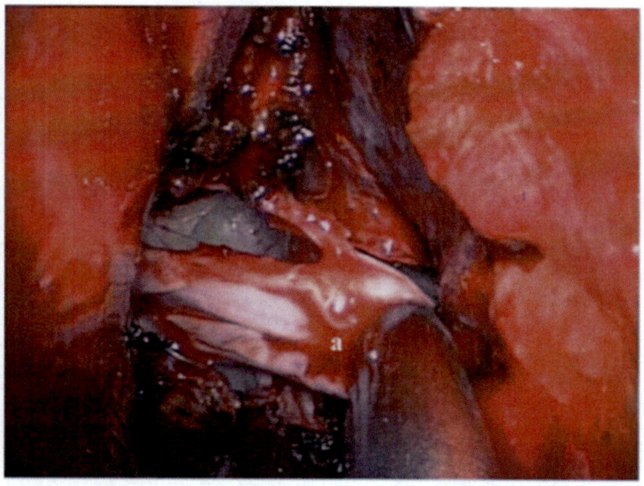

(A)

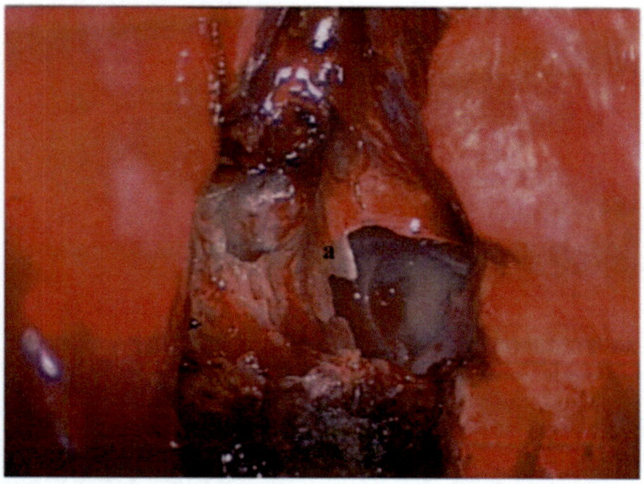

(B)

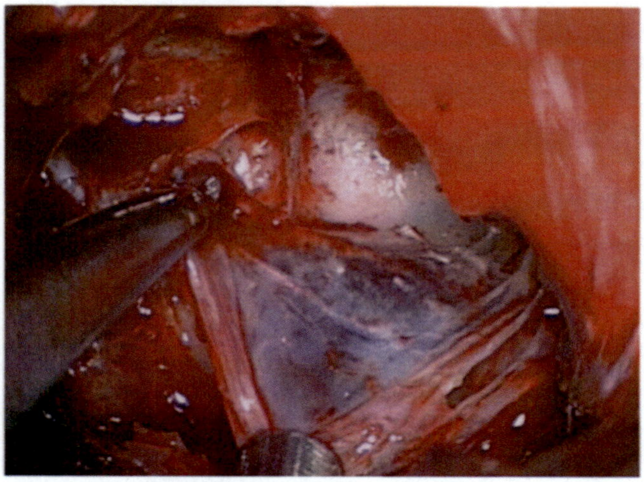

(C)

Fig. 7 (A)–(C) Sellar exposure. (A) *a* Mucosal lining of sphenoid sinus. (B) *a* Intersphenoidal septum.

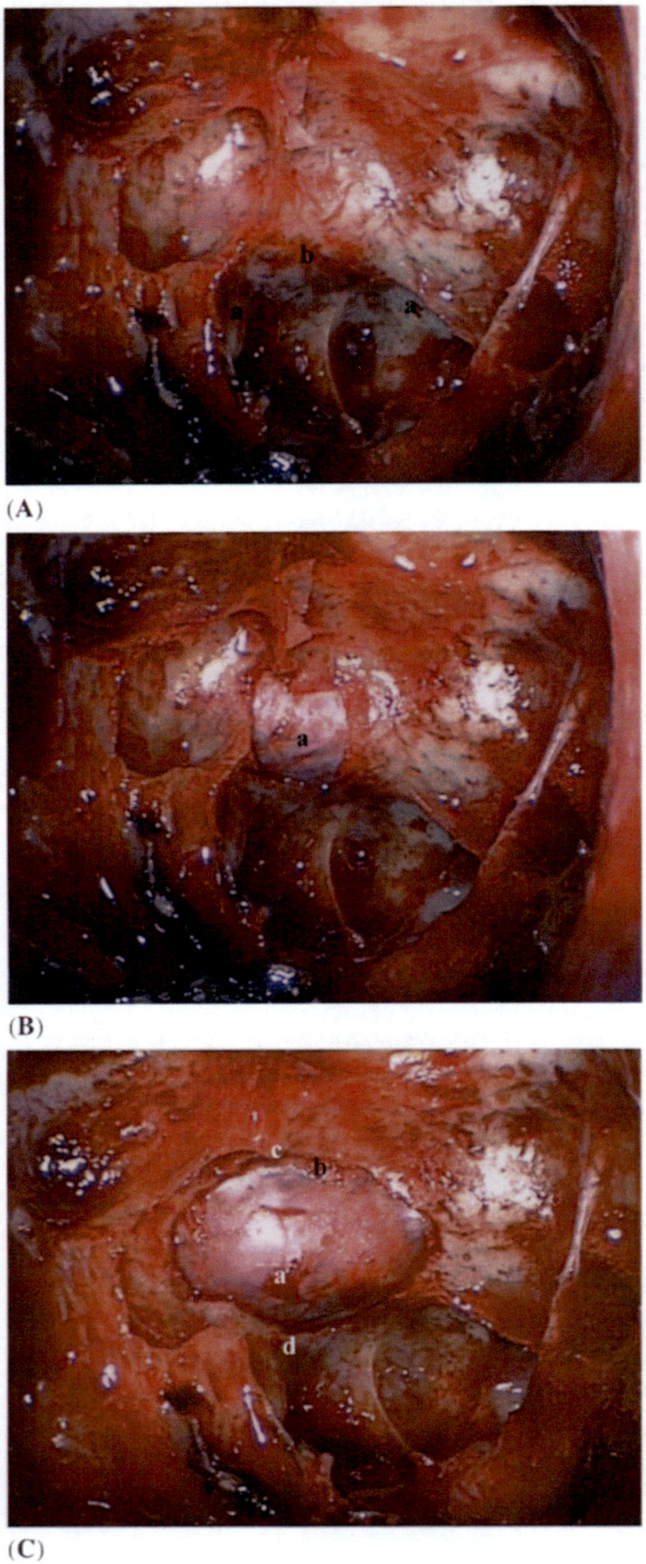

Fig. 8 (A)–(C) Sellar opening. (A) *a* Carotid protuberances. *b* Sellar floor. (B) *a* Sellar dura. (C) *a* Sellar dura. *b* Arachnoid membrane junction. *c* Planum sphenoidale. *d* Upper clivus.

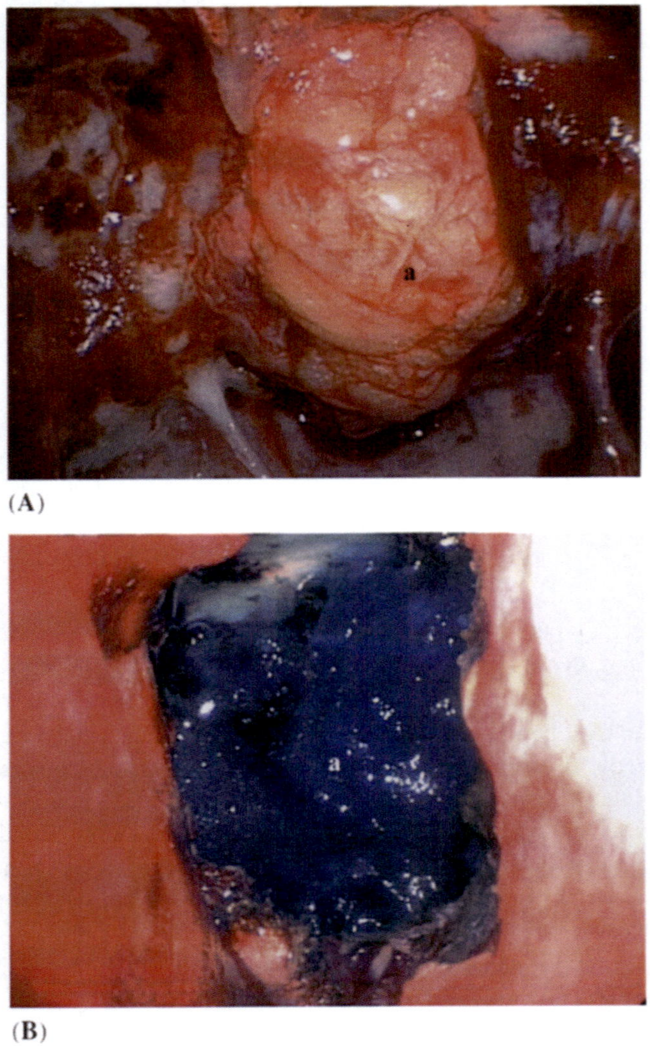

Fig. 9 (A) and (B) Closure. (A) *a* Fat graft. (B) *a* Dural sealant.

7. ILLUSTRATIVE CASES

7.1. PITUITARY MICROADENOMA

7.1.1. Background Pituitary tumors less than 10 mm in diameter (microadenomas) may be secretory or nonsecretory and may be discovered only incidentally or at autopsy. Of the secretory adenomas, the most common are prolactinomas. Other secretory tumors may secrete corticotropin (ACTH), causing Cushing's disease; growth hormone, causing acromegaly; gonadotropins, causing disturbance in the level of sex hormones; or, rarely, thyroid-stimulating hormone (TSH), causing hyperthyroidism. In most cases, magnetic resonance imaging (MRI) can be used to locate the microadenoma, and treatment options are based on the location and symptoms that a microadenoma is causing. Although some microadenomas can be treated with medication, many require surgery.

7.1.2. Approach After the sphenoid sinus is opened and its septae and mucosa are removed, the sellar floor is identified, and a small quadrangle of bone overlying the microadenoma is outlined and in-fractured with a chisel and then removed with the pituitary rongeur. The opening is enlarged as needed, the underlying dura is electrocoagulated and opened, and the microadenoma within the pituitary gland is identified. Using the curved pituitary microscissors, a plane is created between the microadenoma and the normal pituitary gland, after which the microadenoma is resected. A 1-mm margin is also resected circumferentially around the tumor bed to prevent recurrence.

7.1.3. Cases

7.1.3.1. Microadenomectomy for a Left Pituitary Microadenoma (Fig. 10A–J)

7.1.3.2. Microadenomectomy for a Pituitary Microadenoma (Fig. 11A–H)

7.1.3.3. Left One-Third Hypophysectomy for a Pituitary Microadenoma (Fig. 12A–K)

7.2. PITUITARY MACROADENOMA (FIG. 13)

7.2.1. Background Pituitary tumors exceeding 10 mm in diameter (macroadenomas) are usually nonsecretory tumors that present with mass effect causing visual disturbances, such as bitemporal hemianopsia from compression of the optic chiasm, headache from direct stretching of the dura, hydrocephalus from obstruction of the foramen of Monro, or hypopituitarism from compression of the pituitary gland itself. Some macroadenomas may be asymptomatic, while others are secretory and may produce distinct clinical syndromes as a result of hormonal overproduction, such as acromegaly, Cushing's disease, or hyperprolactinemia. Hyperprolactinemia can also be caused by direct pituitary stalk compression by an enlarging macroadenoma regardless of hormone activity.

Panhypopituitarism may present with a deficiency of all the pituitary hormones, but often some are spared. The larger the macroadenoma, the more likely it is to affect pituitary hormones. Pituitary apoplexy, a medical emergency, may result from infarction or sudden hemorrhage within the tumor; this complication tends to occur with macroadenomas but not with microadenomas. MRI studies can be used to define the boundaries of a pituitary macroadenoma and depict any partial descent of the adenoma into the sphenoid sinus.

7.2.2. Approach (Fig. 14) The bone of the sellar floor is removed in a piecemeal fashion to expose the dura overlying the pituitary gland. A cruciate incision is used to open the sellar dura. The dura is freed from the underlying tumor capsule and pituitary

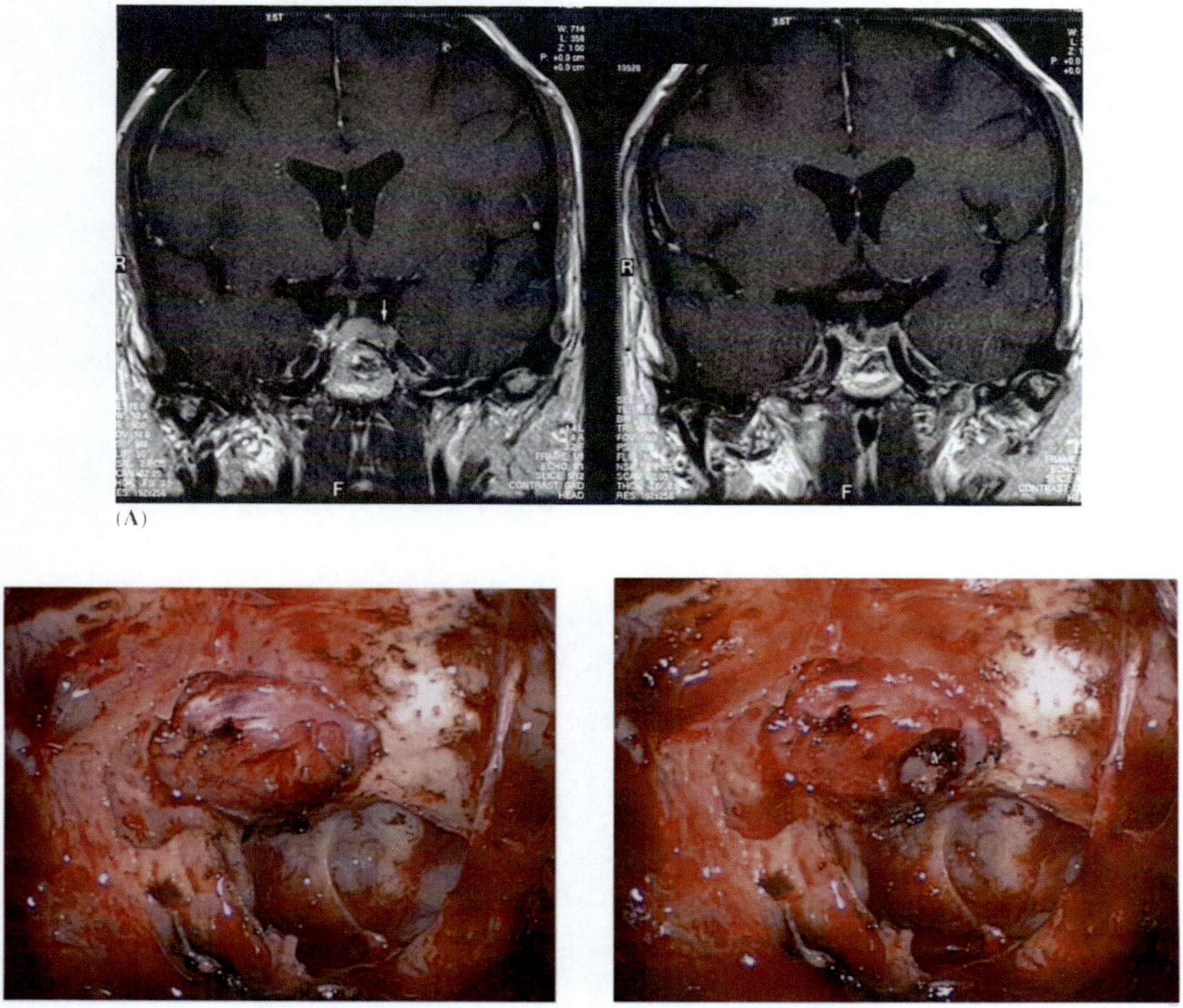

(A) (B) (C)

Fig. 10 (**A**) T_1-weighted coronal contrasted MRIs showing a pituitary microadenoma. (**B**) and (**C**) Opening of the dura and initial exposure of pituitary microadenoma. (**C**) *a* Adenoma. (**D**)–(**F**) Intraoperative endoscopic view showing microadenomectomy. (**D**) *a* Adenoma. *b* Ring curette. (**G**)–(**I**) Intraoperative endoscopic view after complete resection removal of a pituitary microadenoma. (**H**) *a* Adenoma cavity. *b* Normal pituitary. *c* Arachnoid membrane junction. *d* Planum sphenoidale. (**I**) *a* Fat graft. (**J**) Postoperative contrast-enhanced coronal MRIs.

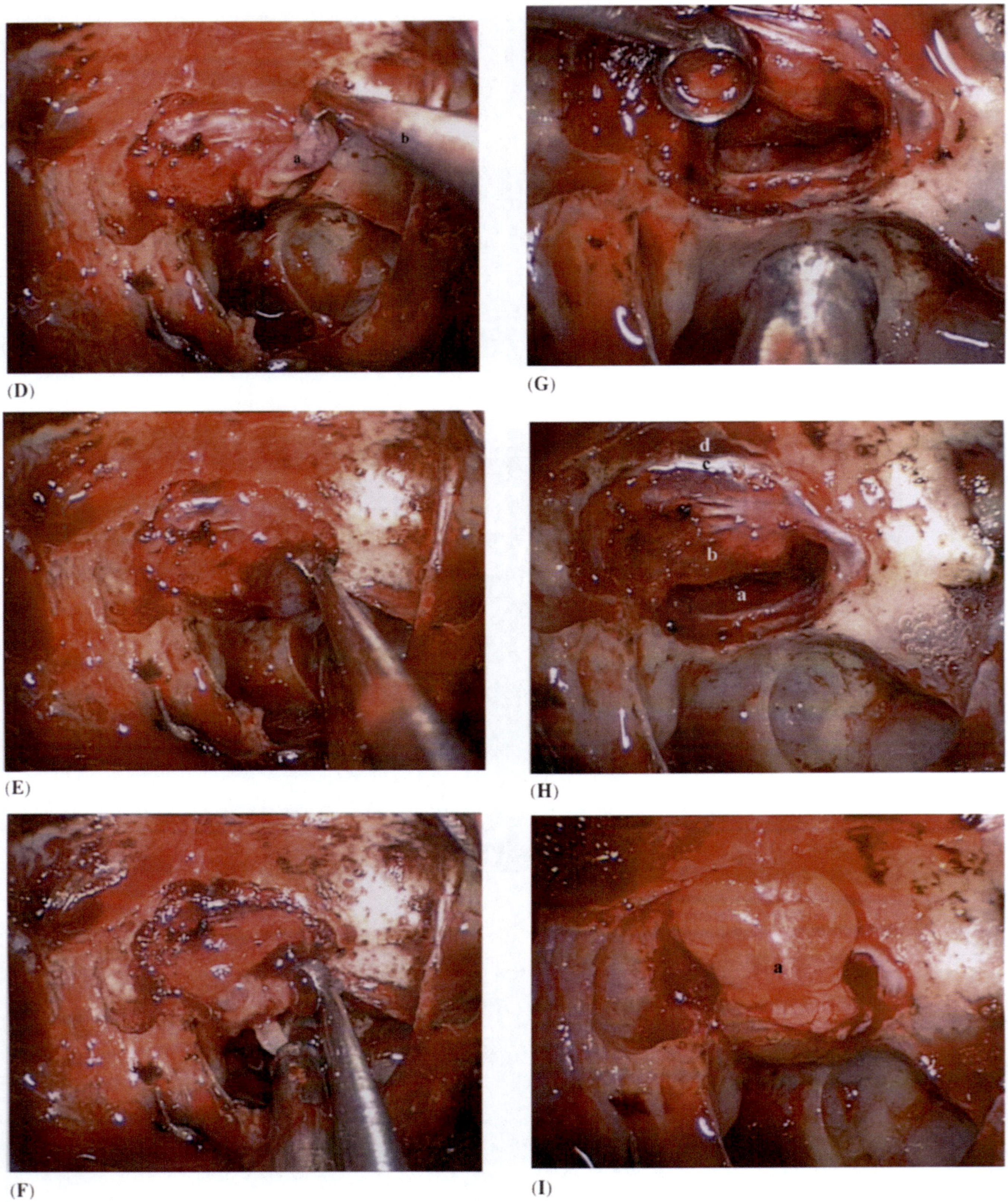

Fig. 10 (continued)

gland using the curved dissector; the pituitary gland and tumor are thus exposed. A biopsy from the tumor is initially obtained to confirm the diagnosis, and then the tumor is internally debulked using ring curettes and gentle suction. Tumor is carefully dissected laterally from the medial walls of the cavernous sinuses and internal carotid arteries under direct endoscopic visualization. Using a blunt ring curette, any tumor from the area of the tuberculum sellae that is hidden from direct view is then removed. The Valsalva maneuver can be used if necessary to force the suprasellar component of the tumor into the operative field. The 0° endoscope is then withdrawn, and the 30° endoscope is inserted to survey for any residual tumor superiorly, inferiorly, or laterally.

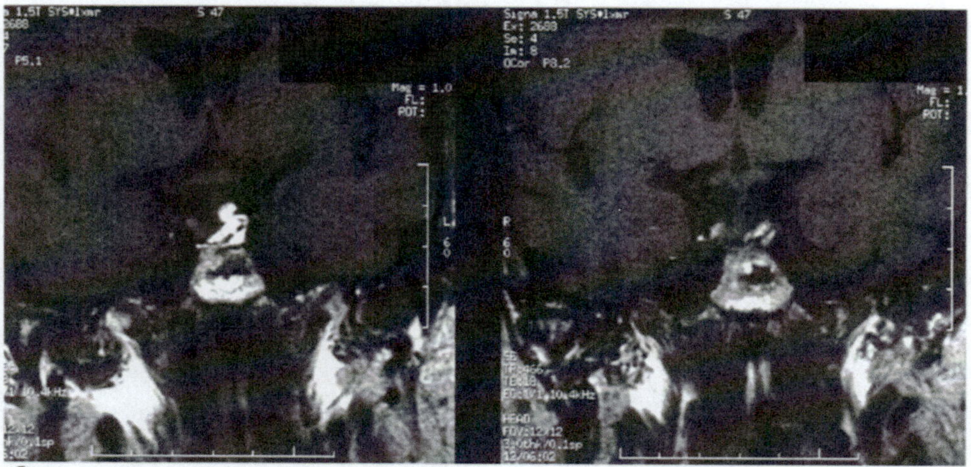

(J)

Fig. 10 (continued)

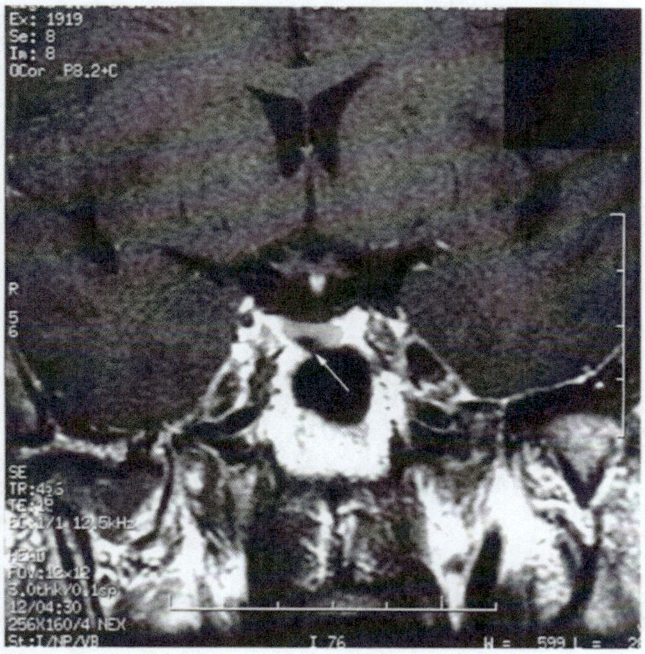

(A)

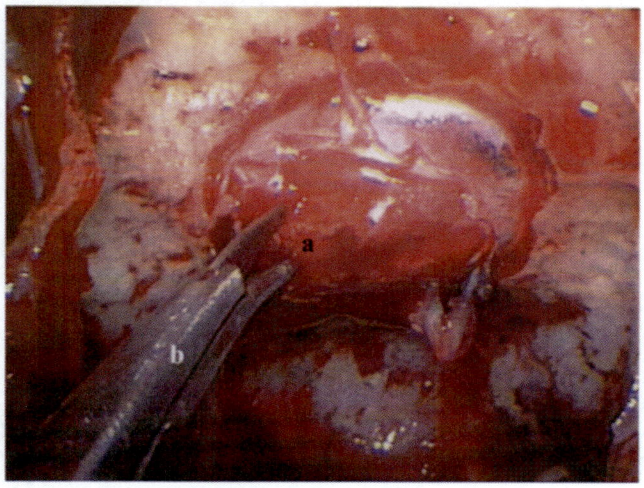

(C)

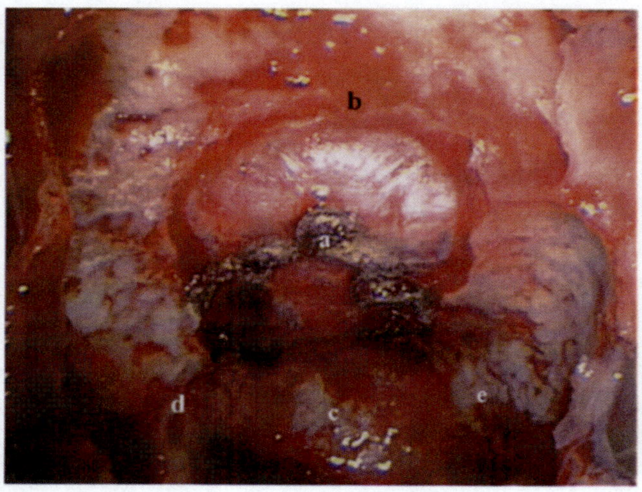

(B)

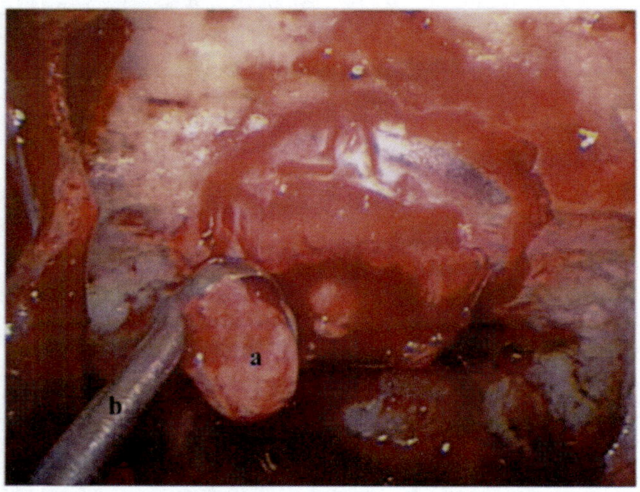

(D)

Fig. 11 (**A**) T_1-weighted coronal contrasted MRI showing pituitary microadenoma. (**B**) and (**C**) Opening of the dura for resection of pituitary microadenoma. (**B**) *a* Sellar dura cauterized. *b* Planum sphenoidale. *c* Clivus. *d* Right carotid protuberance. *e* Left carotid protuberance. (**C**) *a* Adenoma bulge. *b* Sharp dissection of adenoma. (**D**)–(**F**) Intraoperative endoscopic view showing microadenomectomy and fat graft

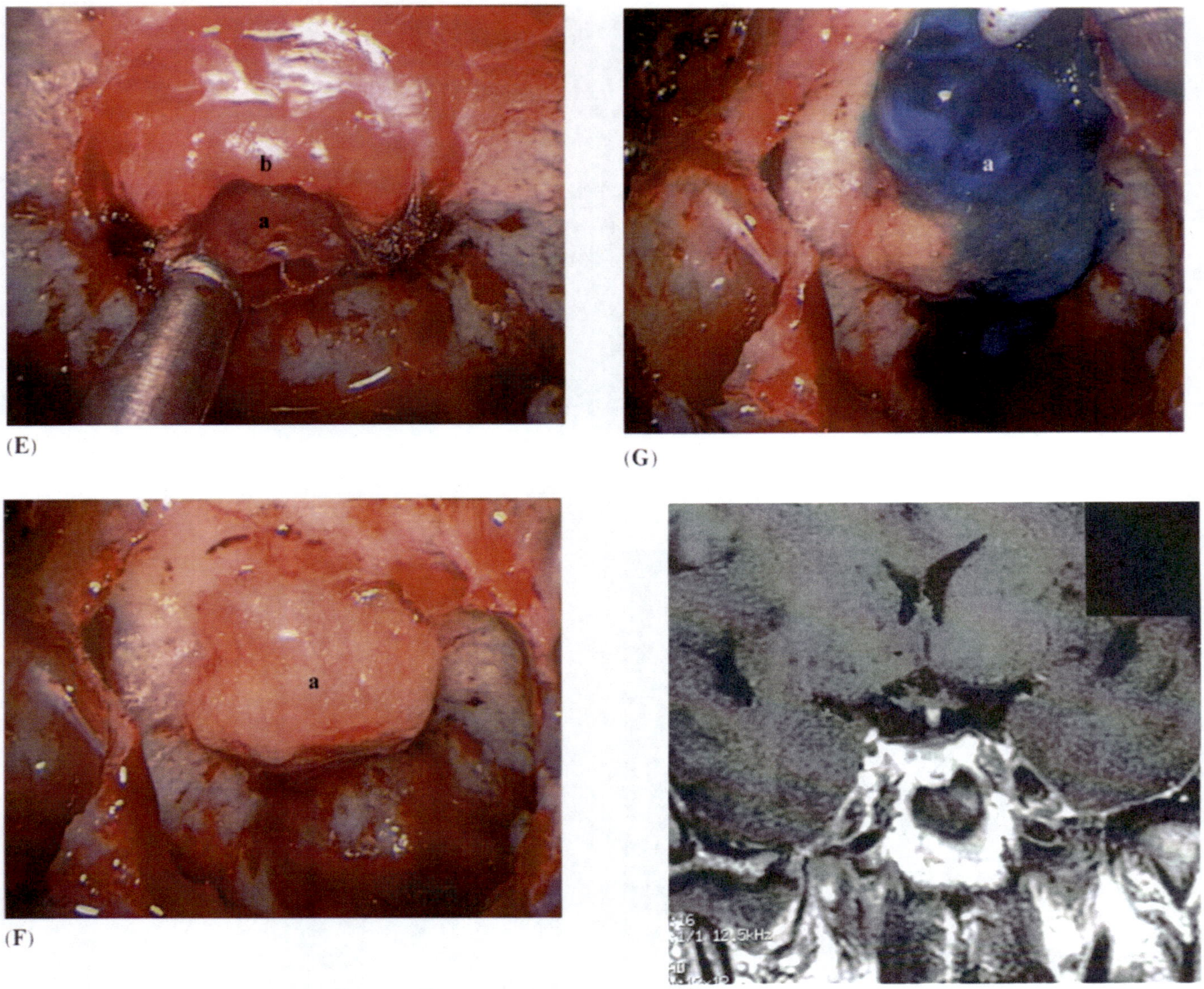

(E) (G) (F) (H)

Fig. 11 (continued) placement. (**D**) *a* Adenoma. *b* Ring curette. (**E**) *a* Adenoma cavity after compete resection. *b* Normal pituitary. (**F**) *a* Fat graft. (**G**) *a* Dural sealant. (**H**) Postoperative contrast-enhanced coronal MRI.

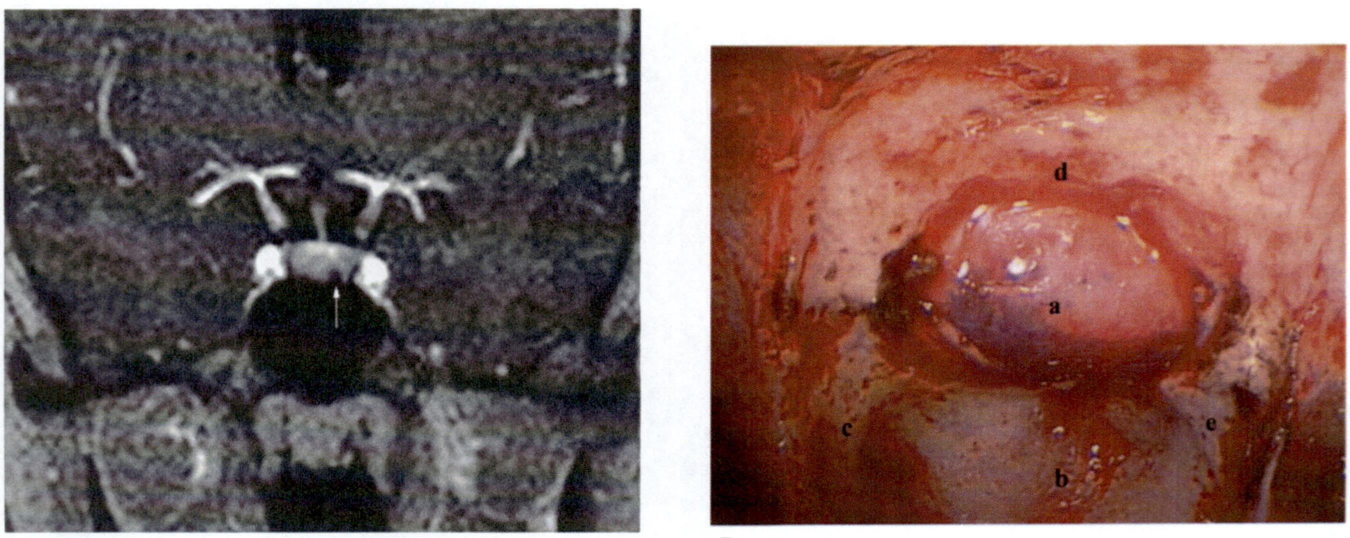

(A) (B)

Fig. 12 (**A**) T_1-weighted coronal contrasted dynamic MRI showing a pituitary microadenoma. (**B**)–(**K**) Intraoperative endoscopic view showing one third left pituitary hypophysectomy and fat graft placement. (**B**) *a* Pituitary. *b* Clivus. *c* Right carotid protuberance. *d* Planum sphenoidale. *e* Left carotid protuberance. (**C**) *a* Straight microscissors. (**F**) *a* Microadenoma. *b* Remaining normal pituitary. (**G**) *a* Medial wall of left cavernous sinus. *b* Remaining normal pituitary. (**J**) *a* Fat graft. (**K**) *a* Dural sealant.

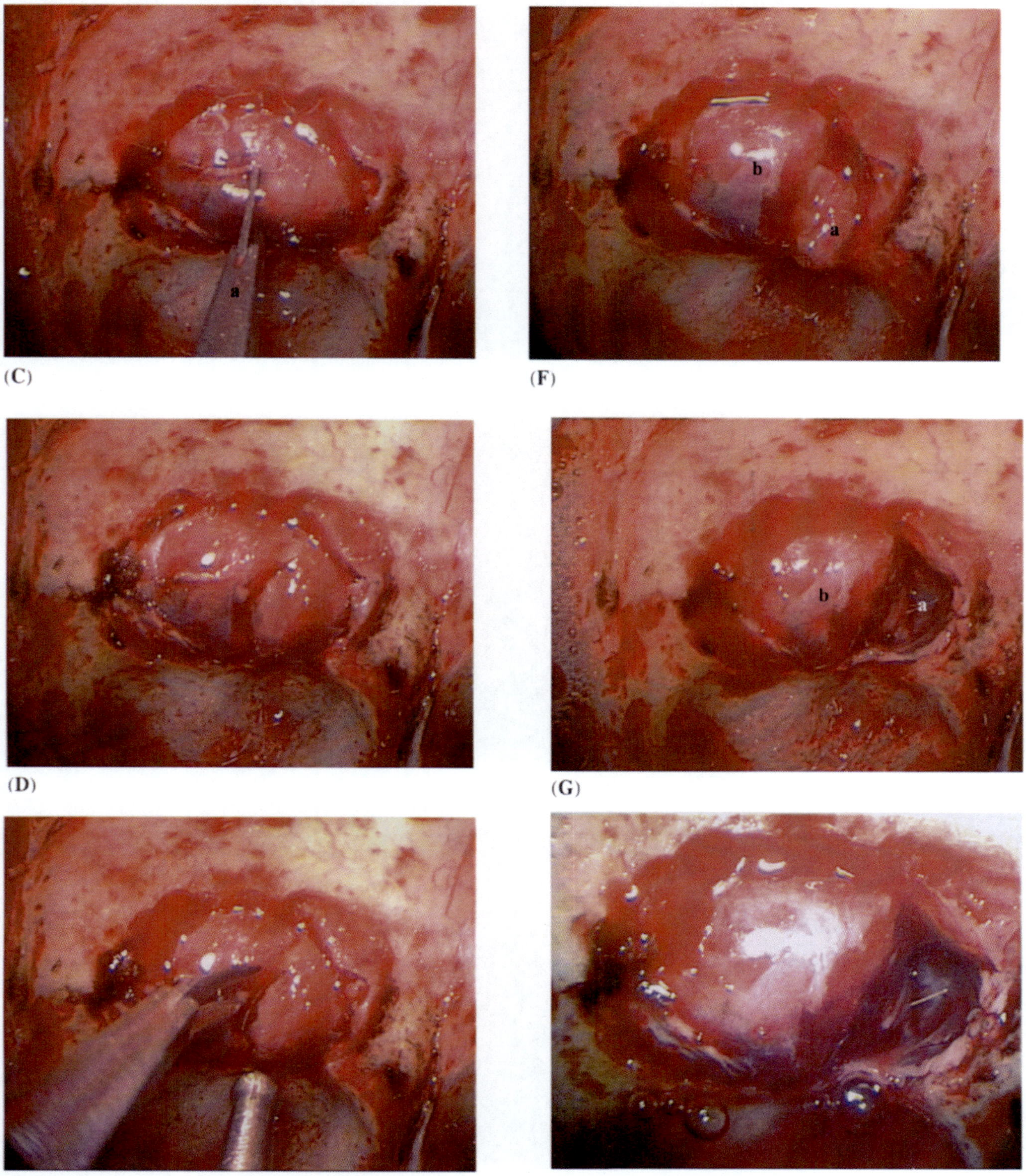

(C) (F) (D) (G) (E) (H)

Fig. 12 (continued)

7.2.3. Cases

7.2.3.1. Pituitary Macroadenoma (Fig. 15A–O)

7.2.3.2. Pituitary Macroadenoma (Fig. 16A-N)

7.2.3.3. Pituitary Macroadenoma (Fig. 17A–X)

7.3. Periclival Tumors

7.3.1 Background A variety of lesions occur in and around the clival region, including the anterior foramen magnum. Meningiomas, chordomas, and neurofibromas are the most common tumors. Other pathologies include chondrosarcomas, tuberculomas, epidermoids, and others. These tumors, whether extra- or intradural, occur in a critical area of the skull base and may pose unique diagnostic and management challenges. The progressive growth of such tumors often results in compression and invasion of important neighboring structures. Associated symptoms are typically nonspecific and may persist chronically before acute or focal neurological findings develop. Tumors

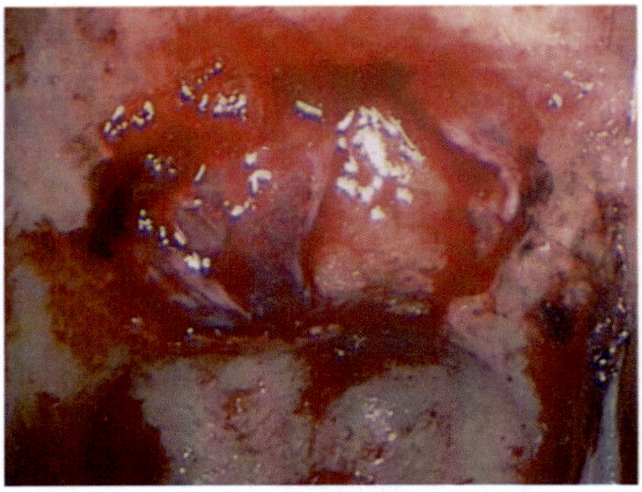

(I)

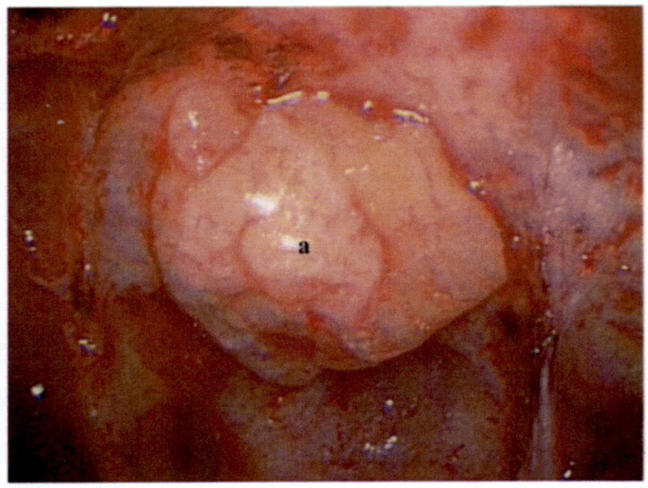

(J)

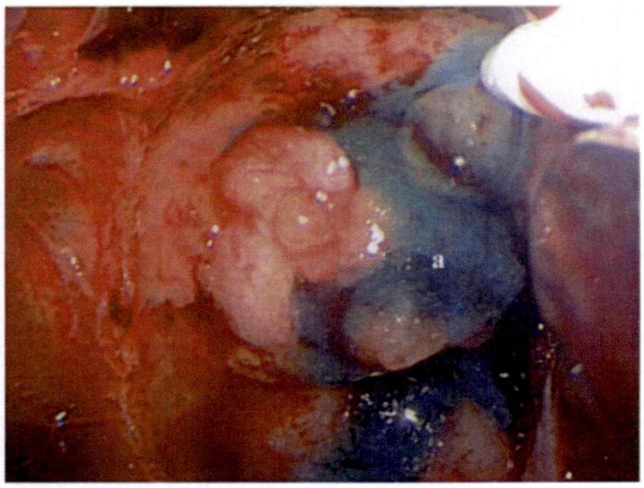

(K)

Fig. 12 (continued)

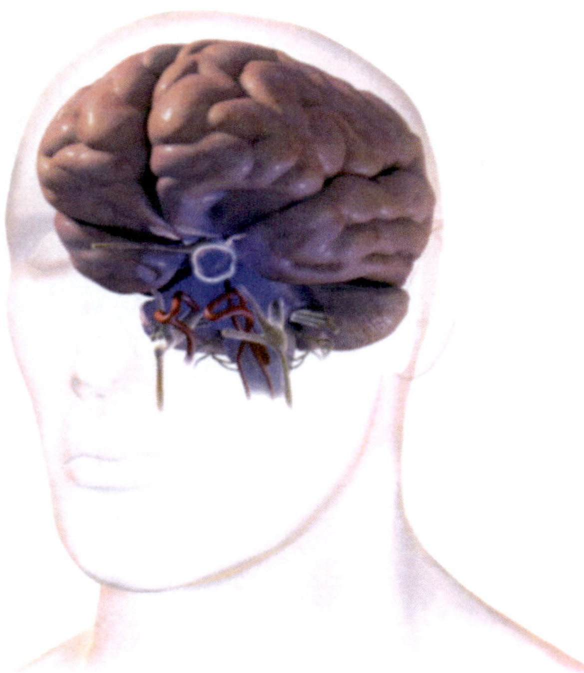

Fig. 13 Pituitary macroadenoma.

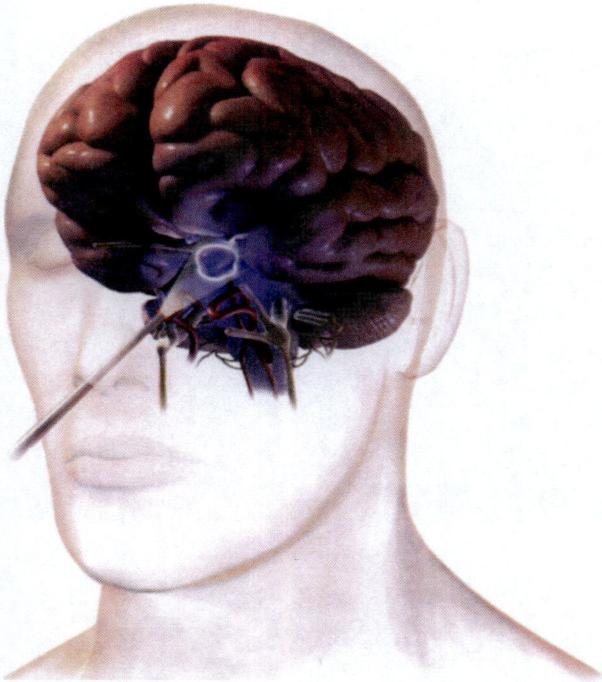

Fig. 14 Approach to pituitary macroadenoma.

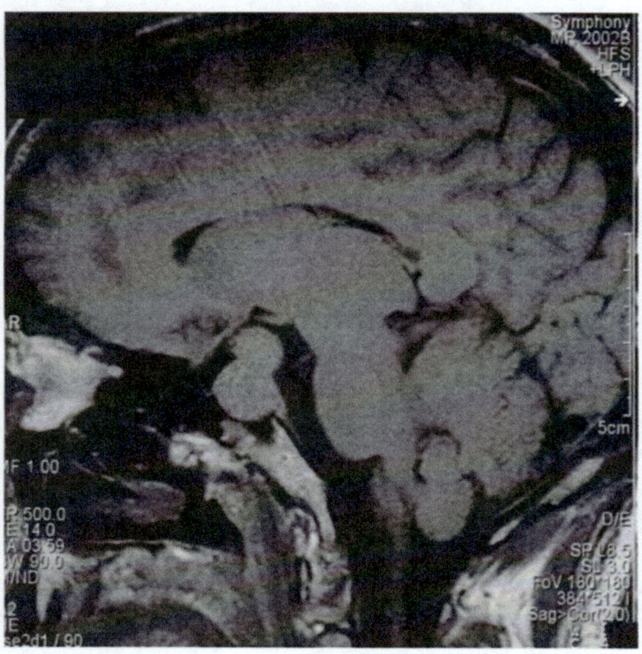

(A)

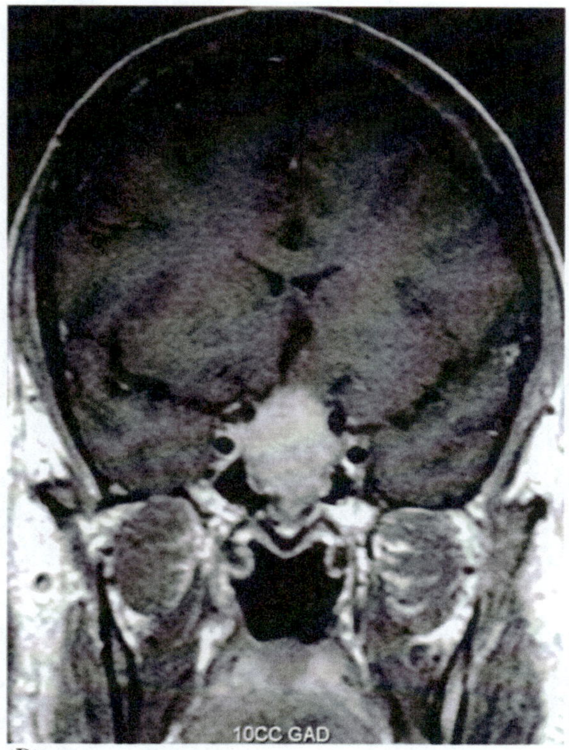

(B)

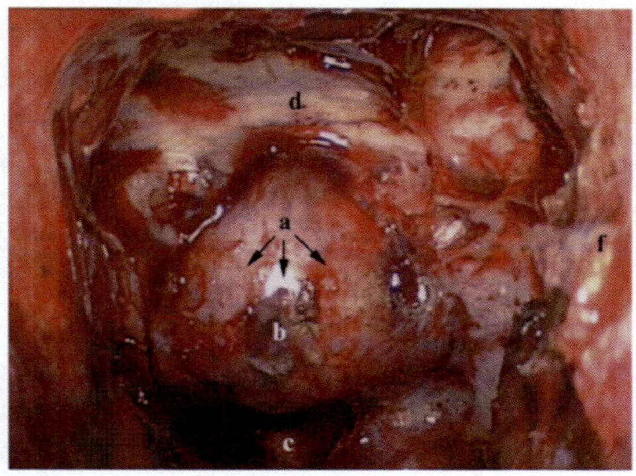

(C)

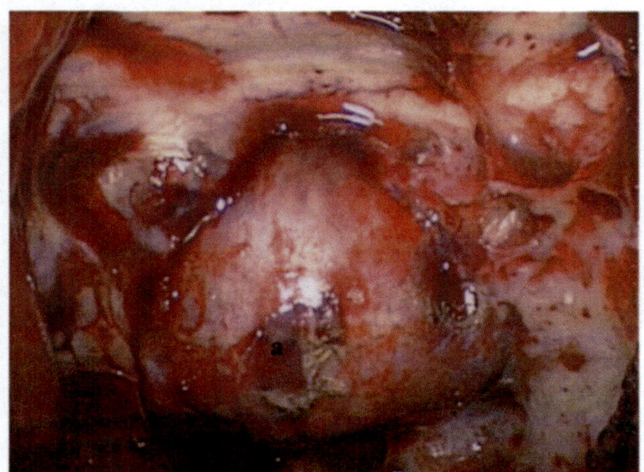

(D)

Fig. 15 (**A**) T_1-weighted sagittal MRI showing a pituitary macroadenoma. (**B**) T_1-weighted coronal contrast-enhanced MRI showing a pituitary macroadenoma. (**C**) and (**D**) Intraoperative endoscopic view showing initial exposure of pituitary macroadenoma. (**C**) *a* Macroadenoma bulge. *b* Eroded sellar dura. *c* Clivus. *d* Planum sphenoidale. (**D**) *a* Close-up view showing dural erosion by tumor.

(continued)

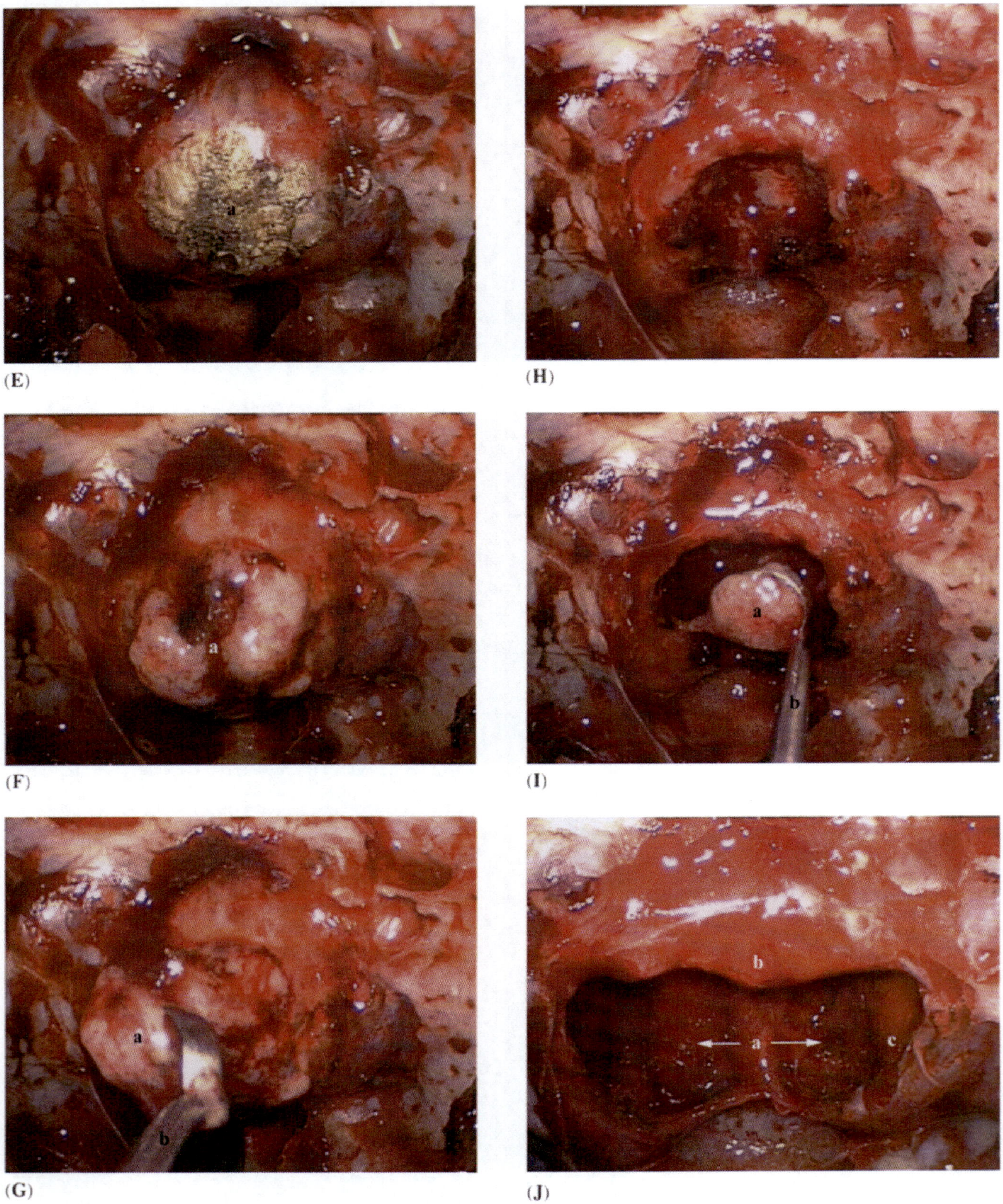

Fig. 15 (continued) **(E)–(I)** Intraoperative endoscopic view showing gradual resection of pituitary macroadenoma. **(E)** *a* Cauterized sellar dura. **(F)** *a* Adenoma. **(G)** *a* Adenoma. *b* Ring curette. **(I)** *a* Final portions of adenoma. *b* Ring curette. **(J)–(M)** Intraoperative endoscopic view following complete resection of pituitary macroadenoma. **(J)** *a* Close-up view of adenoma cavity after complete tumor removal. *b* Pituitary. *c* Medial wall of left cavernous sinus.

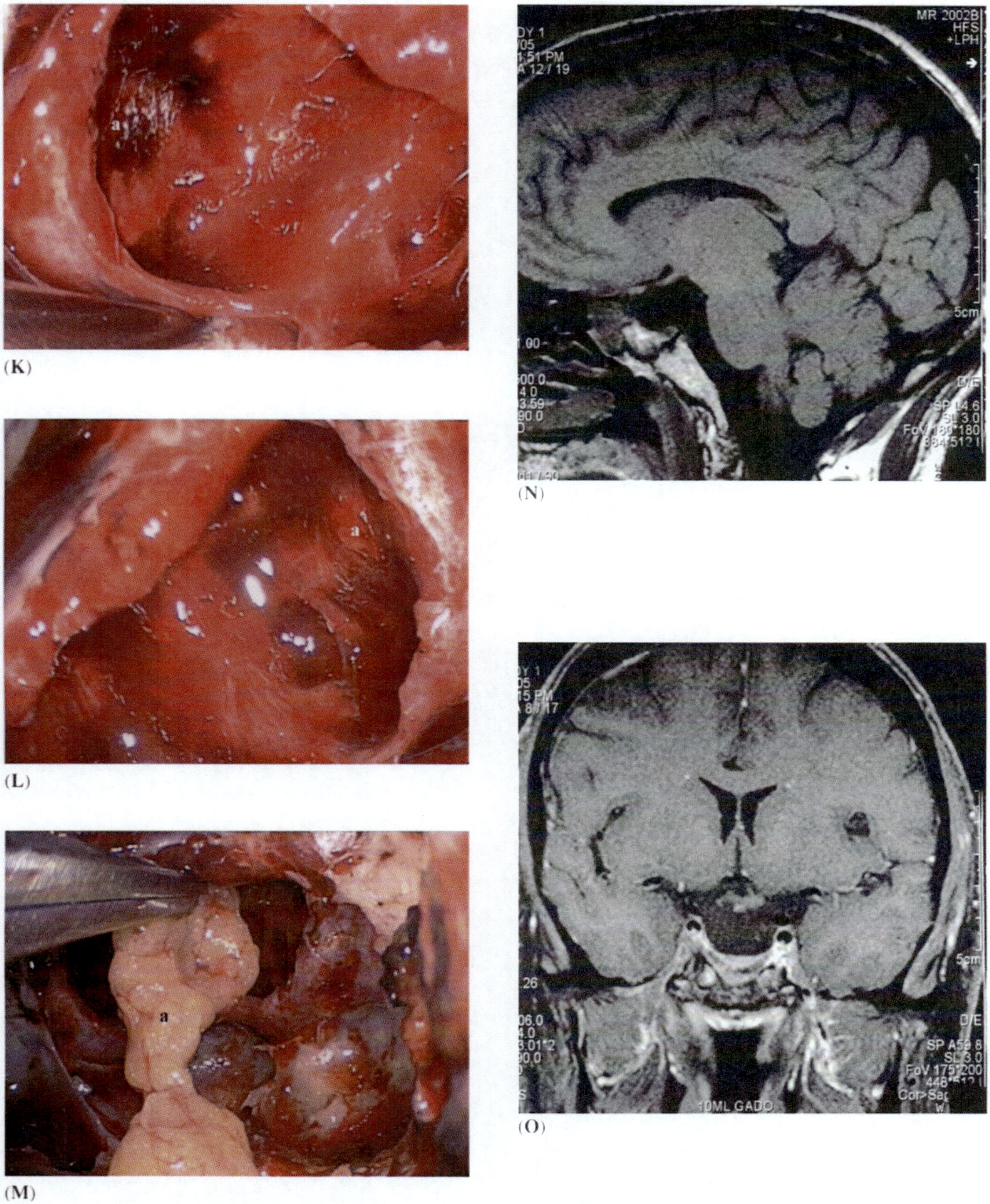

Fig. 15 (continued) (**K**) *a* Close-up view of right medial cavernous sinus wall using 30° endoscope. (**L**) *a* Close-up view of left medial cavernous sinus wall using 30° endoscope. (**M**) *a* Fat graft. (**N**) Postoperative contrast-enhanced sagital MRI. (**O**) Postoperative contrast-enhanced coronal MRI.

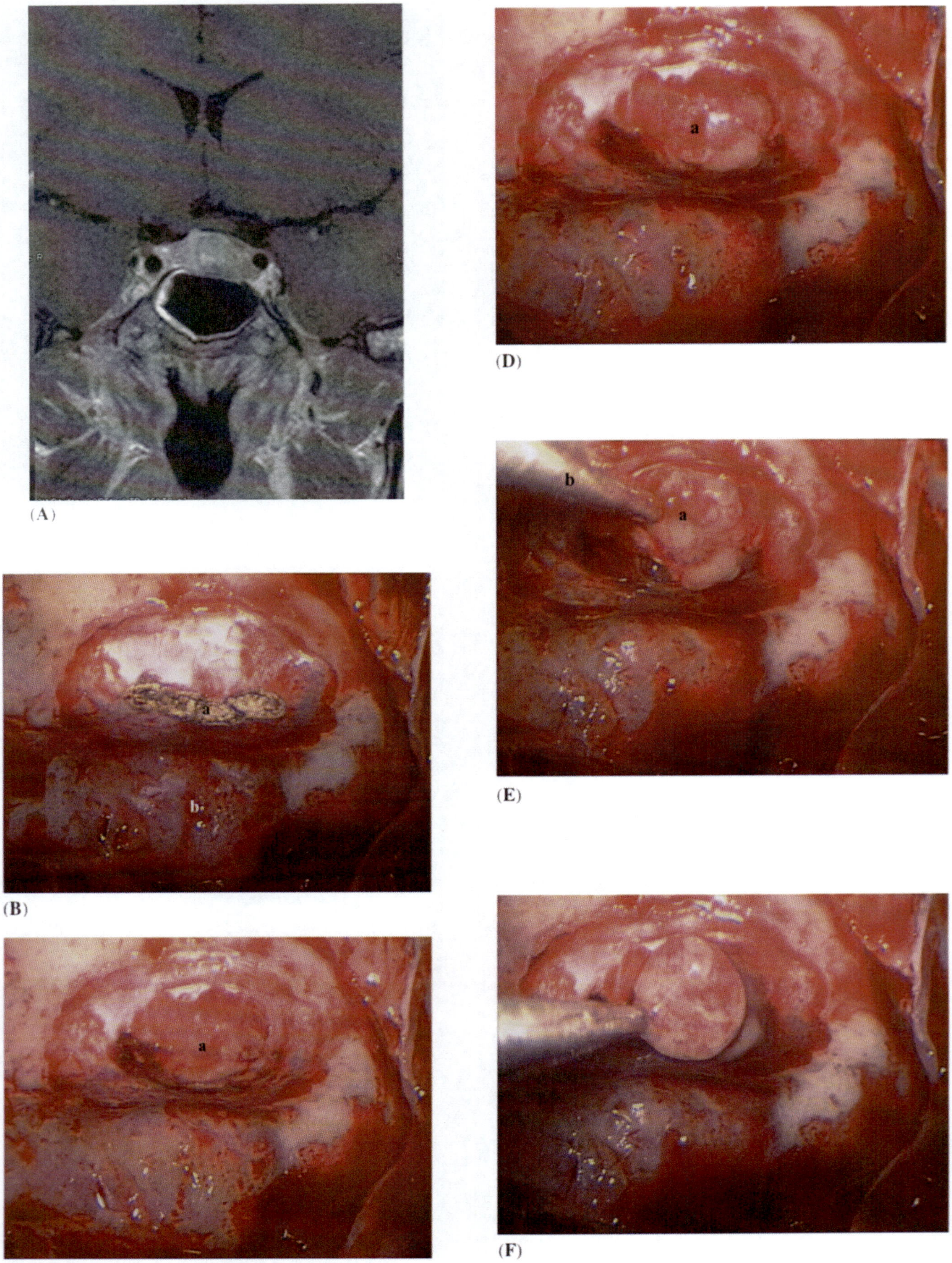

Fig. 16 (**A**) T_1-weighted coronal contrast-enhanced MRIs showing a pituitary macroadenoma. (**B**)–(**D**) Intraoperative endoscopic view showing initial exposure for pituitary macroadenoma. (**B**) *a* Cauterized sellar dura. *b* Clivus. (**C**) *a* Adenoma. (**D**) *a* Close-up view of adenoma. (**E**)–(**J**)

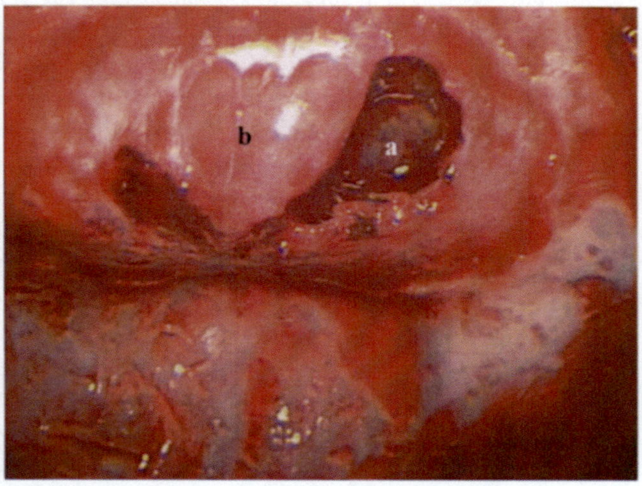

(G)

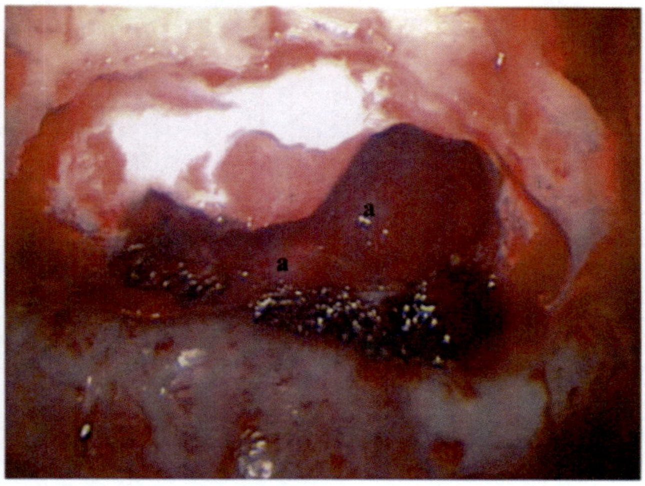

(J)

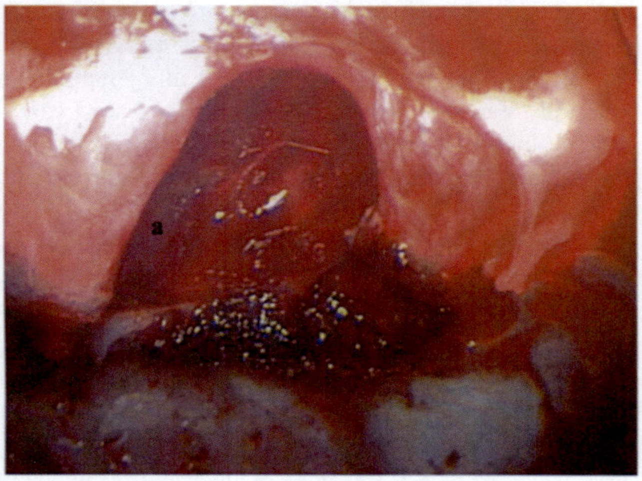

(H)

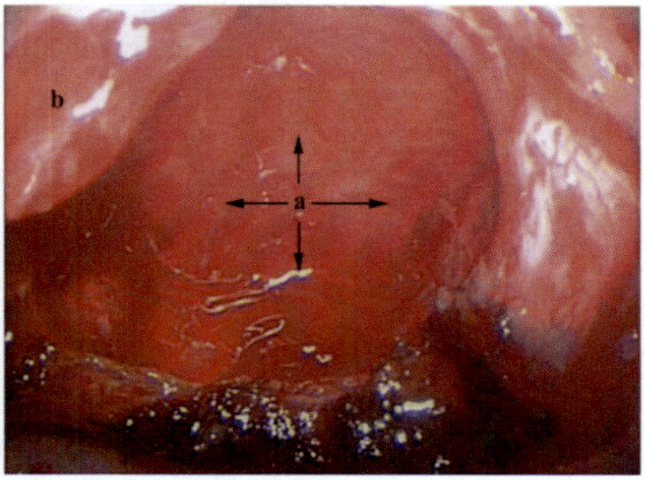

(K)

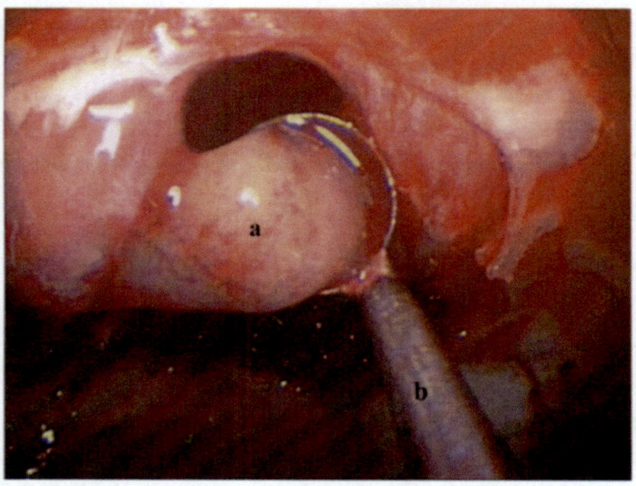

(I)

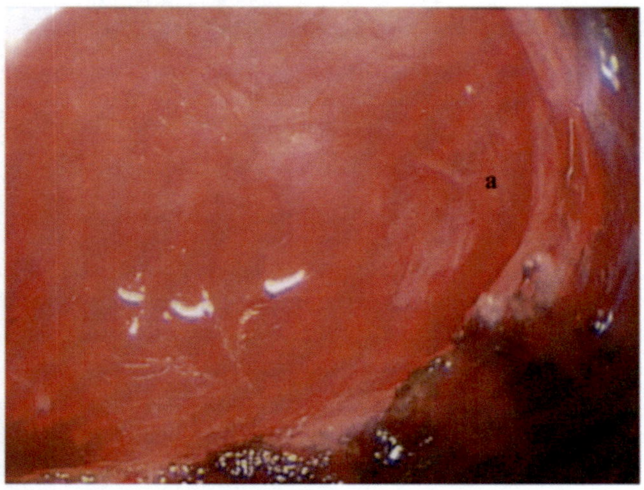

(L)

Fig. 16 (continued) Intraoperative endoscopic view showing gradual resection of pituitary macroadenoma. (**E**) *a* Adenoma. *b* Ring curette. (**G**) *a* Adenoma. *b* Normal anterior pituitary. (**H**) *a* Residual adenoma. (**I**) *a* Adenoma. *b* Ring curette. (**J**) *a* Final remnants of adenoma. (**K**) and (**L**) Intraoperative endoscopic view following complete resection of pituitary macroadenoma. (**K**) *a* Close-up view of adenoma cavity. *b* Pituitary. (**L**) *a* Close-up view of left medial cavernous sinus wall using 30° endoscope. (**M**) *a* Fat graft. (**N**) Postoperative contrast-enhanced coronal MRI.

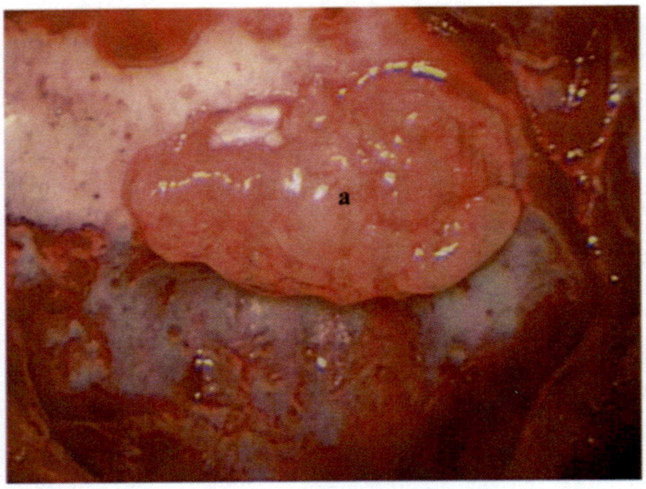

(M)

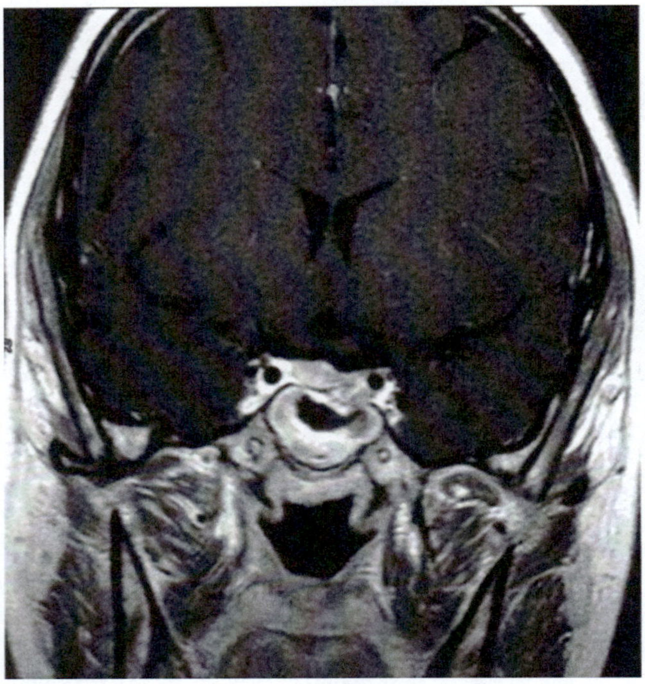

(N)

Fig. 16 (continued)

such as clival chordomas may invade the surrounding cranial nerves, causing clinical signs that include headache and cranial nerve deficits. The cranial nerve involved most often is cranial nerve VI (abducent); other signs may include dysphagia, facial pain, facial paresis, visual loss, hearing loss, and ataxia.

Many operative techniques and approaches have been utilized in the surgical management of periclival tumors; the choice among different approaches usually depends on the location and extent of the tumor. Nevertheless, the clivus along with the posterior surface of the petrous bone constitute the most anatomically complex area of the skull base and the most difficult to access surgically. A plethora of transfacial approaches, including the transbasal, transnasal, and transoral approaches, along with several transcranial approaches such as the suboccipital, subtemporal, and transcondylar approaches, have provided vast experience in the treatment of these previously unresectable tumors. Whether using a single or staged approach or whether using endoscopic techniques or more traditional open microsurgical techniques, no single technique can provide an exposure adequate for all clival and periclival lesions.

7.3.2. Approach The endoscopic endonasal approach offers a minimally invasive, anatomically direct route for resection of clival and retroclival tumors and obviates the need for brain retraction. To approach the clivus or the retroclival region, the endoscope is advanced toward the sphenoid sinus, and its mucosa and any septae are removed in the usual manner. On entering the sphenoid sinus, the tumor may be immediately visualized in some cases, such as in chordomas of the upper third of clivus. In these cases, the clivus typically has a diseased "moth-eaten" appearance and is resected as thoroughly as possible. In retroclival tumors, a transclival approach is performed by which the entire length of the clivus can be drilled using cutting and diamond burrs to obtain direct access to the prepontine region. For intradural prepontine lesions, the dura is sharply incised, taking great care to avoid any injury to the basilar artery immediately posterior, and the underlying tumor is first identified and subsequently resected.

The surgical principles that are followed include obtaining a frozen section analysis of the tumor to confirm the histopathologic diagnosis and resecting the tumor piecemeal using a combination of dissecting microinstruments, micro-CUSA, and microbipolar. Resection of any tumor extensions into the sphenoid sinus, the sella turcica, or the anterior clivus is performed. Following the resection, the 0° endoscope is slowly withdrawn from the surgical field, and a 30° endoscope is placed to confirm gross removal of all tumor remnants. A small Teflon-coated pledget is then placed in the region of the clivus to mark the limits of surgical resection if a second-stage procedure is planned. Small dural defects should be avoided at all cost in case of extradural lesions. If the dura is incised open to access an intradural prepontine lesion, it is closed with a double layer of fat graft and a collagen dural substitute followed by application of fibrin or dural sealant. The clival defect is obliterated with a hydroxyapatite bone substitute.

7.3.3. Case

7.3.3.1. Prepontine Epidermoid Tumor (Fig. 18A–Z)

8. POTENTIAL COMPLICATIONS

Potential complications of the fully endoscopic endonasal approach include the following:

- Bleeding, infection, cerebrovascular accident, and death (these are also potential complications associated with traditional transcranial and transspheoidal approaches to the pituitary gland).
- Endocrine complications include anterior pituitary insufficiency (this is typically detected postoperatively and may involve one or more of the pituitary axes) and posterior pituitary insufficiency, leading to complications such as transient

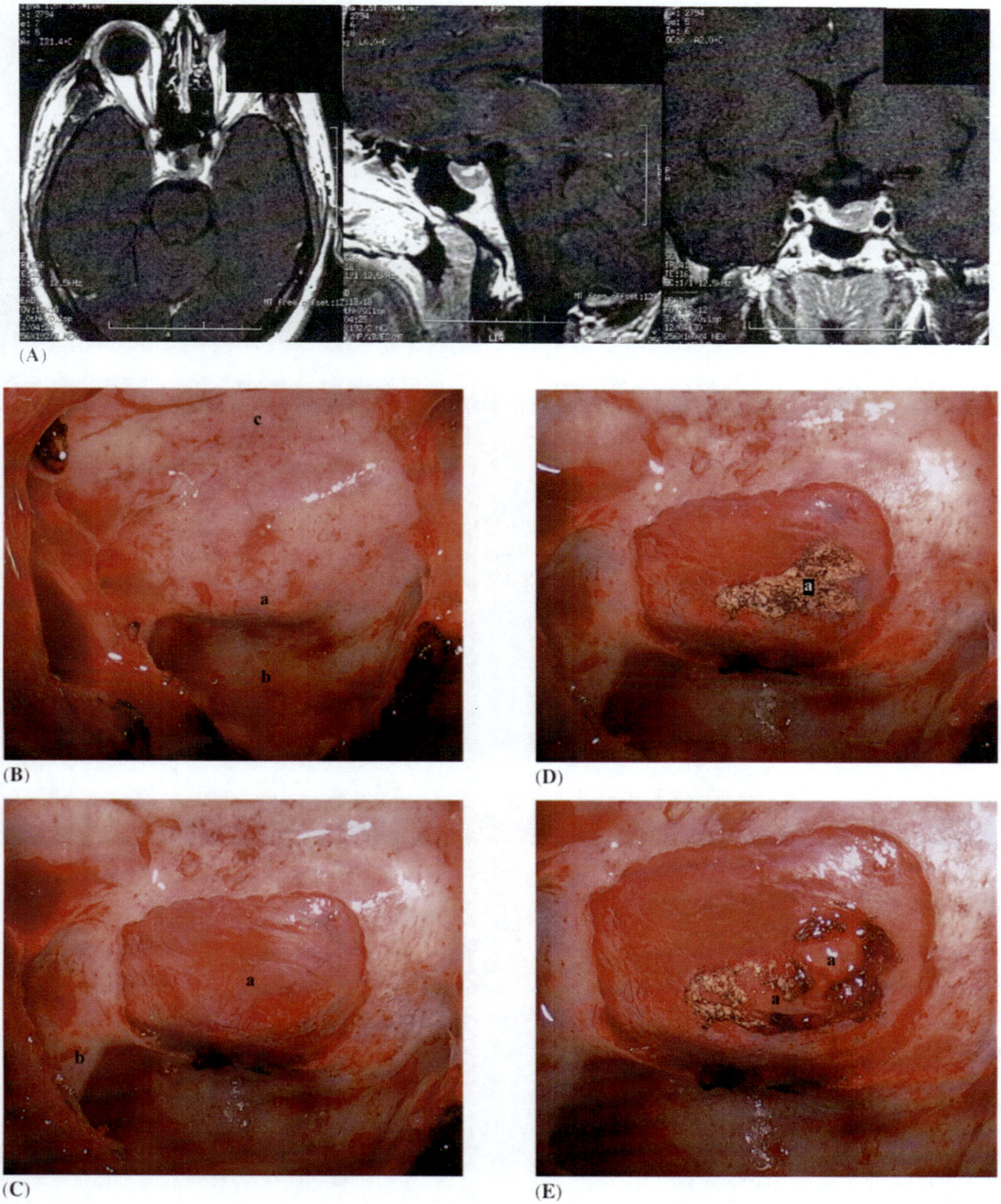

Fig. 17 (**A**) T_1-weighted axial, sagittal and coronal contrast-enhanced MRIs showing a pituitary macroadenoma. (**B**)–(**F**) Intraoperative endoscopic view showing initial exposure for pituitary macroadenoma. (**B**) *a* Sellar floor. *b* Clivus. *c* Planum sphenoidale. (**C**) *a* Sellar dura. *b* Right carotid protuberance. (**D**) *a* Cauterized sellar dura. (**E**) *a* Adenoma. (**G**)–(**R**) Intraoperative endoscopic view showing gradual resection of pituitary macroadenoma. (**G**) *a* Adenoma. *b* Ring curette. (**K**) *a* Adenoma. *b* Normal anterior pituitary. (**M**) *a* Adenoma. *b* Ring curette. *c* Atraumatic suction. (**Q**) *a* Final portions of adenoma. *b* Normal anterior pituitary. (**R**) *a* Close-up view showing final portions of adenoma. *b* Normal anterior pituitary. *c* Arachnoid. (**S**)–(**W**) Intraoperative endoscopic view following complete resection of pituitary macroadenoma. (**S**) *a* Close-up view of adenoma cavity. *b* Normal anterior pituitary. *c* Arachnoid. *d* Medial wall of left cavernous sinus. (**T**) *a* Close-up view of right medial cavernous sinus wall using 30° endoscope. *b* Arachnoid. (**U**) *a* Close-up view of left medial cavernous sinus using 30° endoscope. *b* Arachnoid. (**V**) *a* Fat graft. (**W**) *a* Dural sealant. (**X**) Postoperative contrast-enhanced axial, saggital, and coronal MRIs.

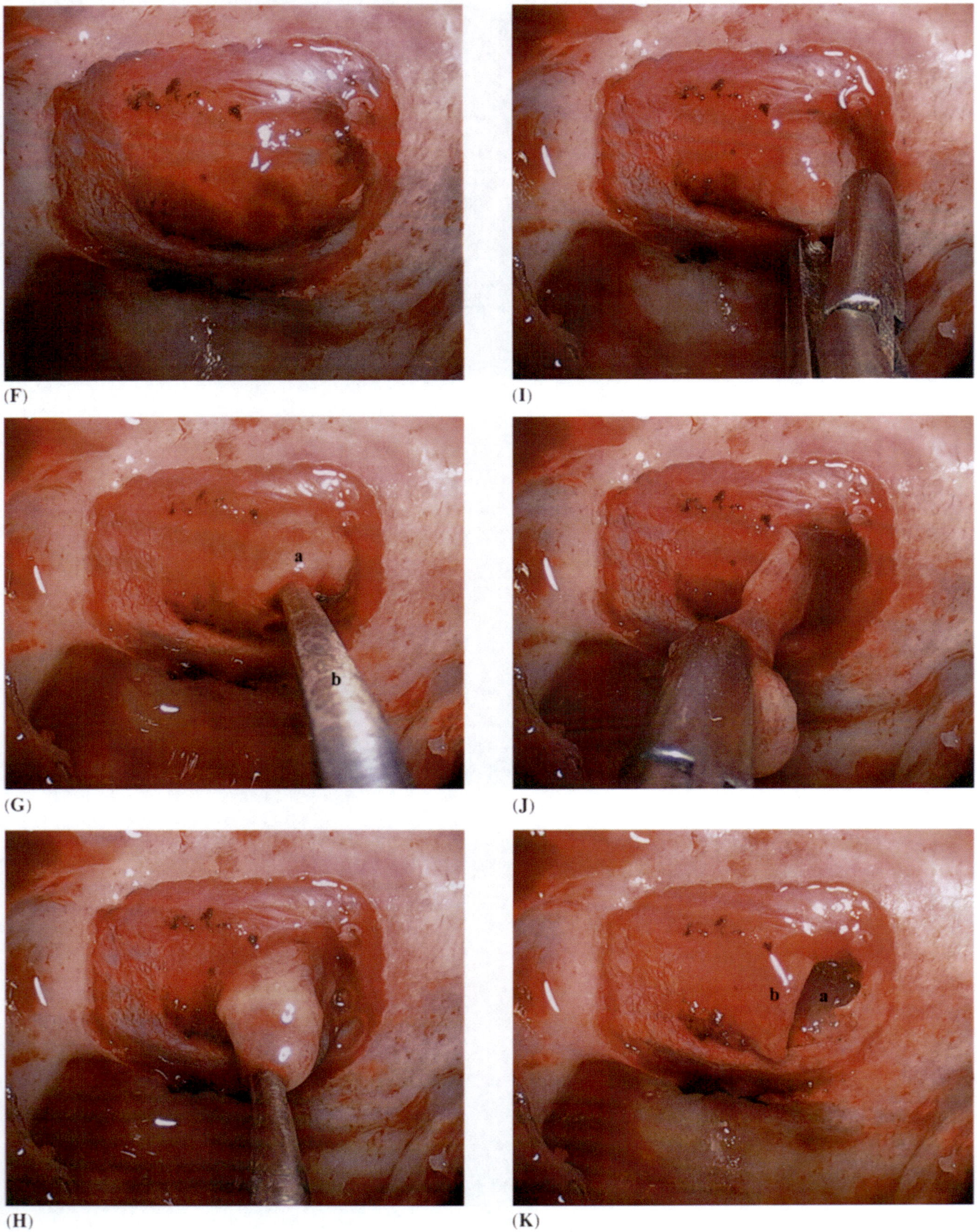

Fig. 17 (continued)

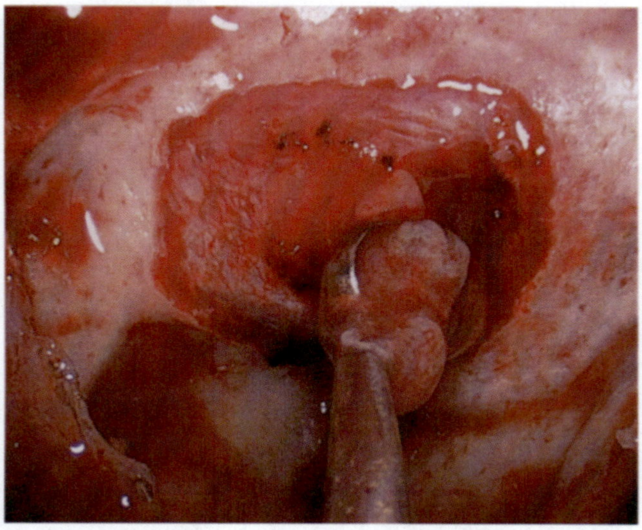
(L)

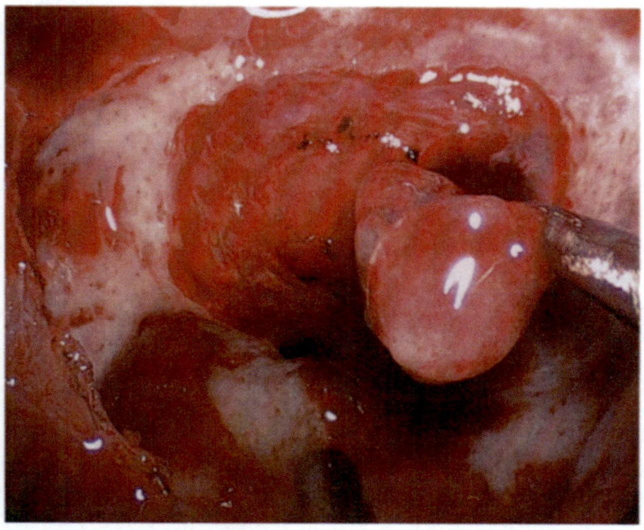
(O)

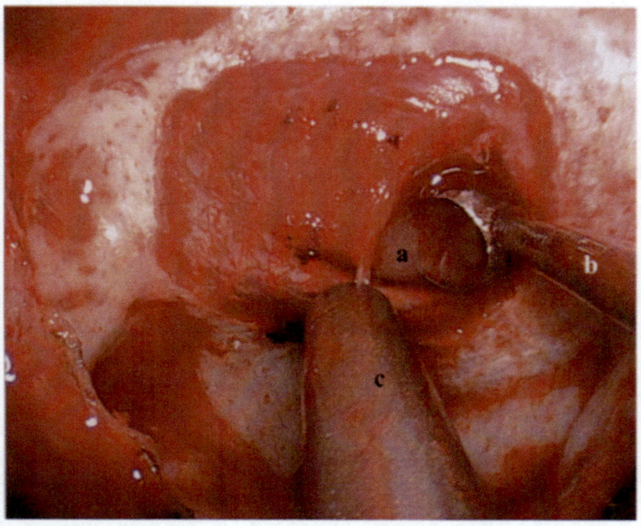

(M)

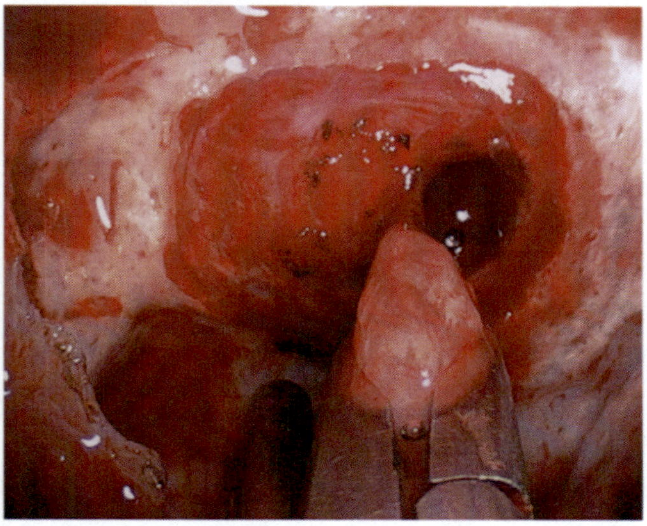
(P)

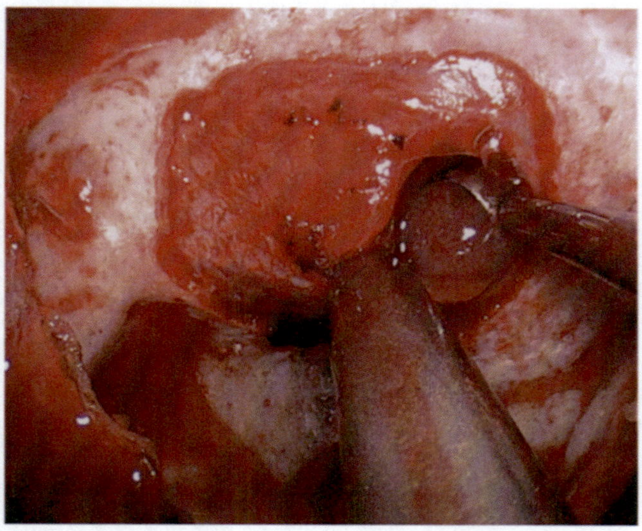
(N)

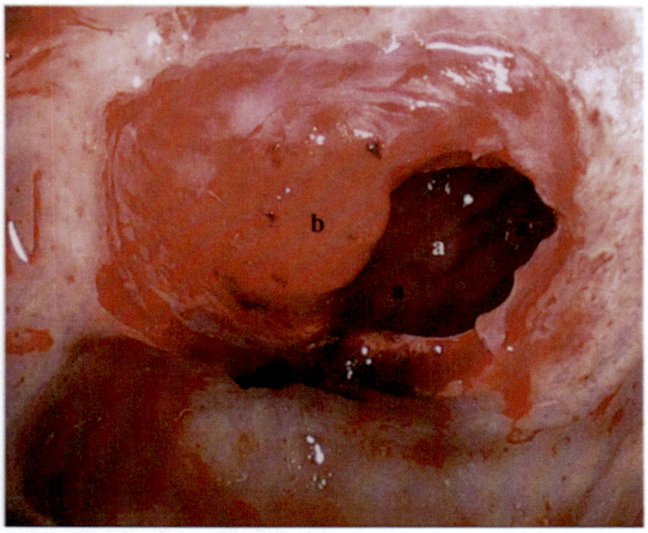

(Q)

Fig. 17 (continued)

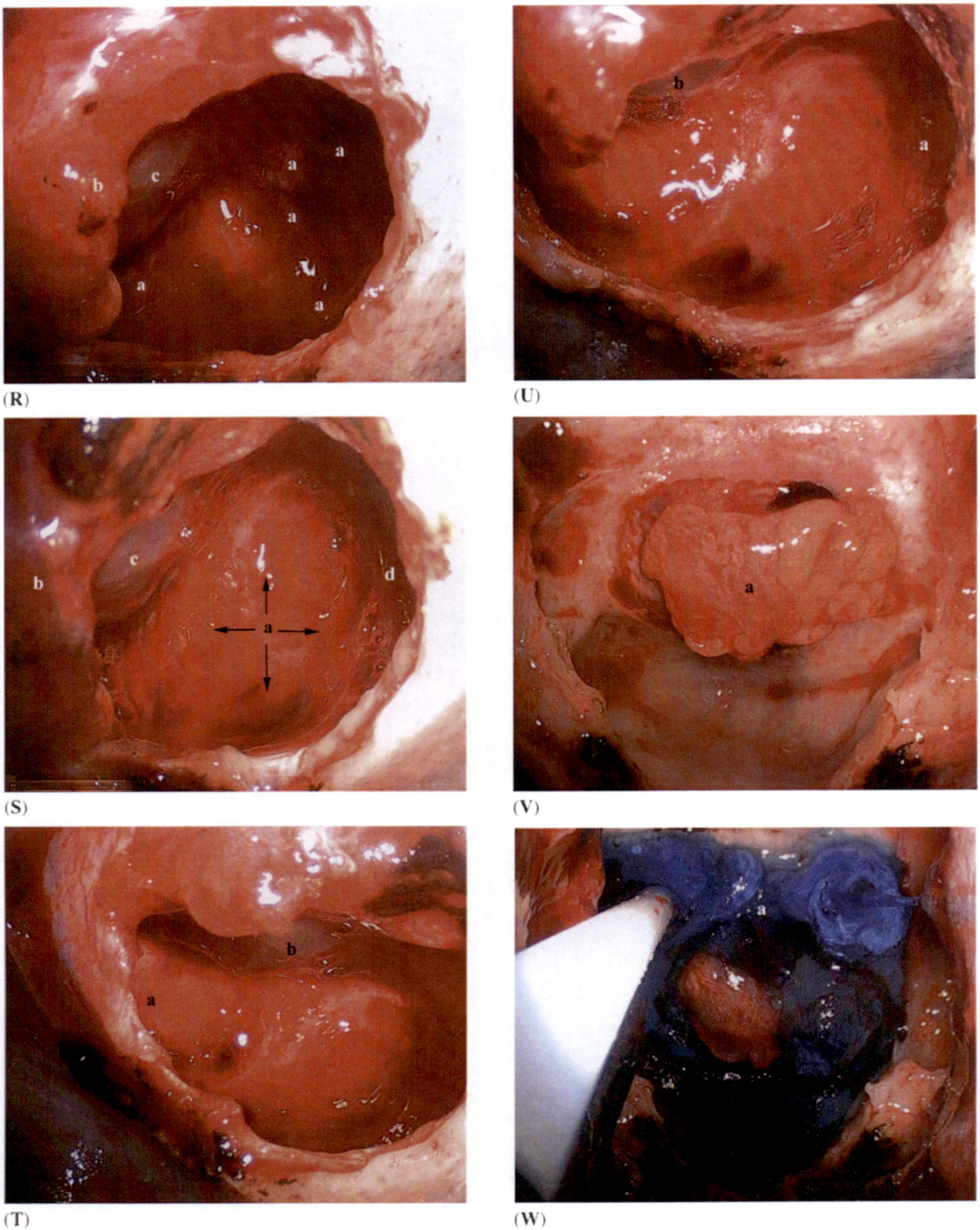

Fig. 17 (continued)

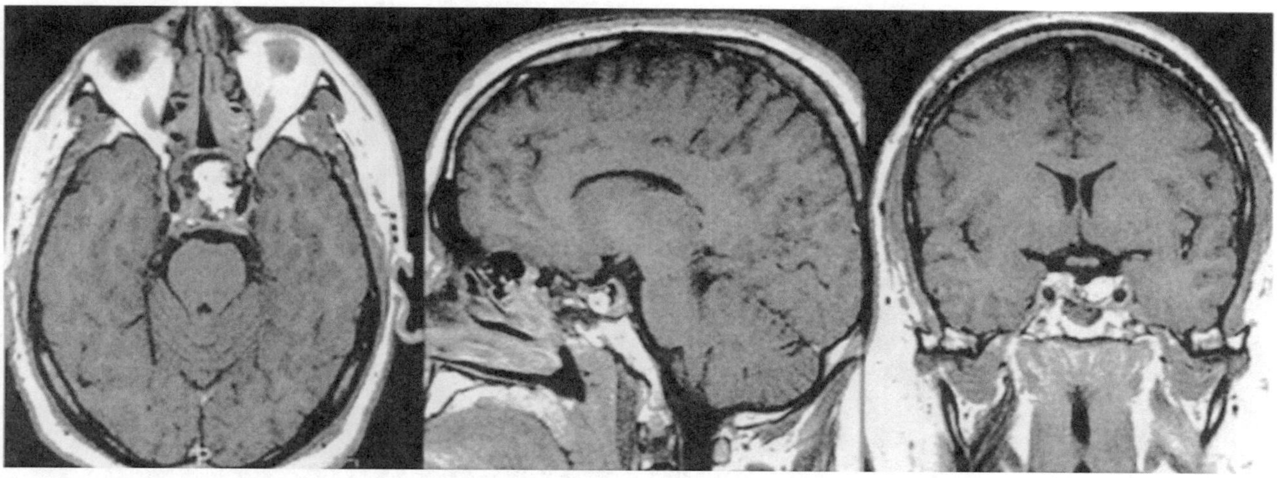

(X)

Fig. 17 (continued)

or persistent diabetes insipidus (DI).

- CSF leak, meningitis.
- Direct neurovascular injuries can occur to the optic apparatus, cranial nerves, carotid artery, hypothalamus, or brain.
- Early or delayed postoperative epistaxis, resulting from rupture of a small septal vessel or mucosal branch of the sphenopalatine artery.
- Sphenoid sinus complications include sphenoid sinusitis or mucocele (symptomatic or asymptomatic).
- Direct injuries during the approach may include nasal septal perforations, anosmia resulting from mucosal trauma or dissection, and accidental bone fractures (hard palate, orbital wall, cribriform plate).
- Severe frontal headaches, tension pneumocephalus.

9. AVOIDING COMPLICATIONS IN AUTHOR'S EXPERIENCE

Improved endoscopic visualization allows the surgeon to recognize and avoid injuring the normal pituitary gland, optic apparatus, carotid prominences, cavernous sinuses, and hypothalamus. Thus, many catastrophic complications that were once associated with limited visibility or blind dissection, such as anterior and posterior pituitary insufficiencies, blindness, cranial nerve deficits, and central nervous system injury, are generally avoidable. Transient DI is probably the most common cause of prolonged hospital stay, but rarely does it persist permanently. Generally, all complications occur less frequently than with the traditional transsphenoidal approach.

The completely endonasal approach eliminates the need for extensive mucosal dissection, the use of nasal speculums, and postoperative nasal packing. Therefore, approach-related complications, such as septal perforations or bony injuries, are completely avoidable. A postoperative sphenoid sinus mucocele and sphenoid sinusitis are rare occurrences with the endoscopic approach. Delayed epistaxis is rare; when significant, it is managed with either posterior packing or neuroradiologic embolization.

The anatomy of the sphenoid sinus depends on the age of the patient and the pathology encountered. It may be nonaerated in pediatric patients, multiseptated, completely filled with tumor that has invaded through the floor of the sella, or as in the case of a clival chordoma, protruding from the clivus. Preoperative MRI studies provide useful information on the individual sphenoid anatomy. In addition, it is recommended to revisit the patient's imaging studies during the initial exposure of the sellar areas to keep orientation to the midline and avoid complications that may result from a deviated trajectory.

Violation of the arachnoid membrane during surgery may result in CSF leak, pneumocephalus, or even bacterial meningitis. Our principal surgical rule is to avoid penetrating the arachnoid membrane as this significantly increases the possibility of serious morbidity and can result in injury to the optic nerves and chiasm, carotid artery and its branches, and the hypothalamus and, by definition, will result in an intraoperative CSF leak, creating the possibility of meningitis, subarachnoid hemorrhage, vasospasm, and tension pneumocephalus.

If too much of the pituitary gland is resected during surgery, the patient may need to be placed on hormonal replacement indefinitely. Therefore, these tumors should be resected with minimal trauma to the underlying normal pituitary gland. Total tumor resection is the ultimate goal of surgery. Large macroadenomas with supra- or parasellar extension that is beyond the limits of the endonasal approach should undergo a second-stage endoscopic supraorbital or transglabellar approach.

Tumor resection is considered complete only after a final survey with the angled endoscopes is completed, confirming absence of all tumor. A 70° endoscope may also be used in this examination; however, in most cases, the information obtained by the 30° lens is sufficient to identify any tumor remnants.

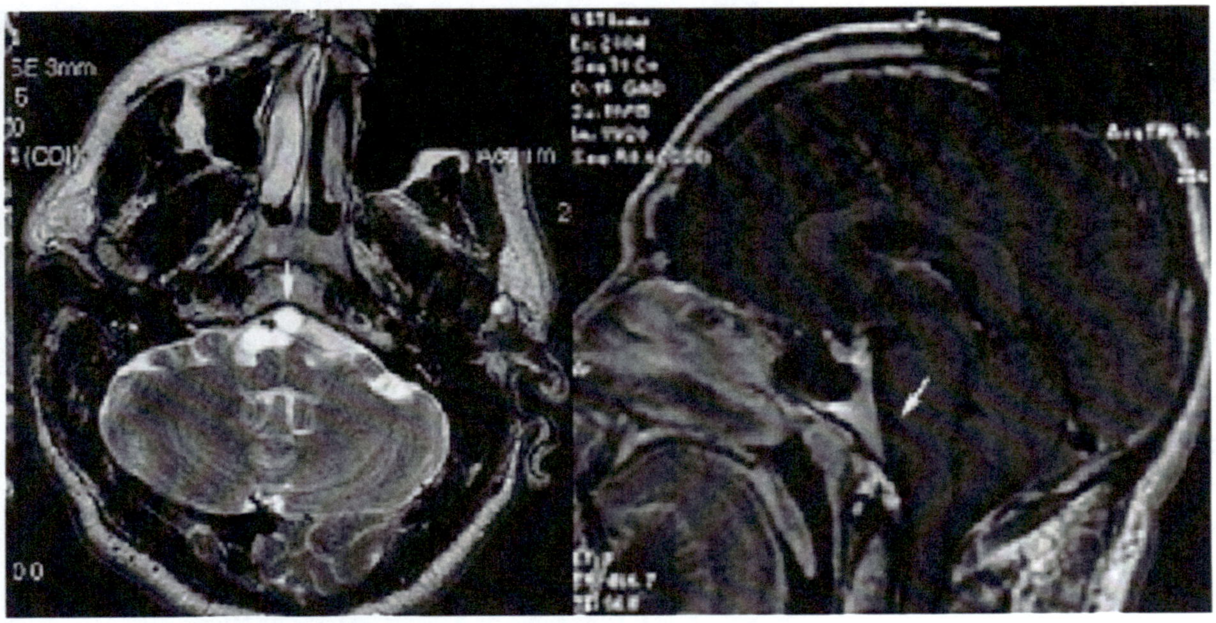

(A)

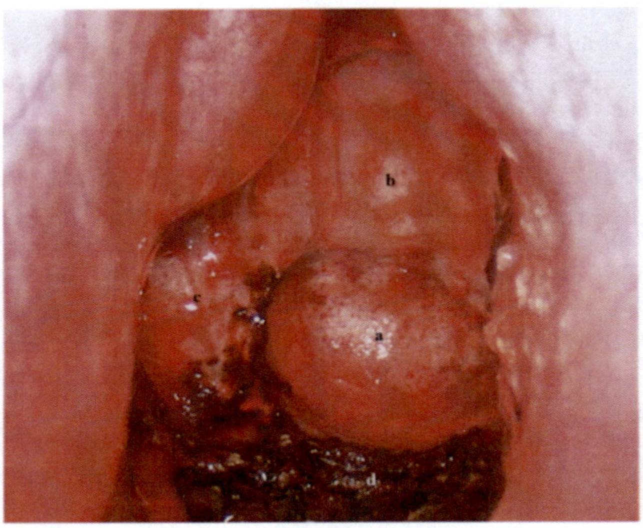

(B)

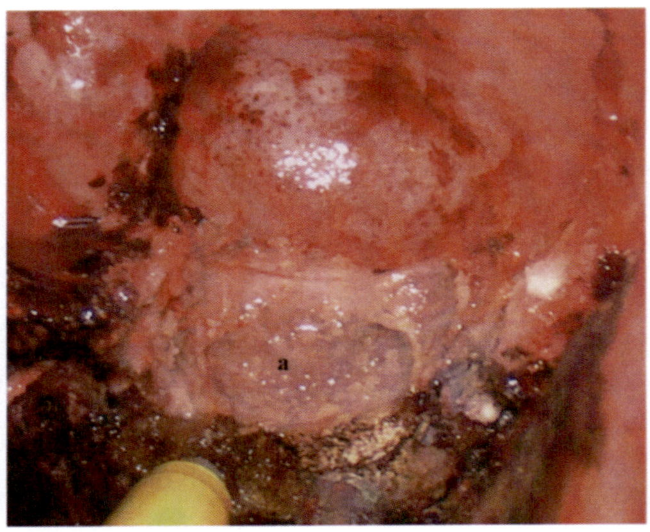

(C)

Fig. 18 (**A**) T_2-weighted axial and T_1-weighted contrast-enhanced saggital MRIs showing a prepontine epidermoid tumor. (**C**)–(**G**) Intraoperative endoscopic view showing transclival exposure for removal of prepontine epidermoid tumor. (**B**) *a.* Clivus. *b* Sella turcica. *c* Right carotid protuberance. (**C**) *a* Drilling through middle third of clivus (cancellous bone of midclivus). (**D**) *a* Dura. *b* High-speed microdrill. *c* Suction. (**E**) *a* Dura hook. *b* Dura. *c* Boundaries of keyhole. *d* Midclival bone. (**F**) *a* Arachnoid. *b* Right-curved microscissors. (**H**)–(**P**) Intraoperative endoscopic view showing gradual removal of prepontine epidermoid tumor. (**H**) *a* Arachnoid. *b* Pearly white shadow of epidermoid tumor. *c* Atraumatic suction. (**I**) *a* Epidermoid tumor. *b* Arachnoid. (**K**) *a* Epidermoid tumor. *b* Left Anterior Inferior cerebellar artery (AICA). (**N**) *a* Epidermoid tumor. *b* Left AICA. (**O**) *a* Basilar artery. *b* Left AICA. *c* Brainstem. *d* Epidermoid tumor. (**P**) *a* Basilar artery. *b* Left AICA. *c* Brainstem. *d* Final remnants of epidermoid tumor. (**Q**)–(**S**) Intraoperative endoscopic view after complete transclival removal of prepontine epidermoid tumor. (**Q**) *a* Basilar artery. *b* Left AICA. *c* Brainstem. *d* Left vertebral artery. (**R**) *a* Close-up view of basilar artery and regional anatomy of prepontine epidermoid tumor. (**S**) *a* Basilar artery. *b* Left AICA. *c* Brainstem. *d* Left vertebral artery. *e* Dura. (**T**)–(**Y**) Intraoperative endoscopic view showing closure after transclival removal of prepontine epidermoid tumor. (**T**) *a* Fat graft (first closure layer). (**U**) *a* Collagen dural onlay graft (second closure layer). (**V**) *b* Fat graft (third closure layer). (**W**) *a* Dural sealant. *b* Fat graft. (**X**) *a* Hydroxyapatite bone substitute. *b* Dural sealant. *c* Fat graft. (**Y**) *a* Hydroxyapatite bone substitute. (**Z**) Postoperative contrast-enhanced T_1-weighted axial and sagittal MRIs.

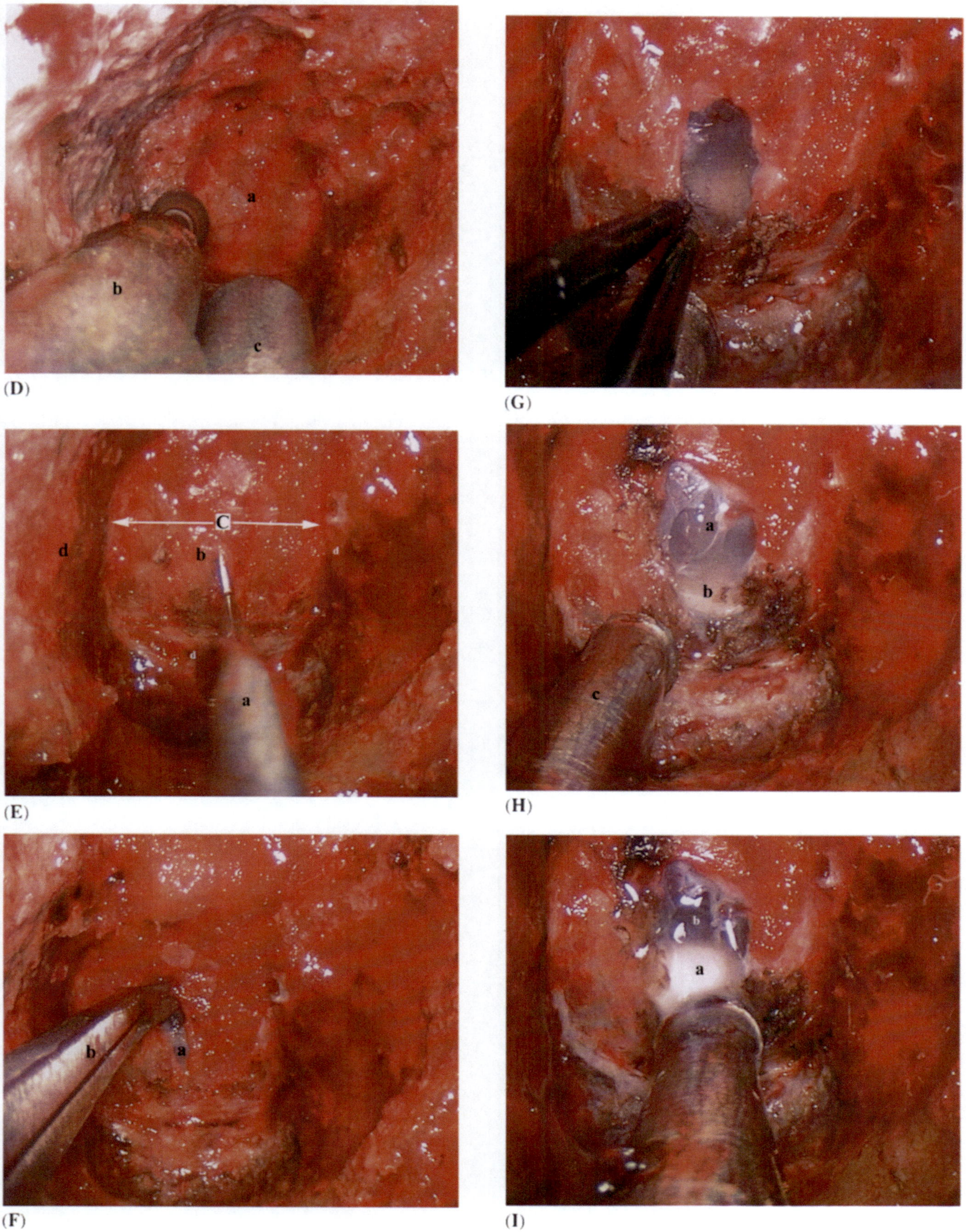

Fig. 18 (continued)

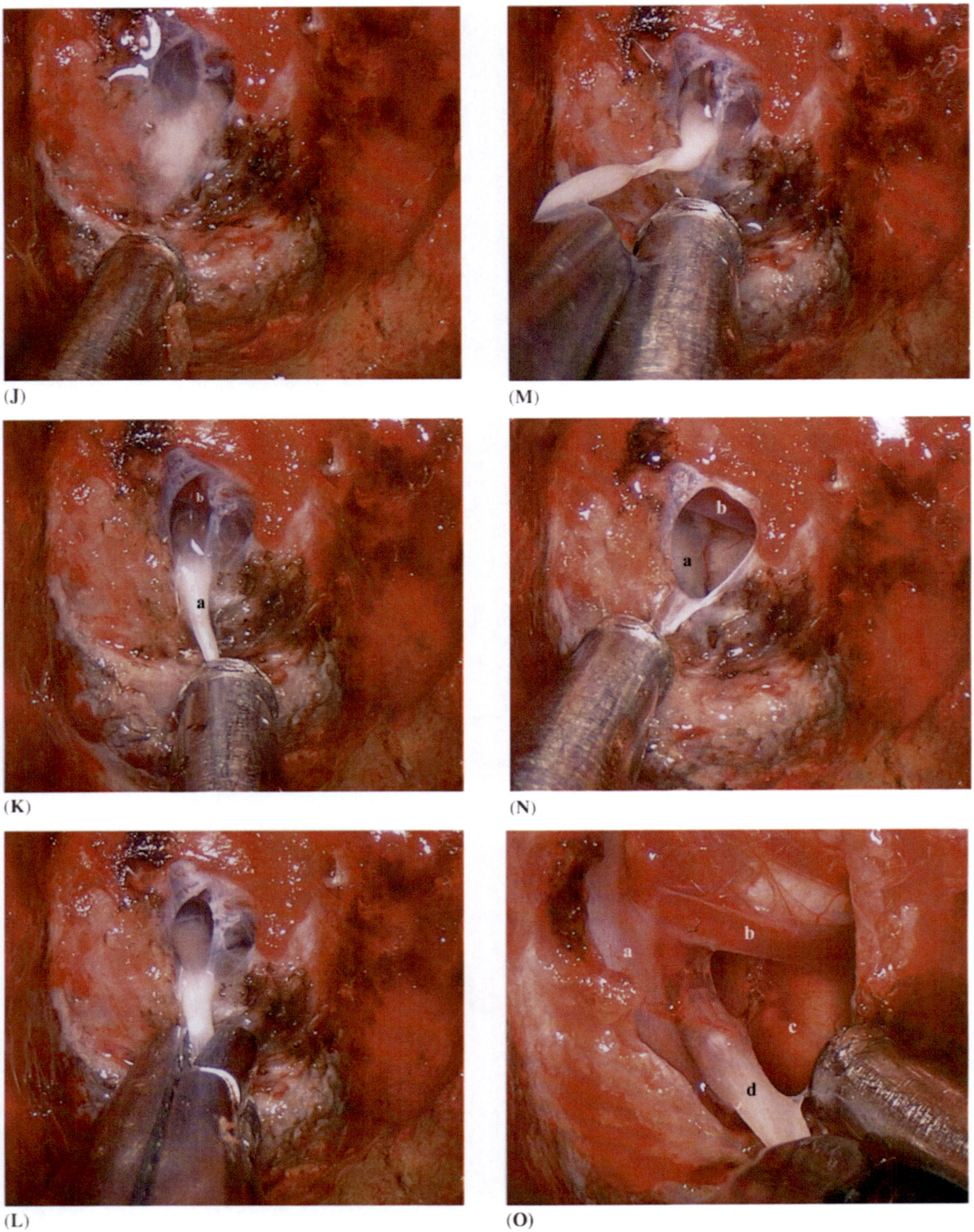

Fig. 18 (continued)

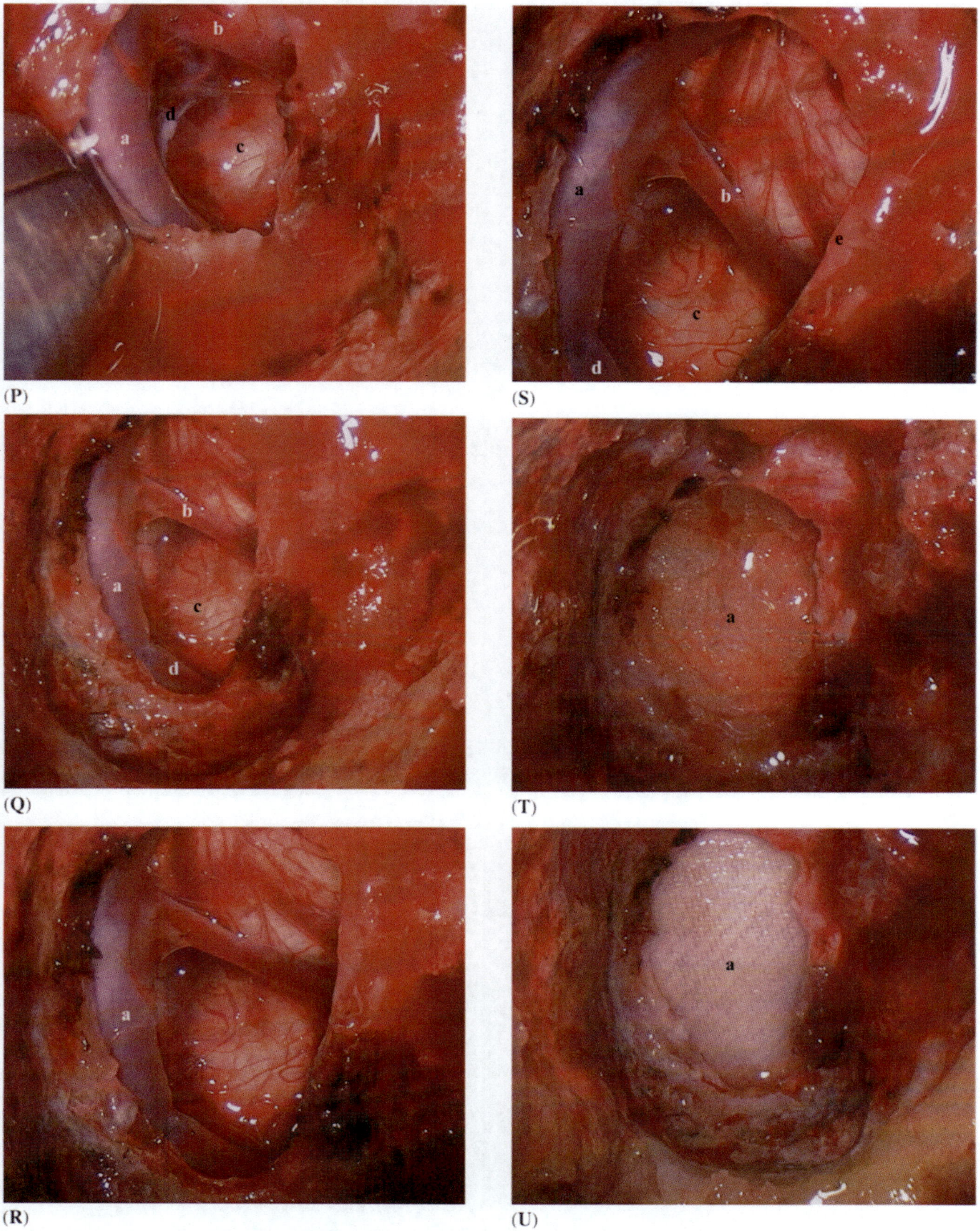

Fig. 18 (continued)

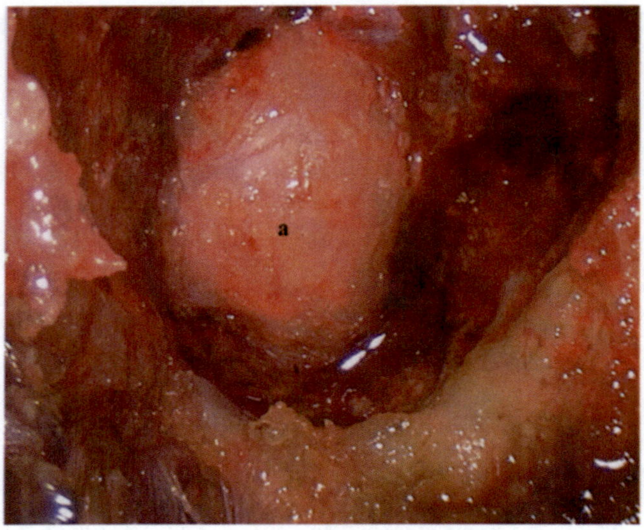

(V)

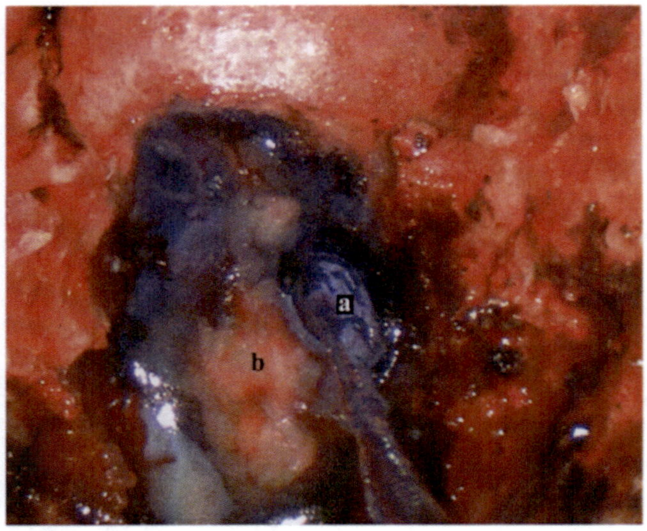

(X)

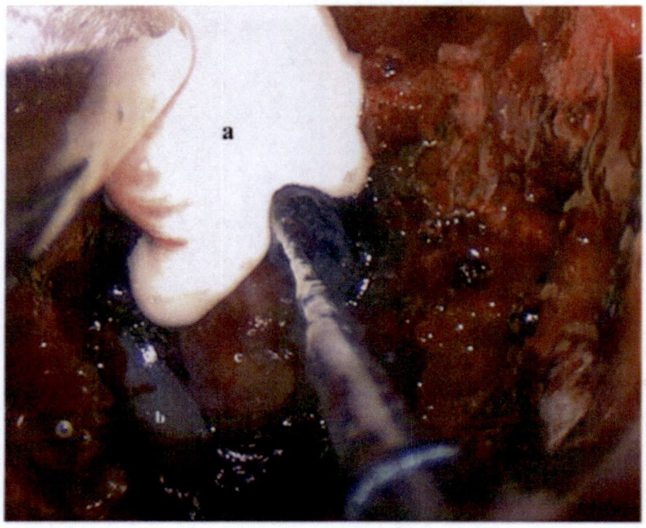

(W)

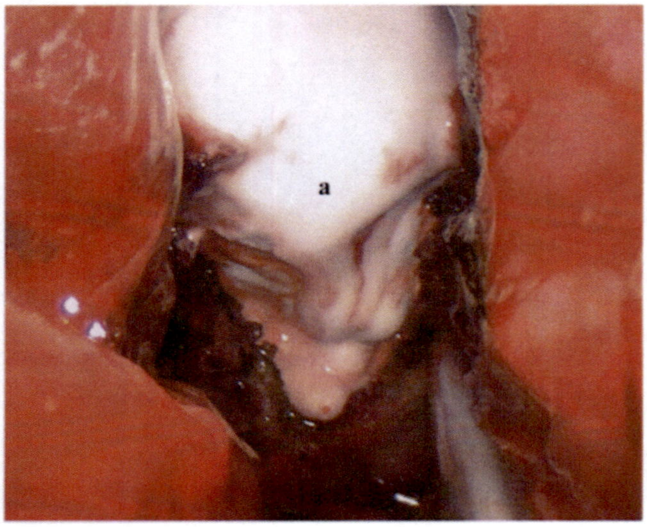

(Y)

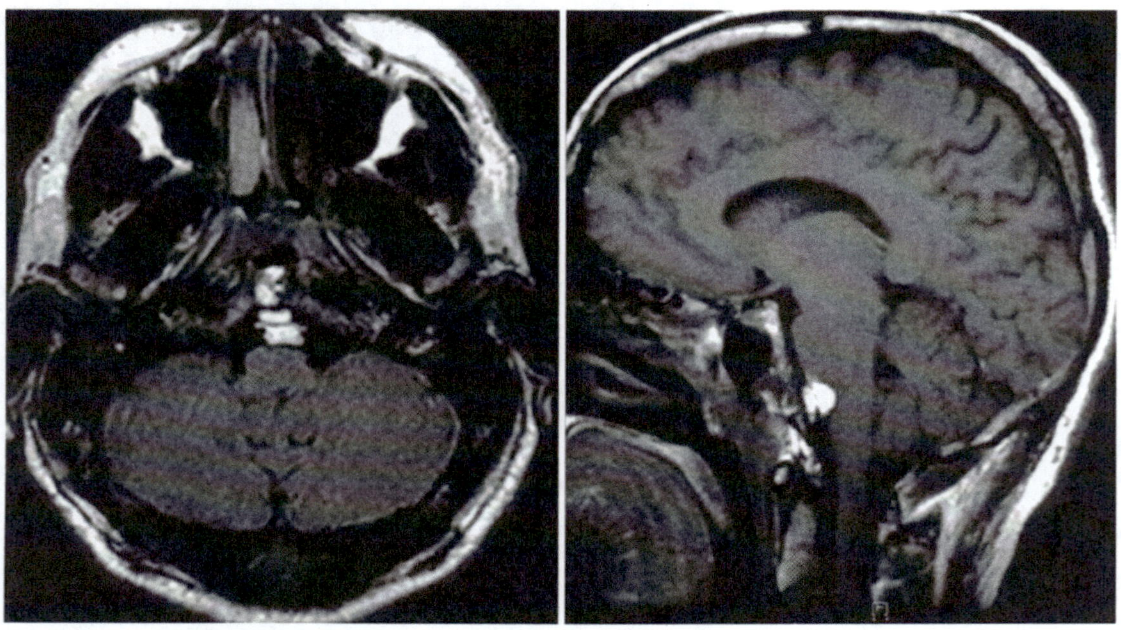

(Z)

Fig. 18 (continued)

Tumor remnants in these areas, constituting the potential sources of recurrence, are effectively removed with a superb visual appreciation of the critical surrounding structures. Inadequate repair of clival dural defects remains the greatest potential complication in clival and transclival tumor resection, and a double-layer closure technique as described is recommended. Lumbar drains are no longer used.

7 The Fully Endoscopic Transglabellar Approach

This chapter discusses the application of the fully endoscopic transglabellar keyhole approach in surgical management of tumors of the anterior cranial base and the suprasellar region. Traditionally, approaches to these tumors have required large frontal craniotomies along with prolonged retraction of the frontal lobes, subjecting patients to undesirable neurological and cosmetic morbidity. In our practice, the endoscopic transglabellar approach has allowed thorough visualization of the anterior fossa, suprasellar region, and all critical structures at the paramedian skull base. Endoscopic imaging thereby facilitates complete tumor resection via a minimally invasive technique that utilizes a small hidden incision that runs in a natural skin crease between the eyebrows. The chapter provides a thorough description of the fully endoscopic transglabellar approach, including indications, operating room setup, patient positioning, operative technique, state-of-the-art illustrative cases, potential complications, and ways to avoid these complications (in the author's experience).

Keywords: Craniopharyngioma; Endoscopic; Keyhole; Macroadenoma; Minimally invasive; Optic chiasm; Optic nerve; Parasellar; Pituitary; Pituitary gland; Pituitary surgery; Sellar; Skull base; Suprasellar; Surgery; Transglabellar.

1. INTRODUCTION

Surgical management of tumors of the anterior cranial base and the suprasellar region has traditionally required large frontal craniotomies with prolonged retraction of the frontal lobes. These wide surgical exposures often subject patients to undesirable neurological and cosmetic morbidity. However, the ease with which endoscopes and instruments can be maneuvered in the space between the frontal lobes and the base of the skull and the ability of rigid endoscopes to overcome the barriers to visualization that a diminutive craniotomy may pose have allowed minimally invasive surgical access to the anterior cranial fossa and suprasellar region with excellent visualization.

Through a transglabellar keyhole approach, the endoscope is advanced directly to the lesion; thus, the effective operating distance is significantly reduced, as is the need for wide skin flaps. The use of 0° and angled endoscopes has allowed unprecedented panoramic views of the anterior cranial fossa, as well as the ability to see around anatomical "corners" that normally would obscure gross and microscopic observation. Therefore, through a limited transglabellar keyhole craniotomy, the floor of the anterior cranial fossa, the paranasal sinuses, the anterior clinoids, and the suprasellar region can all be surgically accessed without the need for wide scalp flaps, large frontal craniotomies, or extensive craniofacial approaches.

2. INDICATIONS

The fully endoscopic transglabellar approach provides minimally invasive access for surgical resection of midline tumors such as craniopharyngiomas, cystic lesions such as Rathke's cleft and arachnoid cysts, dermoids and epidermoids, aneurysms of the anterior circle of Willis, chiasmatic and hypothalamic gliomas, tumors of the pituitary stalk such as hamartomas and germinomas, olfactory groove and suprasellar meningiomas, intracranial extensions of paranasal sinus neoplasms, suprasellar extensions of pituitary tumors, and other tumors of the anterior skull base and suprasellar region.

3. INSTRUMENTATION

The instruments needed to execute this procedure successfully include an endoscopic tower containing a three-chip high-definition digital camera, a xenon or halogen light source, 0° and 30° rigid endoscopes, two endoscope holding arms, endoscope irrigation sheaths, and precision microinstruments.

4. OPERATING ROOM SETUP (FIG. 1)

The patient is placed supine on the operating room table, and the head of the bed is slightly raised. Following the induction of general anesthesia, the airway circuit is extended with

From: *Endoscopic Skull Base Surgery: A Comprehensive Guide with Illustrative Cases.*
Edited by H. K. Shahinian © Humana Press, Totowa, NJ.

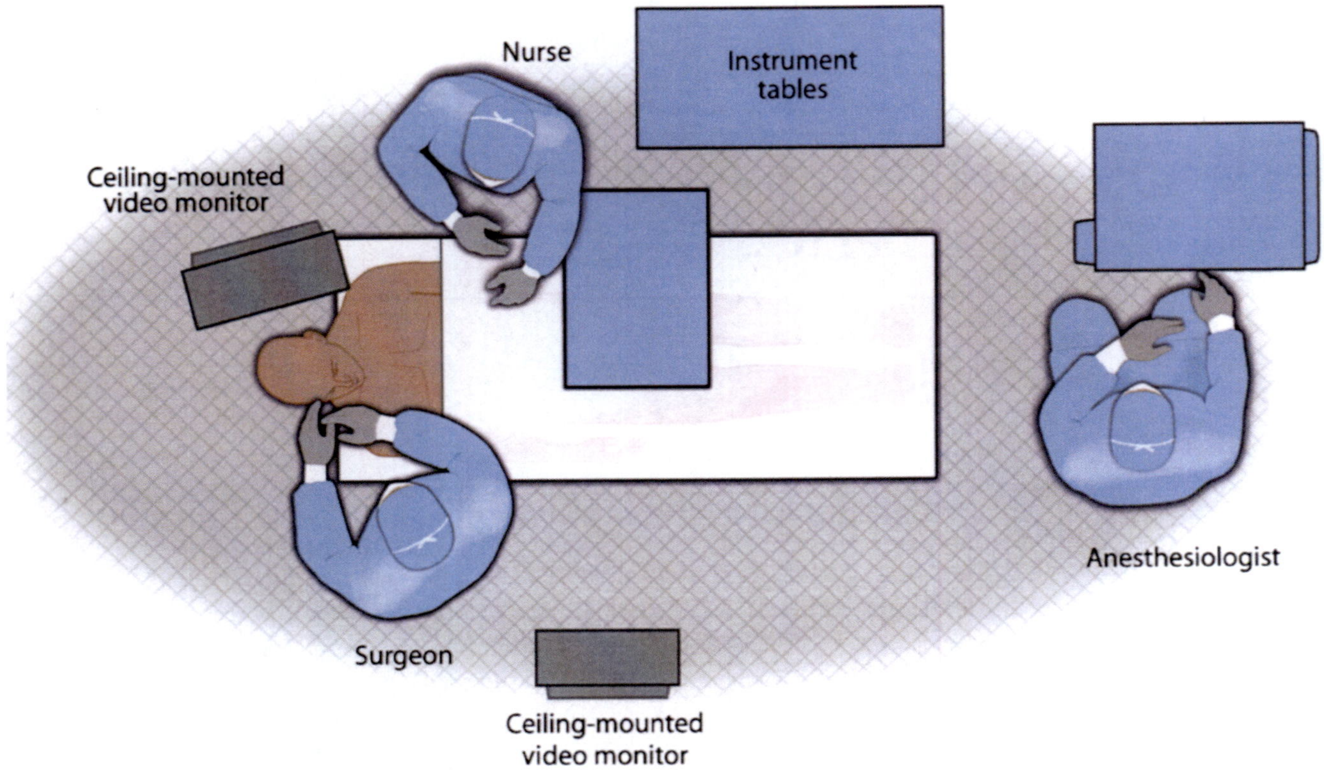

Fig. 1 Operating room setup.

corrugated tubing, and the head is turned 180° away from the anesthesiologist. The endoscopic tower is placed above the patient's head. Two separate pneumatically powered holding arms are affixed to the table, one on each side of the patient, and wrapped in sterile drapes. One holding arm is dedicated to holding the endoscope, and the other is used to hold other endoscopic instruments or soft silicone spatulas.

5. PATIENT POSITIONING (FIG. 2)

The patient is placed supine on the operating room table, and the head of the bed is raised 45° to facilitate venous drainage and a subfrontal trajectory. The patient's neck is then slightly flexed and rotated ipsilaterally approximately 15° to face the surgeon. The patient's head is fixed in position using a three-pin Mayfield clamp. Thus positioned—and with mild hyperventilation, cerebrospinal fluid (CSF) drainage, and intravenous mannitol—the frontal lobes will eventually "relax," enhancing a subfrontal path along which the endoscope is advanced.

6. OPERATIVE TECHNIQUE

Once the patient is under general anesthesia, a color marker is used to define the landmarks of the skin incision, and the frontal and nasal areas are cleansed with an aqueous antiseptic solution and then draped. A 3-cm incision is made between the medial ends of the eyebrows, crossing the nasion in a natural skin crease. The skin flap is developed in a subcutaneous plane and retracted superiorly. The glabellar periosteum is elevated separately and retracted inferiorly for further use as an inferiorly based pericranial flap in reconstructing the skull base (Fig. 3A–C). A small burr hole is placed in the frontal bone, and the outer table of the frontal sinus is osteotomized. Once the sinus cavity is exposed, its mucosa is stripped, and both nasofrontal ducts are obliterated.

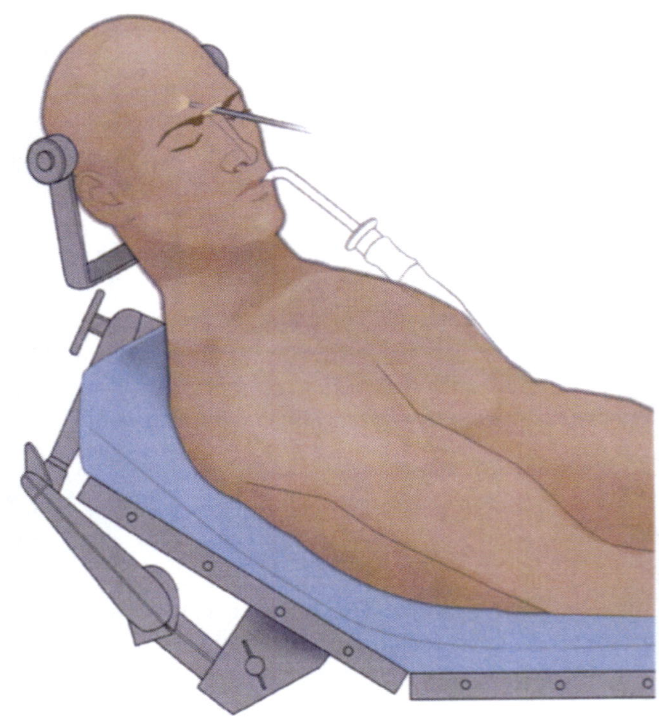

Fig. 2 Patient positioning.

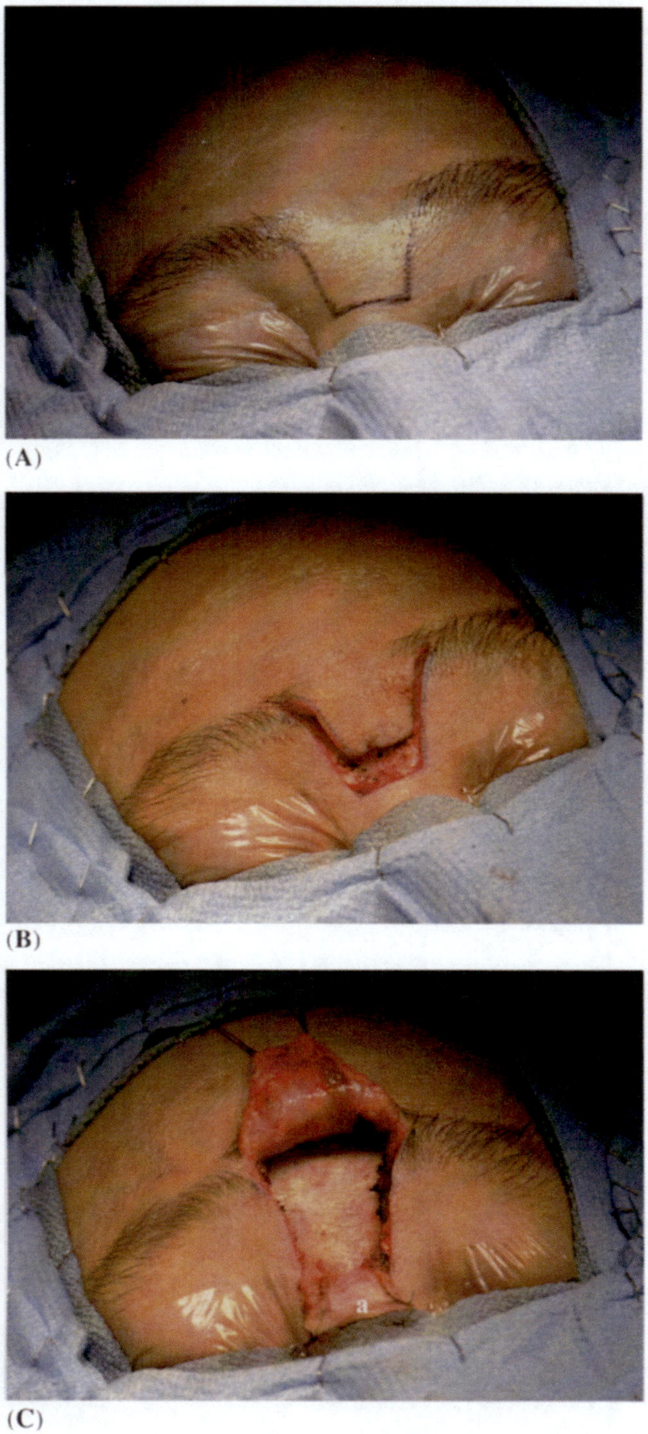

Fig. 3 (**A**) Marking and draping, (**B**) and (**C**) skin incision. *a* Pericranium reflected inferiorly.

A burr hole is then placed in the posterior wall of the sinus, and a second bone flap is removed, revealing the underlying dura. The craniotomy can be extended laterally over the orbital roofs as dictated by the pathological anatomy (Fig. 4A–D). A curved dural incision is then made and reflected superiorly; the falx cerebri is divided at its anterior attachment to the crista galli of the ethmoid bone, and CSF is liberally drained to relax the frontal lobes (Fig. 5A,B). The endoscope is then slowly advanced posteriorly between both olfactory tracts to the level of the pathology. A preliminary endoscopic survey can then be conducted to reveal the degree of intracranial tumor spread. A combination of a custom-designed bipolar electrocautery

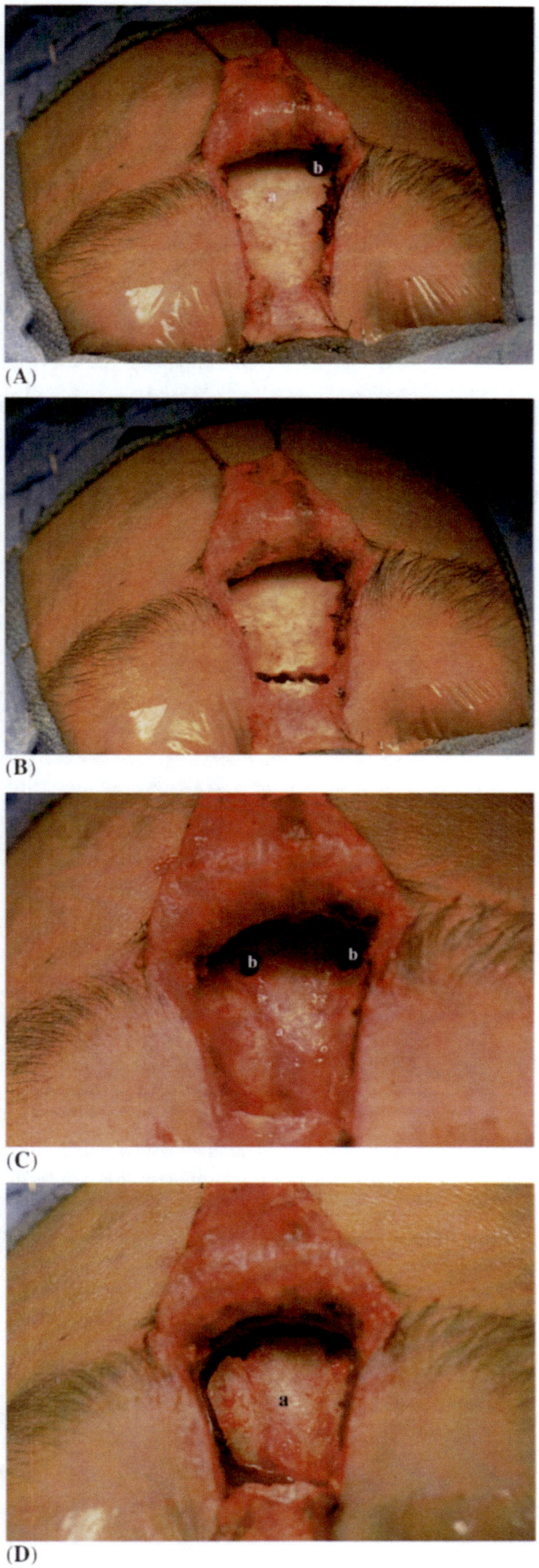

Fig. 4 (**A**)–(**D**) Burr hole and keyhole craniotomy. (**A**) *a* Outer table of frontal sinus. *b* Burr hole. (**C**) *a* Inner table of frontal sinus. *b* Burr holes. (**D**) *a* Keyhole bone flap.

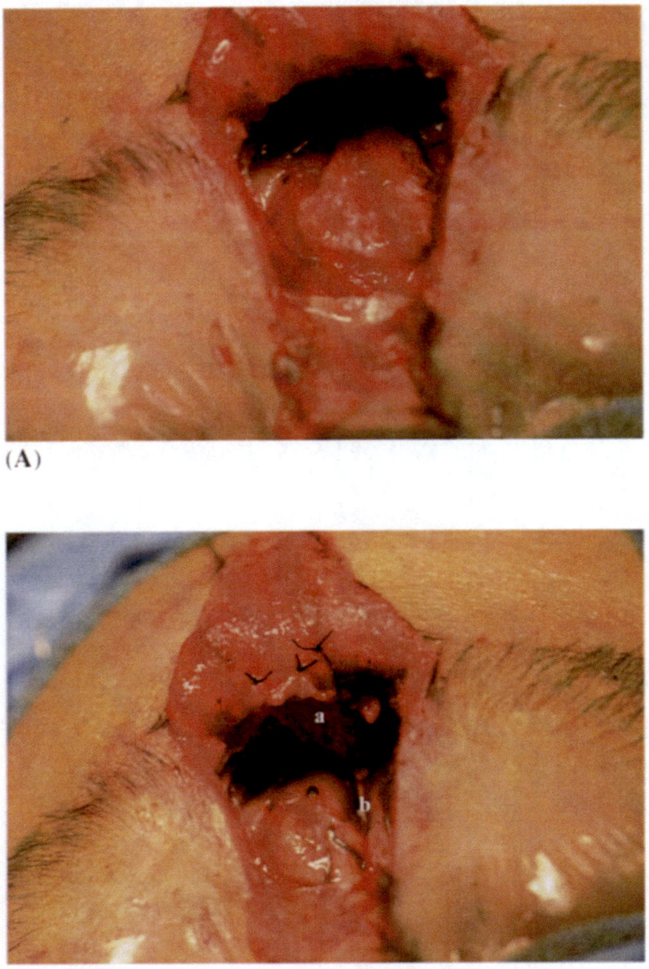

(A)

(B)

Fig. 5 (**A**) and (**B**) Dural opening. (**B**) *a* Superiorly reflected dura. *b* Anterior attachment of falx cerebri.

system, micro-Cavitron ultrasonic surgical aspirator (micro-CUSA), and dissecting instruments are utilized to gradually resect the tumor.

Following tumor removal, strict hemostasis, and copious irrigation of the surgical field, the endoscope is gradually withdrawn. A second survey of the entire region is conducted using a 30° endoscope. The dura is then closed in a watertight fashion, and the pericranial flap is sutured to its lower margin in a single layer. A collagen dural substitute membrane is then applied to the sutured dura, and the entire area is covered with a dural sealant (Fig. 6A–C). The nasoglabellar bone flap, constituting the outer table of the frontal sinuses, is then repositioned and secured in place by absorbable microplates and screws; a hydroxyapatite bone substitute is also applied to completely fill bone defects (Fig. 7A,B). The subcutaneous tissues and skin are closed in layers with careful attention to the aesthetic repair, and Steri-Strips followed by an adhesive bandage dressing are applied to the suture line. The patient is then monitored in the intensive care unit (ICU) or a step-down unit overnight. The majority of patients undergoing this procedure are discharged home 48 h postoperatively (Fig. 8A–E).

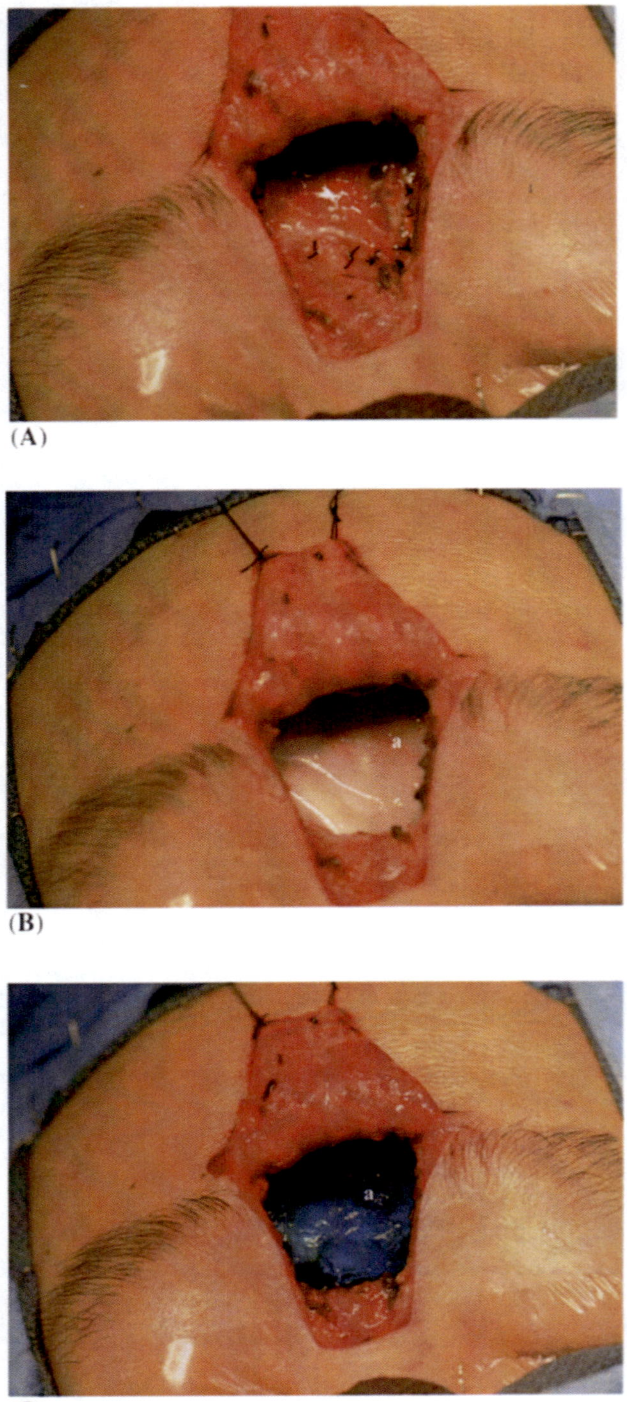

(A)

(B)

(C)

Fig. 6 (**A**)–(**C**) Dural closure. (**B**) *a* Collagen dural substitute (onlay graft). (**C**) *a* Dural sealant.

7. ILLUSTRATIVE CASES

7.1. CRANIOPHARYNGIOMA AND SUPRASELLAR LESIONS

7.1.1. Background Craniopharyngiomas are histologically benign, extraaxial, slow-growing tumors that are more common in children and adolescents and are thought to be derived from squamous cell nests of the hypohyseal stalk. They occur exclusively in the sellar region, starting usually at the junction of the pituitary infundibulum and gland. These tumors can be solid, cystic, or full

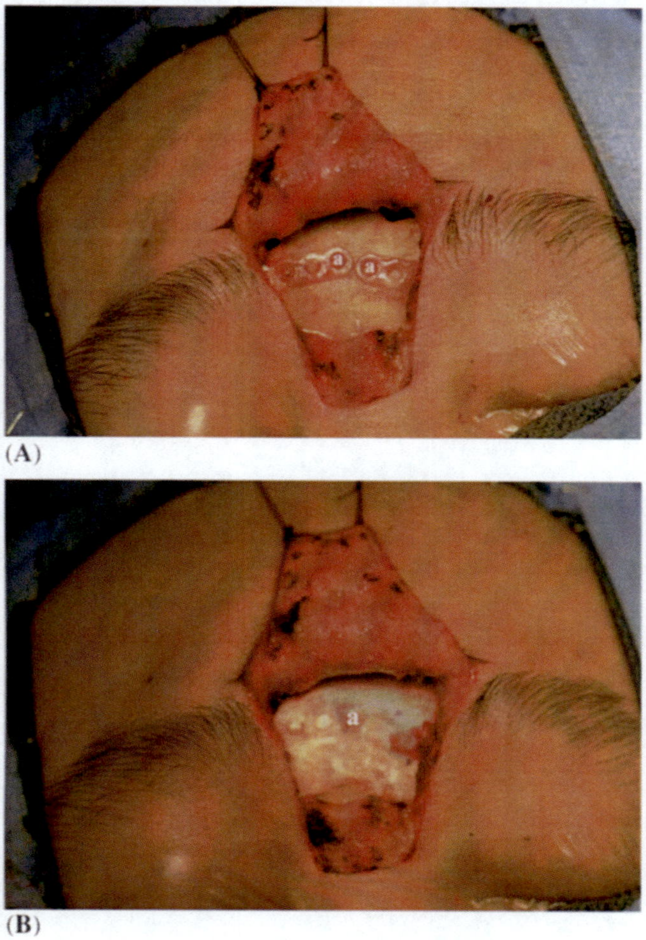

Fig. 7 (**A**) and (**B**) Cranioplasty. (**A**) *a* Absorbable microplates and screws. (**B**) *a* Hydroxyapatite bone substitute.

of debris, and they often show various degrees of calcification or bone formation. Despite their histologic appearance, craniopharyngiomas may rarely behave like malignant tumors and can metastasize. Craniopharyngiomas can be completely asymptomatic, or they may enlarge, causing various endocrine, visual, or psychological disorders. They may cause various degrees of hypopituitarism by compression of the adenohypohysis, pituitary stalk, or the hypothalamus, or they may cause obstructive hydrocephalus by invading the third ventricle.

Pituitary macroadenomas may also enlarge and extend upward to occupy the suprasellar cistern and compress the optic nerves and chiasm. Furthermore, they may cause elevation of the third ventricle, occupy the anterior aspect of the third ventricle, or even extend beyond the foramen of Monro. Lateral extension into the cavernous sinus or parasellar extension lateral to the carotid artery into the middle cranial fossa or projection anteriorly onto the planum sphenoidale and anterior skull base are also possible. In our practice, a large suprasellar tumor component is often approached via an endoscopic transglabellar approach.

Suprasellar cystic lesions are another diverse group of entities, which are often indistinguishable on the basis of clinical and radiographic findings. A diagnosis can often be made only by gross and histologic examination. They include cystic craniopharyngiomas, Rathke's cleft cysts, arachnoid cysts, dermoid and epidermoid cysts, and others. The cysts

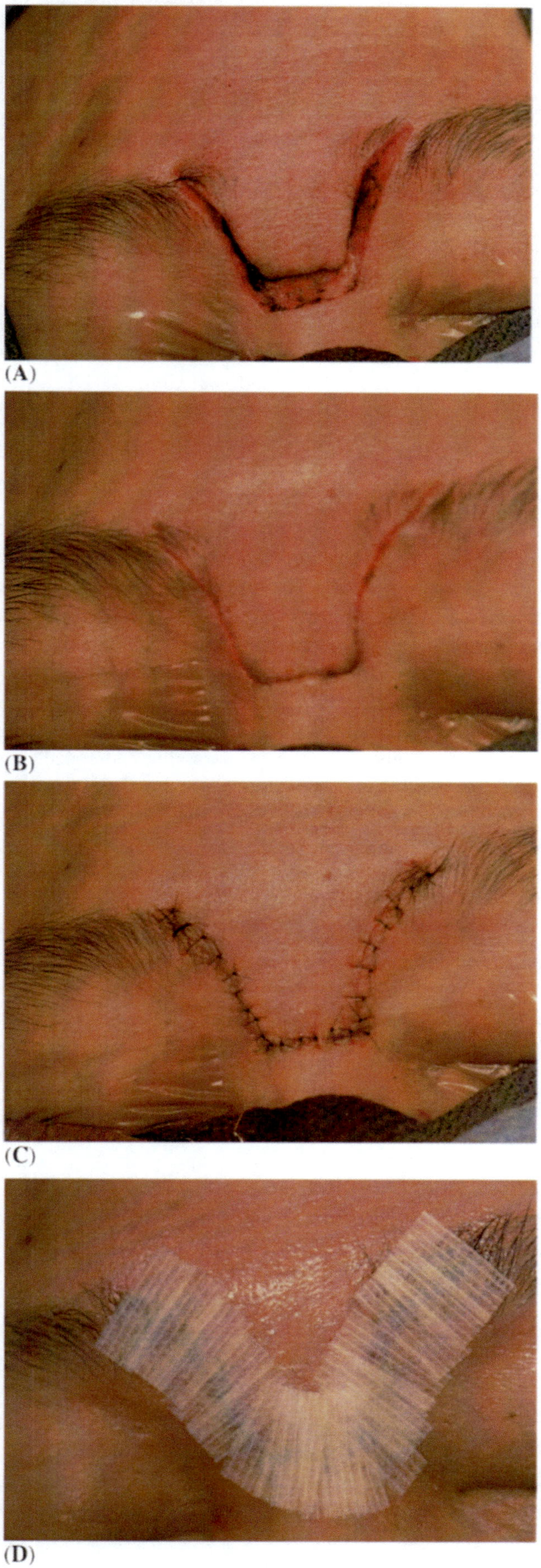

Fig. 7 (continued)

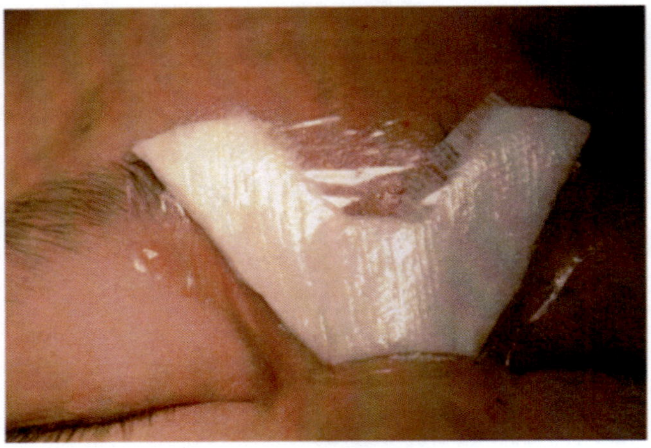

(E)

Fig. 8 (**A**)–(**E**) Skin closure and dressing.

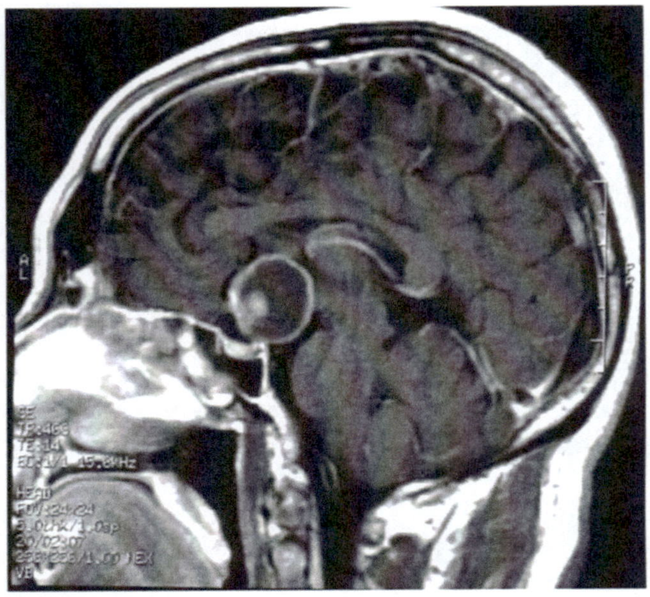

(A)

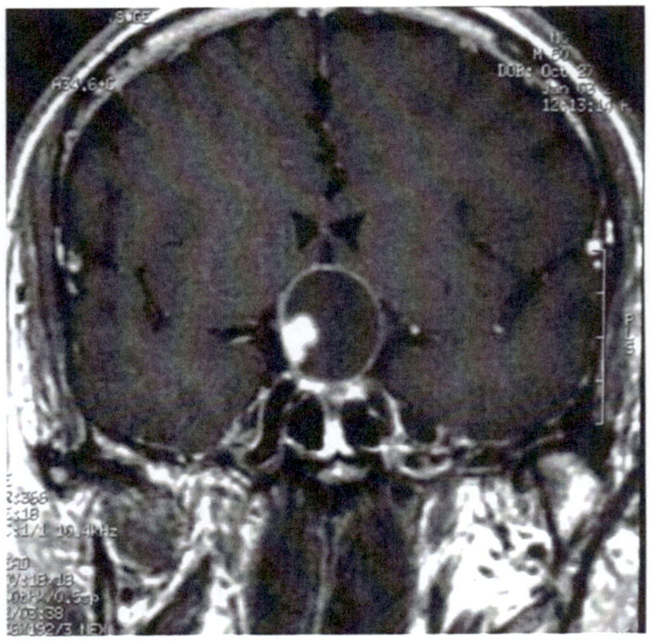

(B)

Fig. 9 (**A**) Sagittal contrasted T_1-weighted MRI showing a craniopharyngioma with a large cystic component. (**B**) Coronal contrasted T_1-weighted MRI showing a craniopharyngioma with a large cystic component. (**C**) and (**D**) Intraoperative endoscopic view showing the

may be completely asymptomatic; alternatively, they can enlarge, causing compression of the pituitary gland, pituitary stalk, optic chiasm, or hypothalamus, producing symptoms that include headaches, visual impairment, and endocrine disorders. In many cases (e.g., Rathke's cysts), the cysts are most commonly treated with transsphenoidal surgery, in which the cyst is partially excised and drained; less commonly, they may be approached through a formal craniotomy. In many cases, simple cyst aspiration is not recommended as the cysts may readily recur. For cysts with a significant suprasellar component, complete cyst removal is achieved by an endoscopic transcranial approach, which can be either transglabellar or supraorbital. The endoscopic endonasal approach is preferred for cysts confined to the sella turcica or with a small suprasellar component

7.1.2. Approach

Following the induction of general anesthesia and after positioning, prepping, draping, initial exposure, and adequate CSF drainage in the previously described manner, the endoscope is advanced posteriorly along the base of the skull between both olfactory tracts toward the optic nerves and chiasm.

For craniopharyngiomas or other suprasellar tumors or tumor extensions such as in large pituitary macroadenomas extending into the suprasellar cistern, the endoscope is advanced all the way to the suprasellar area, and the optic nerves and chiasm are identified. The tumor occupying the suprasellar cistern and typically elevating the optic chiasm is noticed. A small biopsy is then obtained for intraoperative frozen section confirmation of the pathology. Following that and under direct endoscopic visualization and using a combination of the microCUSA, bipolar diathermy, and custom-designed endoscopic instruments, the tumor is gradually debulked. The portion of the tumor adherent to the optic nerves and chiasm is only sharply dissected with straight and angled microscissors. After the tumor is removed, a Teflon sponge is left in the suprasellar cistern as a marker of the extent of suprasellar resection; this is beneficial in the rare cases of massive tumors, for which a combination of an endoscopic endonasal with an endoscopic transglabellar, supraorbital, or subtemporal approach has been planned.

The same essential principles apply for the resection of cystic suprasellar lesions; on advancing the endoscope to the suprasellar region, the thin-walled cyst and the optic nerves and chiasm are visualized. The cyst is incised, and its fluid content is slowly drained; a biopsy of the cyst wall is sent for immediate intraoperative pathology. Following that, the cyst wall is dissected free from the surrounding brain tissue. The part of the cyst adherent to the optic apparatus is dealt with last with sharp dissection from the optic nerves and chiasm.

At the end of the operation, the 0° endoscope is slowly withdrawn from the operative field, and a second survey using an angled 30° or 70° endoscope is performed. Any remaining tumor or residual cyst wall is identified and resected. The entire area is then copiously irrigated, and hemostasis is secured. The dura, bone flap, and skin incision are then repaired in layers as described previously.

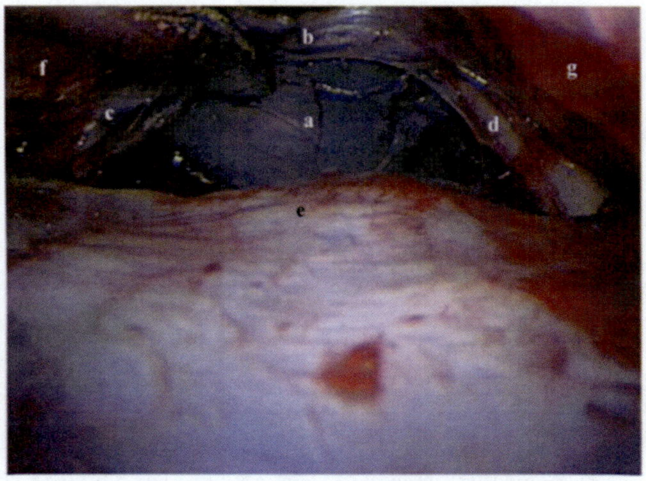

(C)

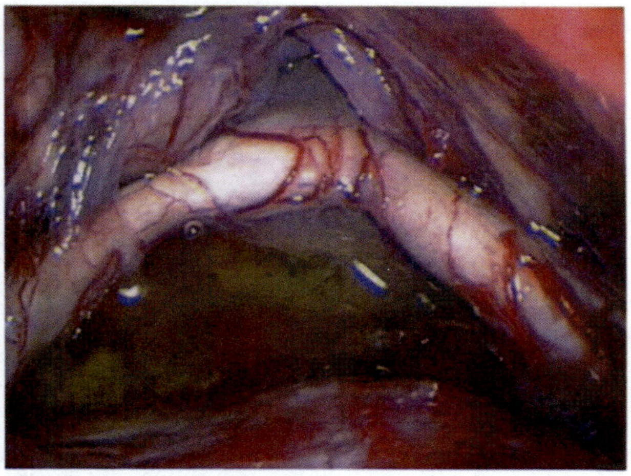

(F)

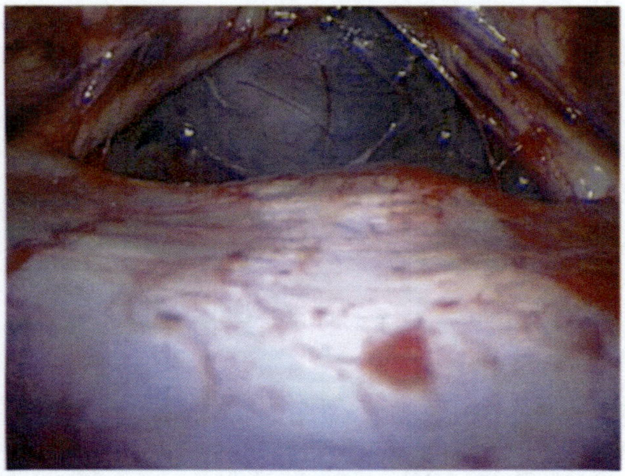

(D)

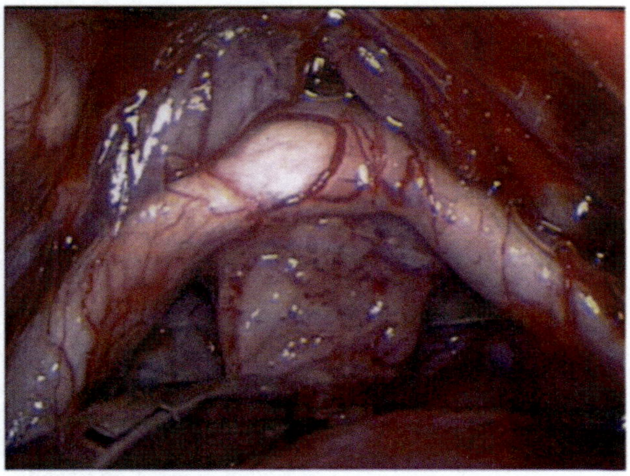

(G)

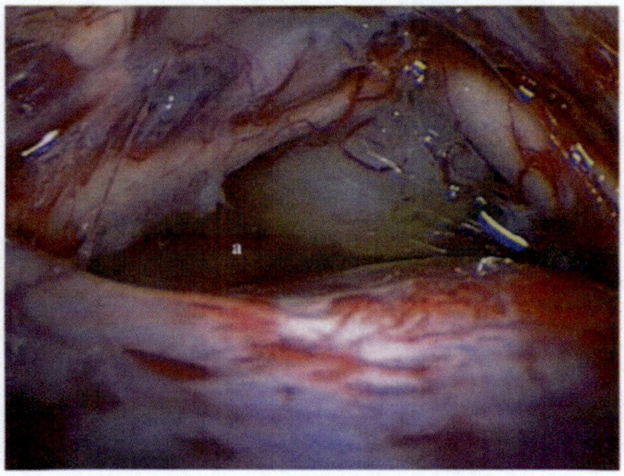

(E)

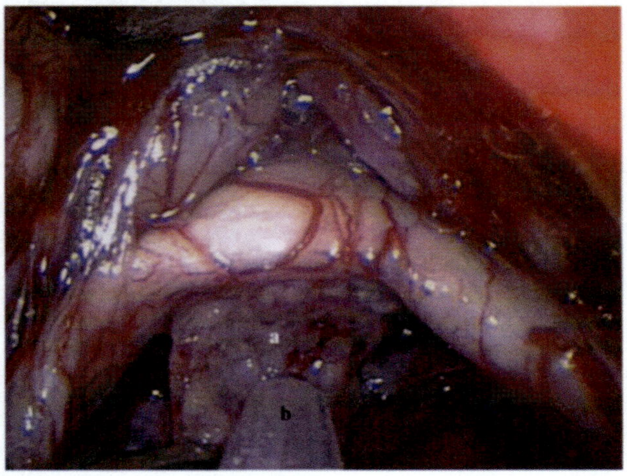

(H)

Fig. 9 (continued) initial exposure of a craniopharyngioma. (**C**) *a* Craniopharyngioma. *b* Elevated optic chiasm. *c* Right optic nerve (II). *d* Left optic nerve (II). *e* Planum sphenoidale. *f* Lower aspect of right frontal lobe. *g* Lower aspect of left frontal lobe. (**E**) and (**F**) Intraoperative endoscopic view showing the gradual evacuation of the cystic component of a craniopharyngioma. (**E**) *a* Craniopharyngioma fluid. (**G**)–(**O**) Intraoperative endoscopic view showing the gradual resection of a craniopharyngioma using a combination of blunt and sharp dissection. (**H**) *a* Craniopharyngioma. *b* MicroCUSA tip. (**J**) *a* Craniopharyngioma adherent to optic chiasm. *b* Sharp dissection using a left-curved microscissors. (**K**) *a* Craniopharyngioma. *b* Pituitary stalk. (**L**) *a* Craniopharyngioma being sharply dissected from optic chiasm. (**M**) *a* Posterior capsule of craniopharyngioma. (**N**) *a* Posterior capsule of craniopharyngioma adherent to optic chiasm. *b* Sharp dissection using a right-curved scissors. (**O**) *a* Final portion of craniopharyngioma adherent to optic chiasm. *b* Pituitary stalk. (**P**)–(**R**) Intraoperative endoscopic view following complete tumor removal and gradual withdrawal of the endoscope. (**P**) *a* Pituitary stalk. *b* Optic chiasm. *c* Right optic nerve (II). *d* Left optic nerve (II). (**R**) *a* Craniopharyngioma cavity after complete resection. *b* Optic chiasm. *c* Right optic nerve (II). *d* Left optic nerve (II). *e* Planum sphenoidale. *f* Medial aspect of right frontal lobe. *g* Medial aspect of left frontal lobe. *h* Right olfactory bulb (I). *i* Left olfactory bulb (I). (**S**) Postoperative T_1-weighted, contrast-enhanced sagittal MRI. (**T**) Postoperative T_1-weighted, contrast-enhanced coronal MRI.

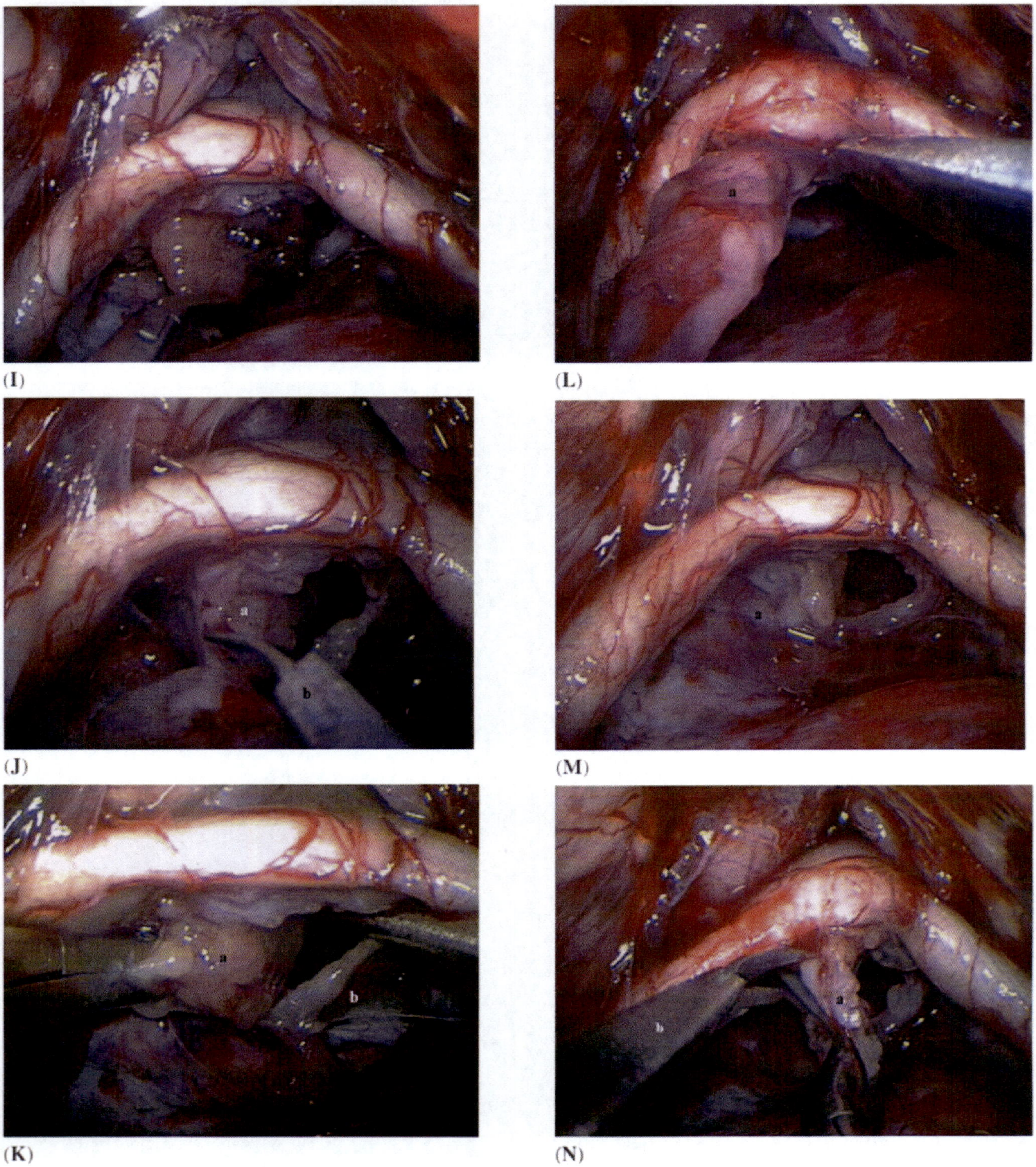

Fig. 9 (continued)

7.1.3. Cases

7.1.3.1. Craniopharyngioma with a Large Cystic Component (Fig. 9A–T)

7.1.3.2. Craniopharyngioma (Fig. 10A–I)

7.1.3.2. Suprasellar Meningioma (Fig. 11A–Y)

8. POTENTIAL COMPLICATIONS

Potential complications of the fully endoscopic transglabellar approach include the following:

- Bleeding (intracerebral/extradural/subdural), wound infection, meningitis, cerebrovascular accident, CSF leak, and death (these are also potential complications associated with open approaches with more extensive dissection).
- Different pathologies have varying degrees of risk for endocrinological morbidity, vascular complications, neuropsychological and behavioral disorders, neurocognitive disorders, and learning disabilities.
- Direct injury can occur to olfactory nerve(s) (anosmia), optic apparatus (visual deficits), cranial nerves, carotid artery or its branches, or pituitary gland or stalk.
- Postoperative severe headache, lethargy, confusion, or slow mentation may occur due to tension pneumocephalus.

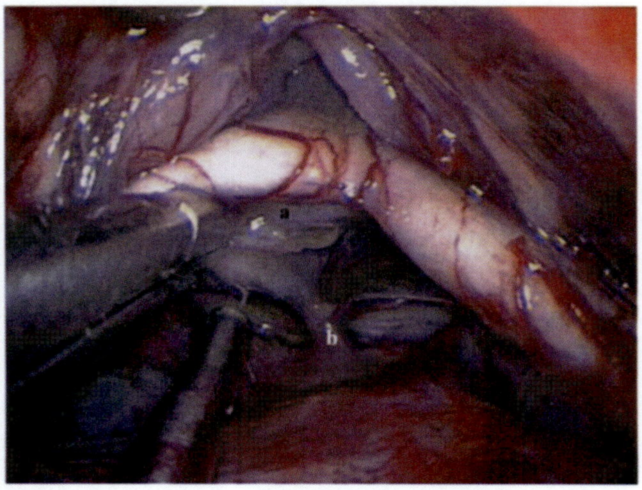

(O)

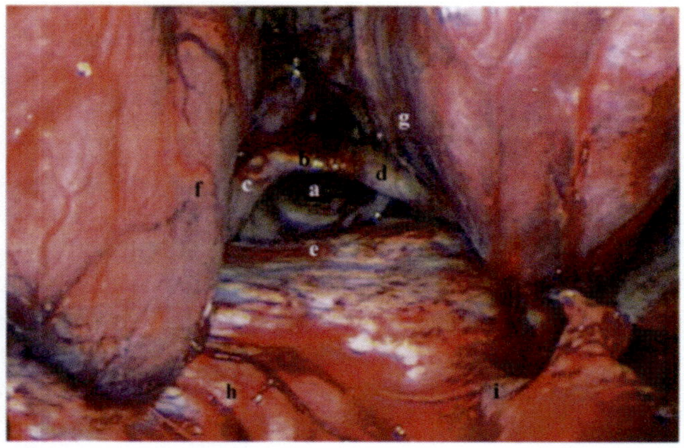

(R)

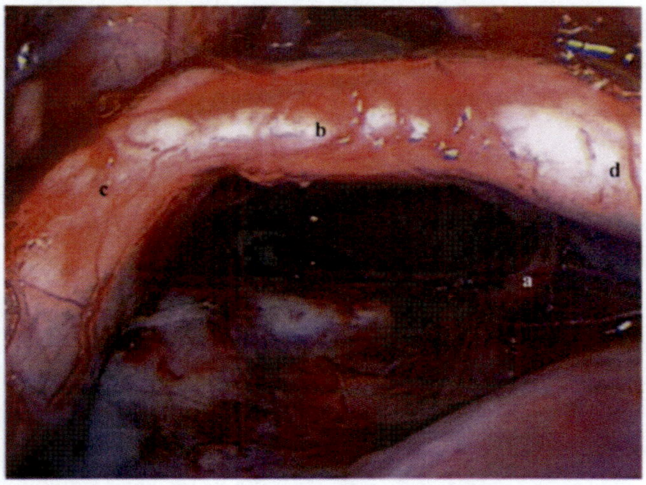

(P)

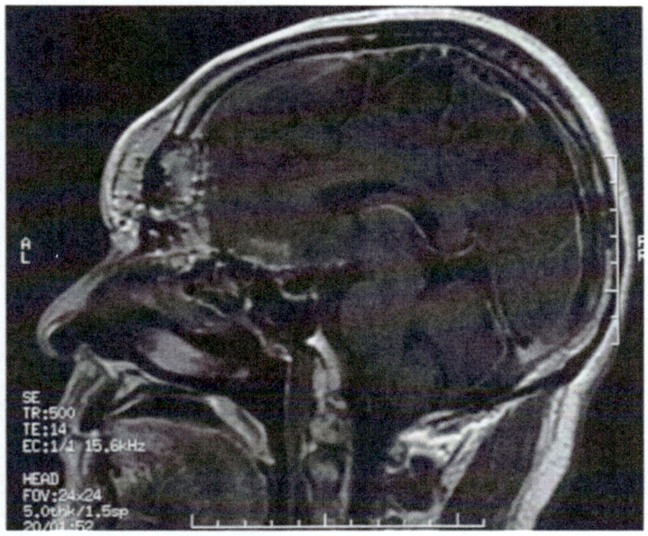

(S)

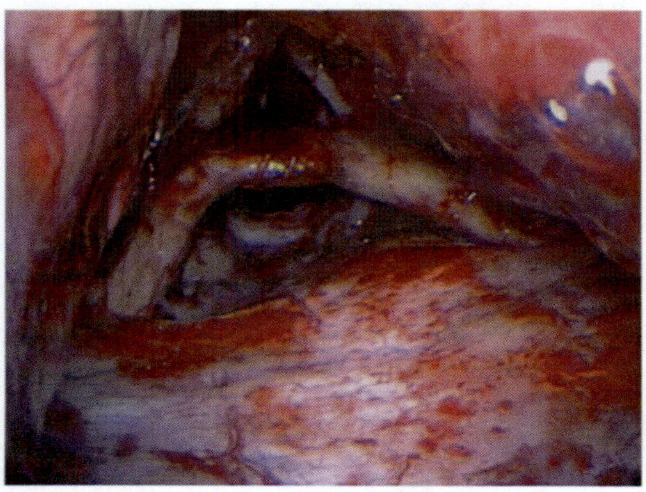

(Q)

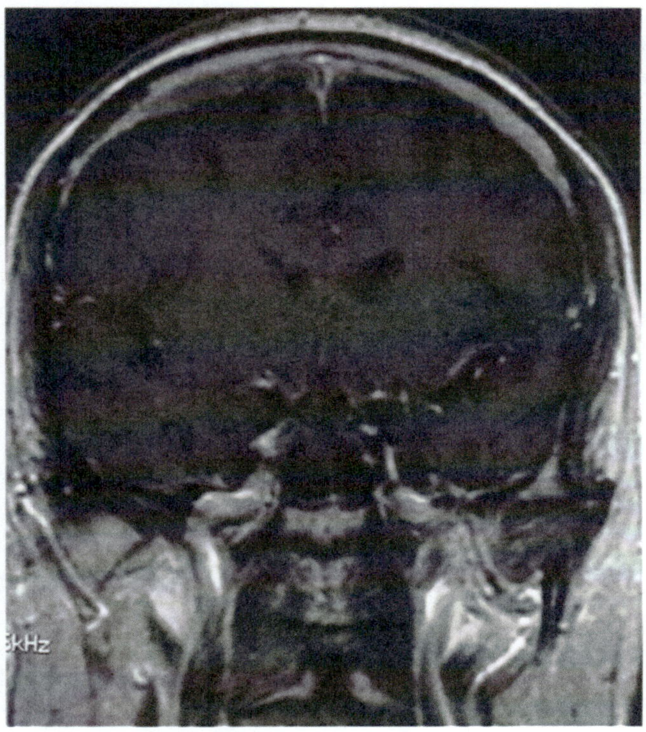

(T)

Fig. 9 (continued)

- Frontal lobe edema, contusion, or direct injury.
- Meningocele, encephalocele.

9. AVOIDING COMPLICATIONS IN AUTHOR'S EXPERIENCE

The most common complications of an endoscopic transglabellar approach result from the consequences of suboptimal reconstruction of the bone flap with inadequate separation of the cranial cavity from the frontal sinuses and nasal cavity. This may potentially lead to CSF rhinorrhea, ascending infection, meningitis, osteomyelitis, and pneumocephalus. Therefore, reconstruction of the skull base should be carried out carefully to avoid these complications. The dura should always be closed in a watertight fashion, and any dural defects or meningeal tears (which may later cause a meningocele or encephalocele) should be sealed with a pericranial graft. The frontal sinus is cranialized to eliminate the dead space, and the nasofrontal ducts are bilaterally obliterated. A dural allograft should be used to further ensure a watertight seal if this is felt to be necessary by the surgeon, and the pericranial flap is interposed between the dura and the paranasal sinuses to reconstruct the base of the skull; no suction drains are used. The nasoglabellar bone flap must be carefully created during craniotomy so that it can easily "fit in" when repositioned at the end of the operation; it is secured in place with absorbable microplates and screws.

Unexpected postoperative visual deterioration is the result of injury to the optic apparatus or its blood supply; ischemia or traction injury to the hypothalamus may lead to diabetes insipidus (DI) and other metabolic and endocrine problems. Frontal lobe edema, hematoma, or direct injury typically results from overenthusiastic brain retraction, which is virtually never used in the described approach. In our experience, minimizing trauma to the brain and careful attention to wound closure with adequate separation of the intracranial cavity from the frontonasal sinus are surgical strategies that have dramatically reduced the incidence of complications. Careful attention to even minor details during the operation can often prevent the most severe complications. As stated above, patients typically have an average hospital stay of 48 h, cosmetic results are excellent, and the skin incision is inconspicuous.

Craniopharyngiomas of the suprasellar region with adhesions to the optic chiasm can occasionally be removed endonasally, but this may cause unnecessary traction on the optic nerves as well as an increased incidence of postoperative CSF leak. They are better approached under direct endoscopic visualization thorough the endoscopic transglabellar approach. This minimally invasive approach is ideal for most craniopharyngiomas since they invariably extend to the suprasellar area and invariably have adhesions to the optic chiasm.

The resection of large suprasellar extensions of pituitary macroadenomas that have a "narrow waist" at the diaphragma sellae from an endonasal approach is not recommended as this imposes traction or even injury to the optic nerves, and it is accompanied by an increased incidence of postoperative CSF leak. It is recommended that these kinds of tumors undergo a two-stage surgical approach for complete tumor resection that involves a combination of an endoscopic endonasal resection of the intrasellar tumor and an endoscopic transglabellar, supraorbital, or subtemporal approach. This can be done simultaneously or can be staged as two separate procedures.

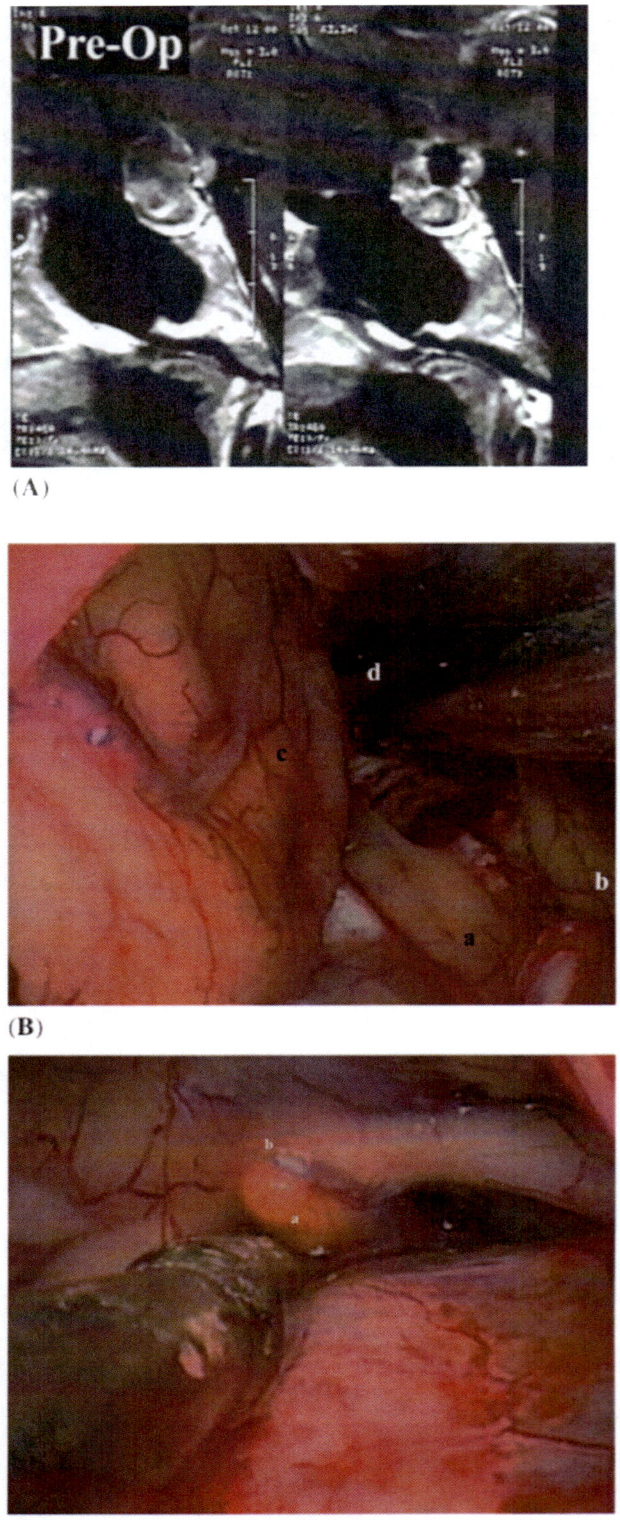

Fig. 10 (**A**) Sagittal contrasted T_1-weighted MRI showing a craniopharyngioma. (**B**)–(**D**) Intraoperative endoscopic view showing the initial exposure for a craniopharyngioma. (**B**) *a* Right olfactory bulb (I). *b* Left olfactory bulb (I). *c* Medial aspect of right frontal lobe. *d* Planum sphenoidale. (**C**) *a* Craniopharyngioma. *b* Elevated optic chiasm. (**E**) and (**F**) Intraoperative endoscopic view showing the resection of a craniopharyngioma using a combination of blunt and sharp dissection. (**E**) *a* Craniopharyngioma partly decompressed. (**F**) *a* Craniopharyngioma adherent to optic chiasm. *b* Sharp dissection using straight microscissors. (**G**) and (**H**) Intraoperative endoscopic view following complete tumor

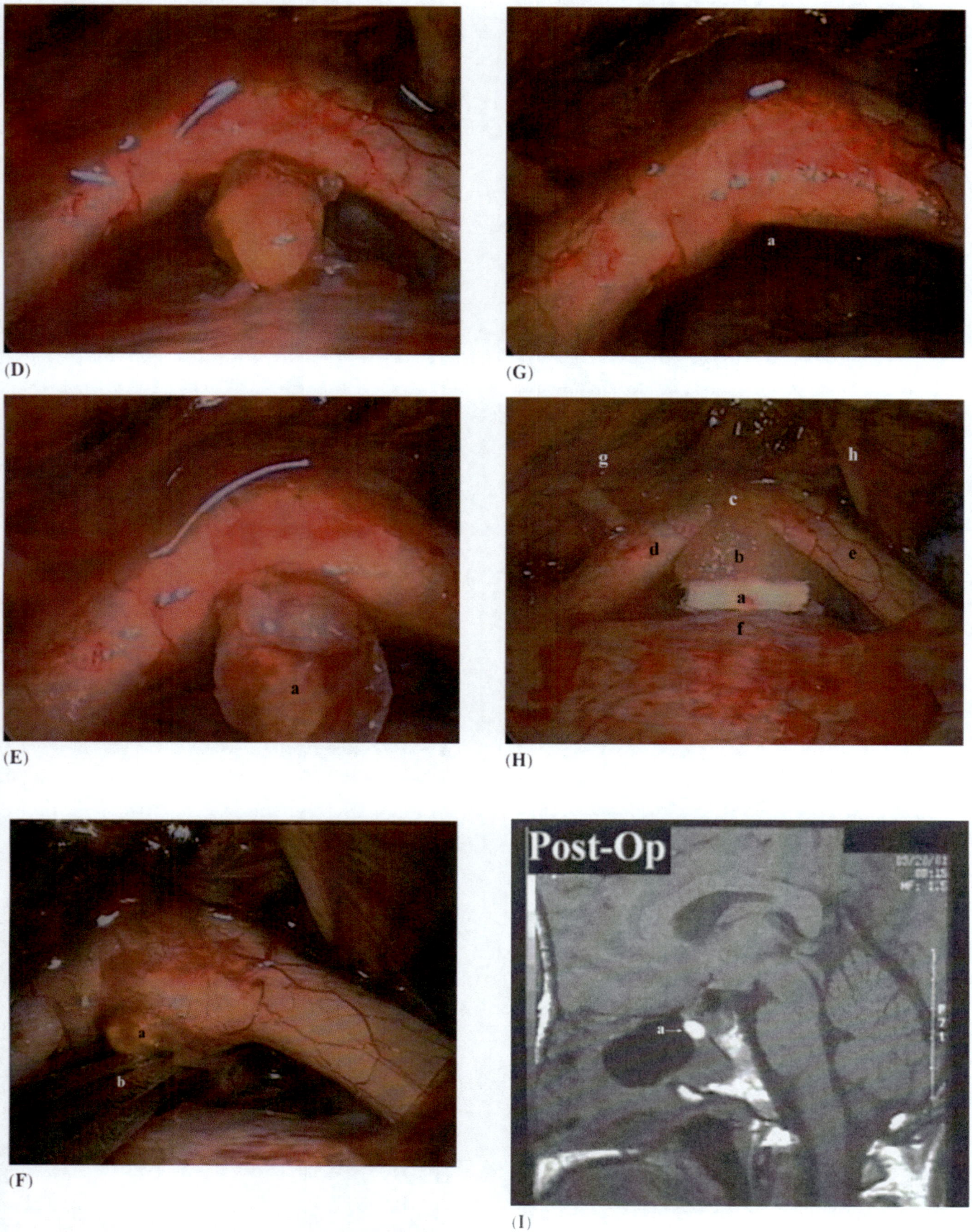

Fig. 10 (continued) removal. (**G**) *a* Craniopharyngioma cavity after complete tumor resection. (**H**) *a* Teflon. *b* Gelfoam. *c* Optic chiasm. *d* Right optic nerve (II). *e* Left optic nerve (II). *f* Planum sphenoidale. *g* Medial aspect of right frontal lobe. *h* Medial aspect of left frontal lobe. (**I**) Postoperative T_1-weighted, contrast-enhanced sagittal MRI. *a* Teflon.

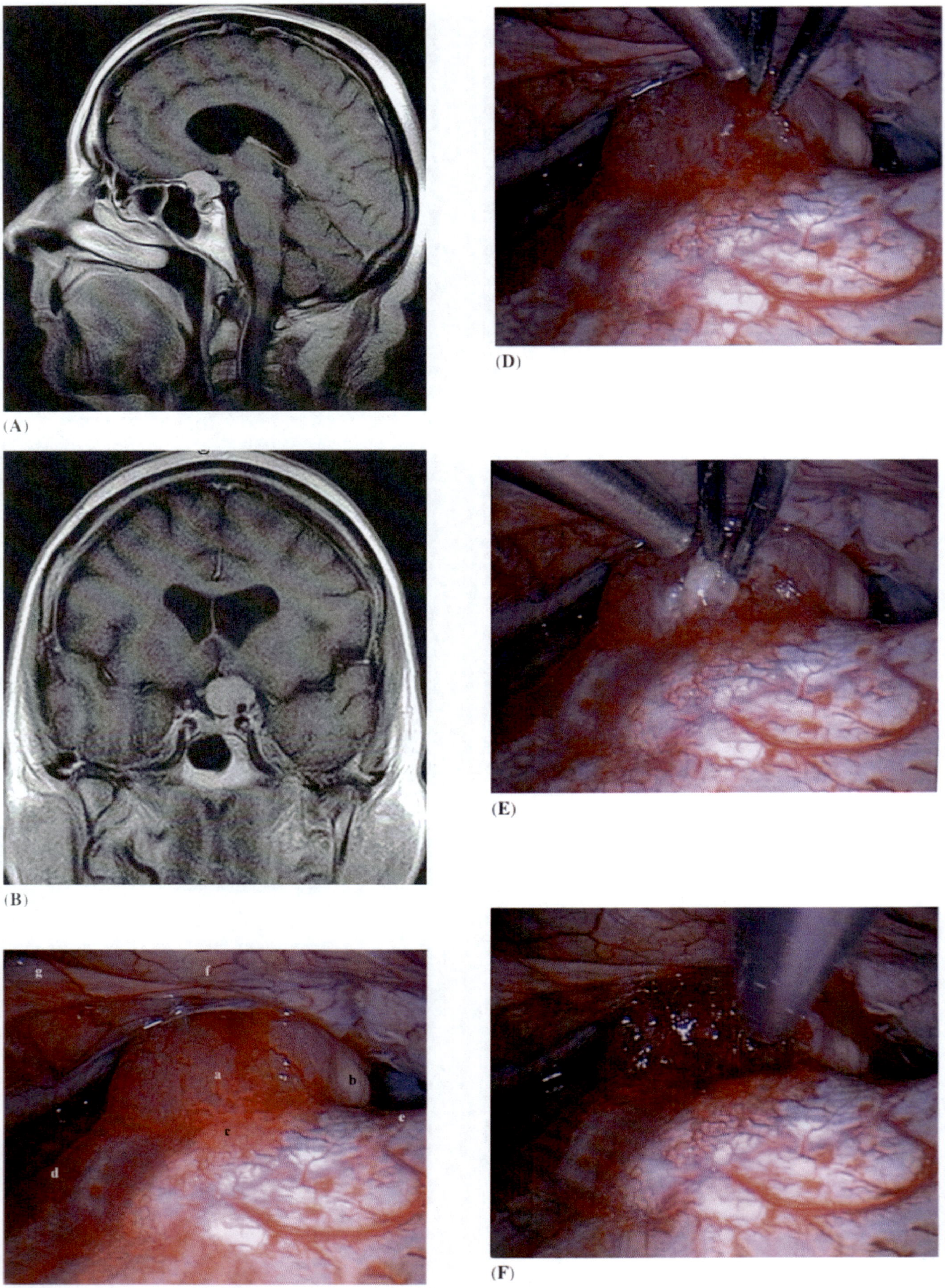

Fig. 11 (**A**) Sagittal contrasted T_1-weighted MRI showing a suprasellar meningioma. (**B**) Coronal contrasted T_1-weighted MRI showing a suprasellar meningioma. (**C**) Intraoperative endoscopic view showing the initial exposure of a suprasellar meningioma. *a* Meningioma. *b* Left optic nerve (II). *c* Planum sphenoidale. *d* Right lesser wing of sphenoid. *e* Left lesser wing of sphenoid. *f* Lower aspect of frontal lobes. *g* Right

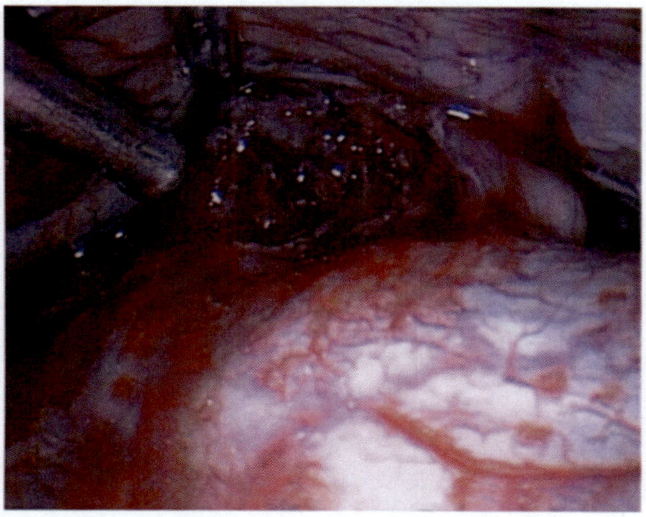
(G)

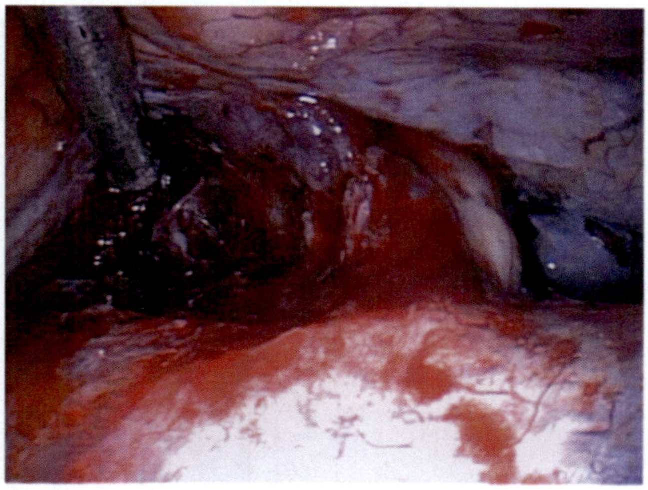
(J)

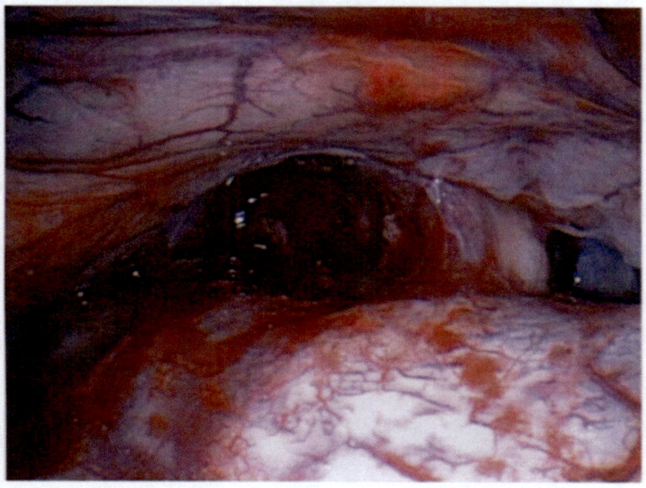
(H)

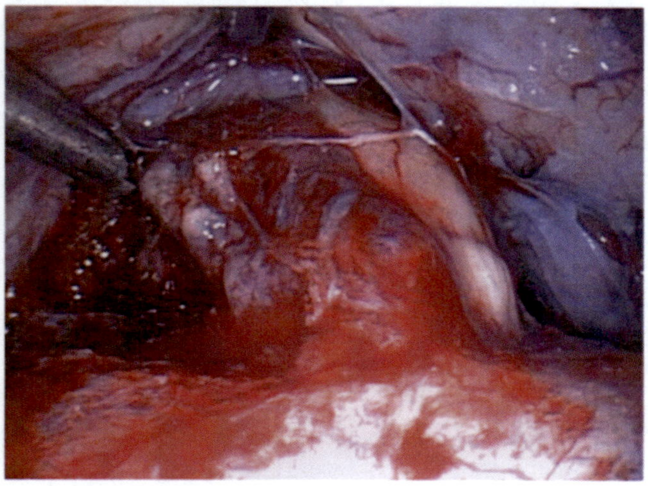
(K)

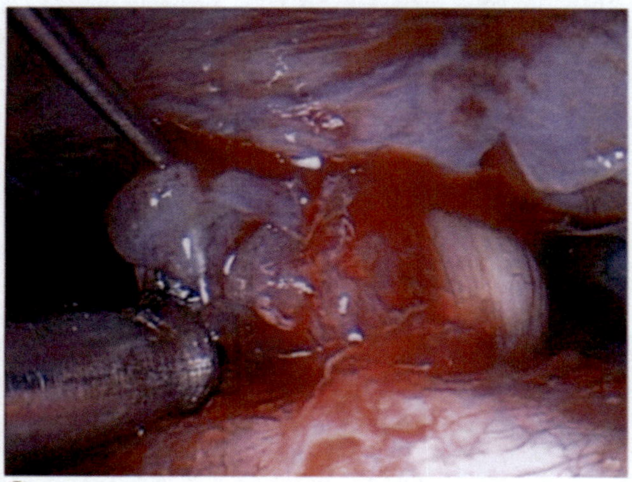
(I)

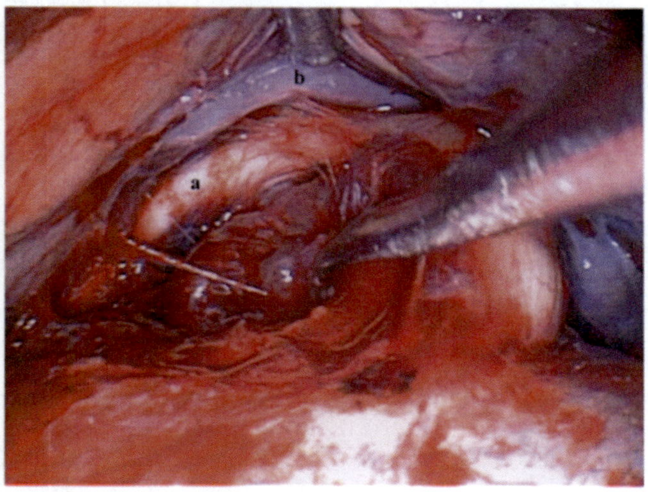

(L)

Fig. 11 (continued) olfactory nerve (I). (**D**)–(**T**) Intraoperative endoscopic view showing the resection of a suprasellar meningioma. (**L**) *a* Right optic nerve (II). *b* Anterior communicating artery. (**M**) *a* Left internal carotid artery. (**O**) *a* Meningioma. *b* MicroCUSA. *c* Left internal carotid artery. (**U**)–(**W**) Intraoperative endoscopic view following complete tumor removal and gradual withdrawal of the endoscope. (**V**) *a* Right optic nerve (II). *b* Left optic nerve (II). *c* Optic chiasm. *d* Tumor cavity following complete resection. (**W**) *a* Meningioma cavity following complete tumor resection. *b* Right optic nerve (II). *c* Left optic nerve (II). *d* Planum sphenoidale. *e* Right lesser wing of sphenoid. *f* Left lesser wing of sphenoid. *g* Right anterior clinoid process. *h* Left anterior clinoid process. *i* Left internal carotid artery. *j* Lower aspect of frontal lobes. (**X**) Postoperative T_1-weighted, contrast-enhanced sagittal MRI. (**Y**) Postoperative T_1-weighted, contrast-enhanced coronal MRI.

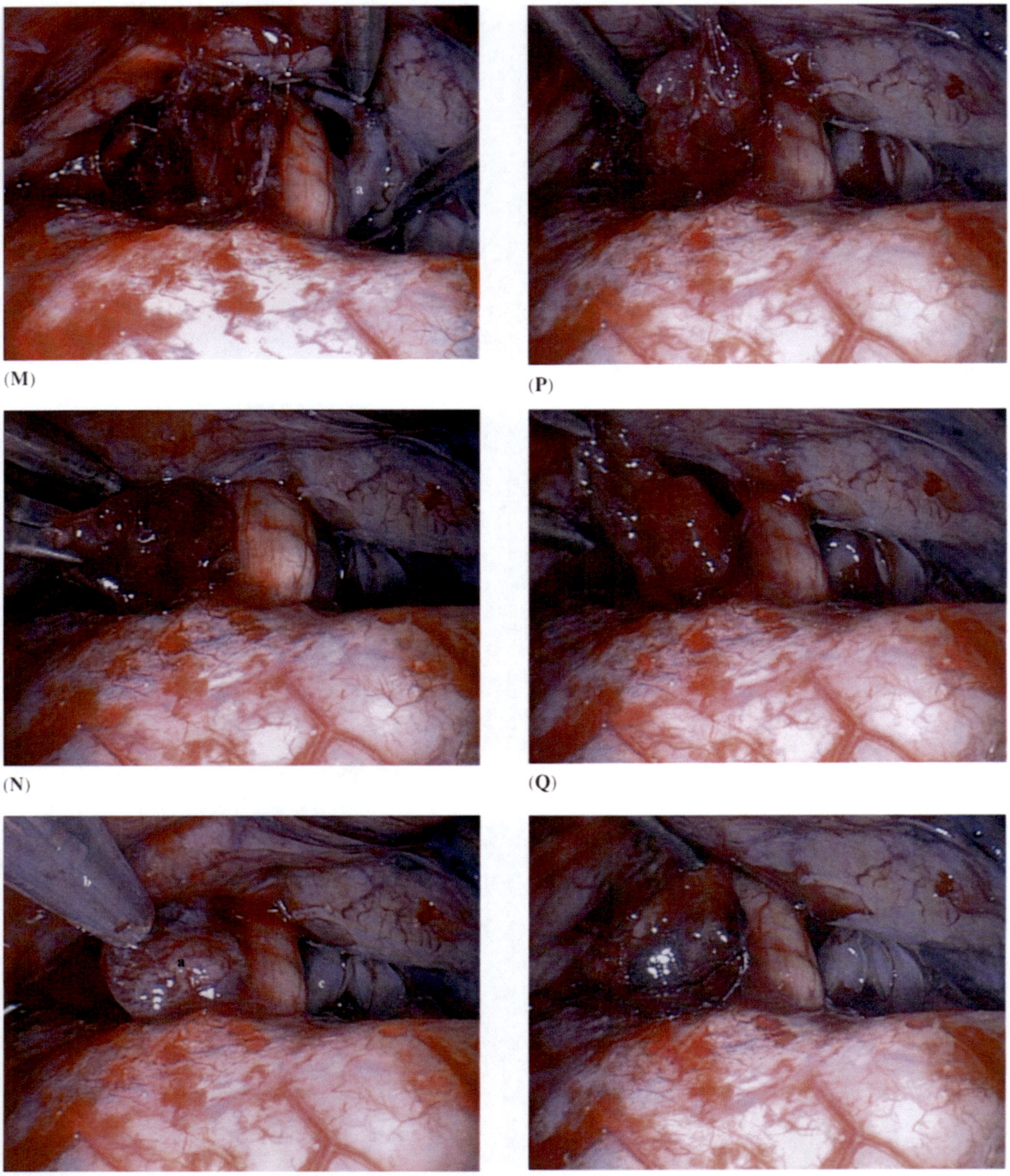

(M) (P)

(N) (Q)

(O) (R)

Fig. 11 (continued)

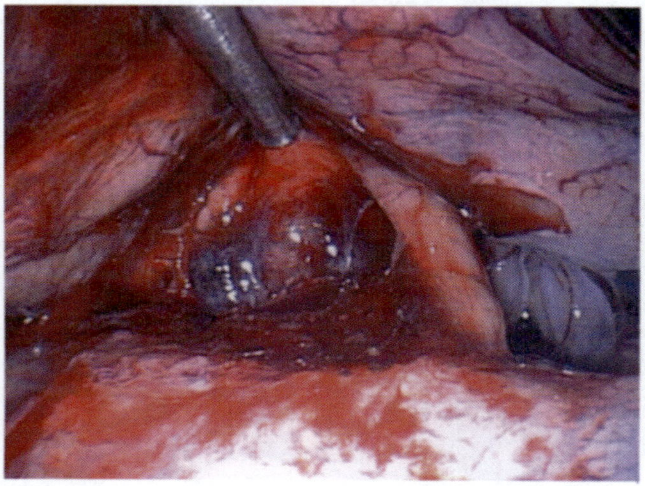
(S)

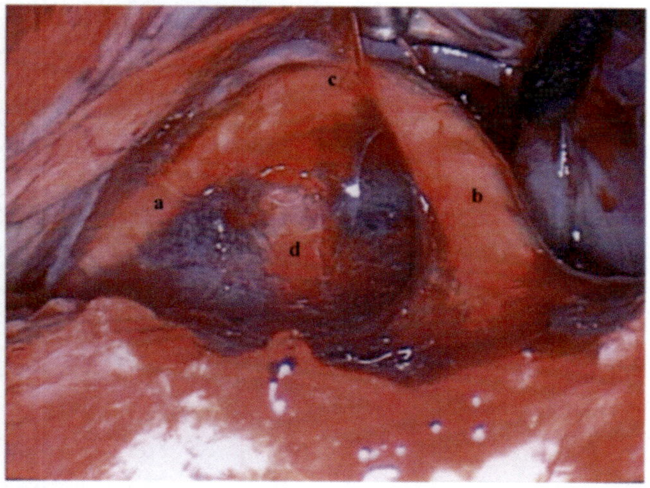

(V)

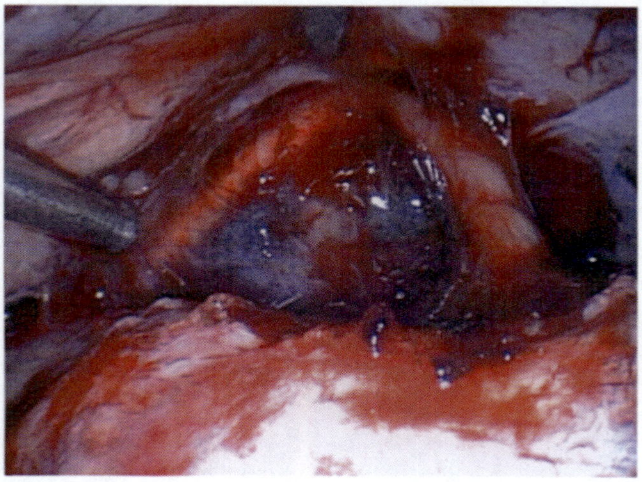
(T)

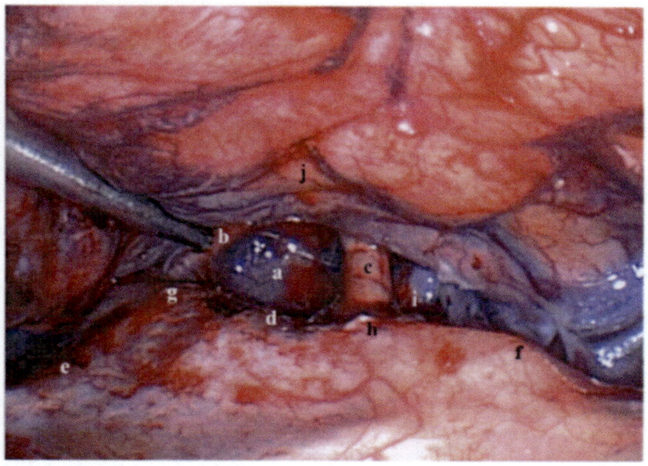

(W)

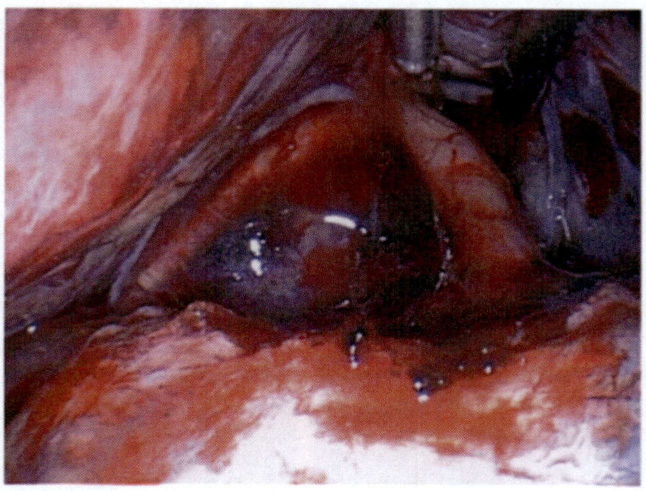
(U)

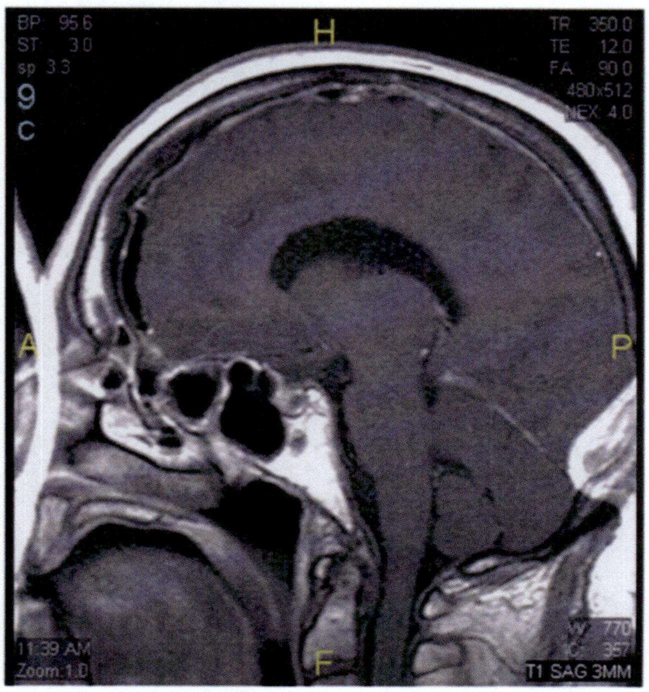

(X)

Fig. 11 (continued)

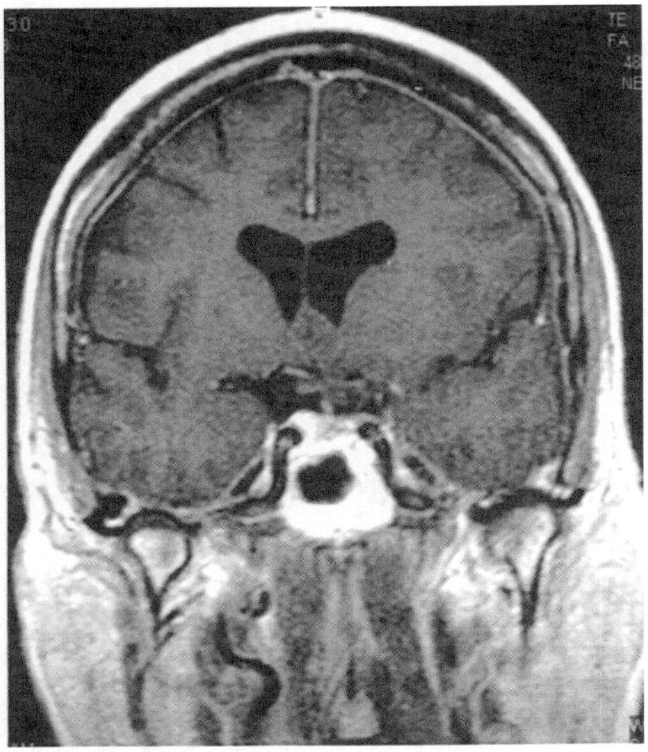

(**Y**)

Fig. 11 (continued)

8 The Fully Endoscopic Supraorbital Approach

This chapter discusses the application of the supraorbital endoscopic keyhole approach to surgery of the anterior and middle skull base. Through a strategically placed keyhole craniotomy, the endoscopic supraorbital approach allows for thorough visualization of critical structures at the median and paramedian skull base without the need for frontal or bifrontal osteotomies, brain retraction, or potentially disfiguring skin incisions. In our experience, we found that the adaptation of rigid endoscopy to the supraorbital approach has broadened the possible surgical exposure with virtually no brain retraction. It minimizes the risk of injury to brain tissue, cranial nerves, and vascular structures and facilitates complete tumor resection due to superior visibility. Other advantages include a more cosmetic, hidden skin incision, within the hair of the eyebrow, and a faster, smoother, and more pleasant postoperative course for the patient. The chapter provides a thorough description of the fully endoscopic supraorbital approach, including indications, operating room setup, patient positioning, operative technique, illustrative cases, potential complications, and ways to avoid these complications (in the authors' experience).

Keywords: Anterior fossa; Craniopharyngioma; Endoscopic; Eyebrow; Keyhole; Macroadenoma; Meningioma; Middle fossa; Minimally invasive; Olfactory groove; Optic chiasm; Optic nerve; Parasellar; Pituitary; Pituitary gland; Pituitary surgery; Planum sphenoidale; Sellar; Skull base; Sphenoid wing; Supraorbital; Suprasellar; Surgery.

1. INTRODUCTION

The application of endoscopic approaches to surgery of the anterior and middle skull base, as well as the parasellar region, can eliminate the need for traditional open craniotomies without compromising surgical success. Wide surgical exposures often come at the expense of a significant degree of brain retraction and craniofacial dissection, frequently resulting in undesirable perioperative morbidity. Through a strategically placed keyhole craniotomy, the endoscopic supraorbital approach has allowed for thorough visualization of critical structures at the median and paramedian skull base without the need for frontal or bifrontal osteotomies, brain retraction, or potentially disfiguring skin incisions. Furthermore, the frontal branch of the facial nerve and the temporalis muscle are not involved in the surgical approach, thus avoiding their injury and allowing for a more cosmetic, hidden, skin incision, within the hair of the eyebrow, and a faster, smoother, and more pleasant postoperative course for the patient.

In our experience, we found that the adaptation of rigid endoscopy to the supraorbital approach has broadened the possible surgical exposure without the introduction of additional dissection or retraction. Endoscopes with varying angles of view have provided a panoramic perspective of the relevant surgical anatomy and allowed for thorough evaluation of the extent of intracranial disease. The maneuverability of the endoscope allows it to be positioned directly at the level of dissection, effectively reducing the viewing and operating distances. Endoscopic imaging thereby facilitates complete tumor resection due to the superior visibility via a minimally invasive technique. We believe that access to the anterior and middle skull base with virtually no brain retraction minimizes the risk of injury to brain tissue, cranial nerves, and vascular structures. The fully endoscopic supraorbital approach has provided extended access to all lesions of the skull base that traditionally have required subfrontal, bilateral subfrontal, transbasal, or pterional approaches.

2. INDICATIONS

The fully endoscopic supraorbital approach provides minimally invasive surgical access to lesions of the midline anterior skull base, such as olfactory groove or planum sphenoidale meningiomas, esthesioneuroblastomas, and transcranial extensions of orbital and paranasal sinus tumors; lesions of the middle skull base, such as medial sphenoid wing meningiomas, schwannomas, neurofibromas, and middle cranial fossa arachnoid

From: *Endoscopic Skull Base Surgery: A Comprehensive Guide with Illustrative Cases.*
Edited by H. K. Shahinian © Humana Press, Totowa, NJ.

cysts; and lesions of the parasellar region, such as anterior clinoid or suprasellar meningiomas, craniopharyngiomas, anterior communicating artery (ACoA) aneurysms, and pituitary macroadenomas with supra- and parasellar extensions.

3. INSTRUMENTATION

The instruments needed to execute this procedure successfully include an endoscopic tower containing a high-definition digital camera, a xenon or halogen light source, digital recording devices, 0° and 30° rigid endoscopes, two endoscope holding arms, endoscope irrigation sheaths and pumps, and precision microinstruments.

4. OPERATING ROOM SETUP (FIG. 1)

The patient is placed supine on the operating room table. Following the induction of general anesthesia, the airway circuit is extended with corrugated tubing, and the head is rotated 180° away from the anesthesiologist, who stands at the foot of the table. The endoscopic tower is placed caudad to the patient's head, directly facing the surgeon, who stands cephalad to the patient's head. The scrub nurse stands to the side of the surgeon ipsilateral to the approach. Two separate pneumatically powered holding arms are affixed to the table, one on each side of the patient, and wrapped in sterile drapes. One holding arm is dedicated to holding the endoscope, and the other is used to hold other endoscopic instruments or soft silicone spatulas.

5. PATIENT POSITIONING (FIG. 2)

The patient is placed supine on the operating room table, and the head of the bed is slightly raised to improve venous drainage. Following the induction of general anesthesia, the patient's neck is extended approximately 30° so that the frontal and temporal lobes relax and retract away from the orbital roof and the floor of the skull base once cerebrospinal fluid (CSF) is drained. The patient's head is maintained at 0° rotation. The head is fixed in place using a Mayfield three-pin clamp. This position enhances surgical access to the anterior and middle cranial fossa from an anterior subfrontal trajectory.

6. OPERATIVE TECHNIQUE

Following general anesthesia, the frontal and paranasal areas are cleansed with an aqueous antiseptic solution and then draped. A standard skin incision is placed within the hair of the eyebrow a few millimeters above the orbital rim. The skin, soft tissue, and pericranium are incised down to the level of the cranium, and small hooks are used to retract these layers superiorly and inferiorly (Fig. 3A–C). The position of the incision will vary slightly according to each patient's individual skull shape.

A small burr hole is then placed laterally and inferiorly within the frontal bone, and a 1.5-cm supraorbital craniotomy is performed with its lower end flush with the skull base (Fig. 4A–D). The dura is then incised curvilinear along the frontal pole and reflected downward, and CSF is slowly drained (Fig. 5A,B). A combination of mild hyperventilation, positioning, and CSF drainage opens a path for the endoscope as the frontal lobe "relaxes" away from the anterior cranial base. The endoscope is introduced through the keyhole craniotomy and advanced between the frontal lobe and the floor of the anterior cranial base (Fig. 6A–C).

From this point, surgery will vary according to the type of pathology being addressed. For lesions of the middle cranial fossa, the endoscope is further advanced over the orbital roof and the lesser wing of the sphenoid bone all the way to the middle cranial fossa. For lesions of the parasellar region or the midanterior skull base, the endoscope is advanced toward

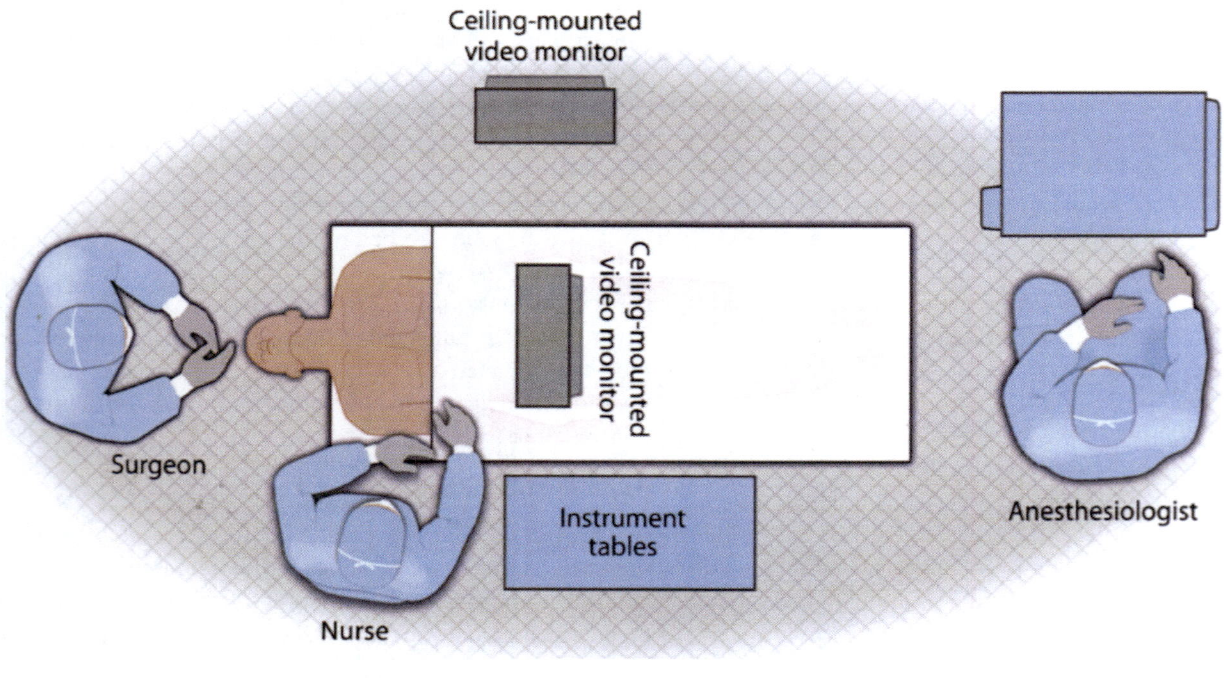

Fig. 1 Operating room setup.

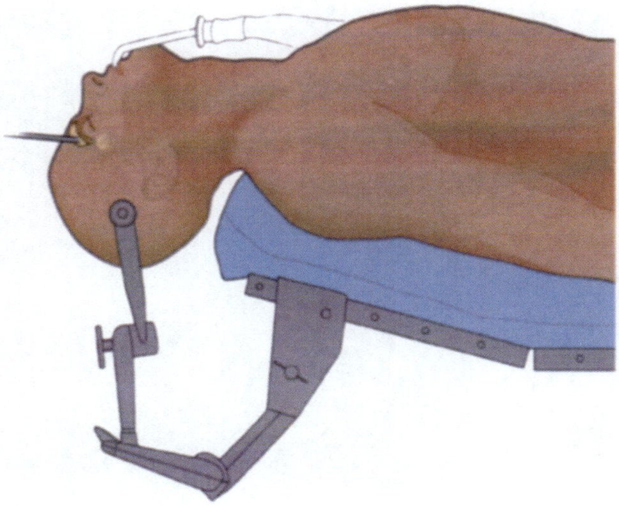

Fig. 2 Patient positioning.

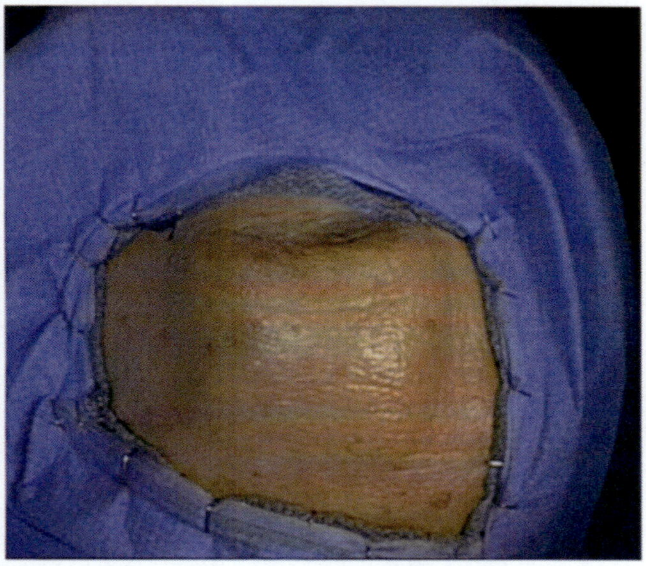

(A)

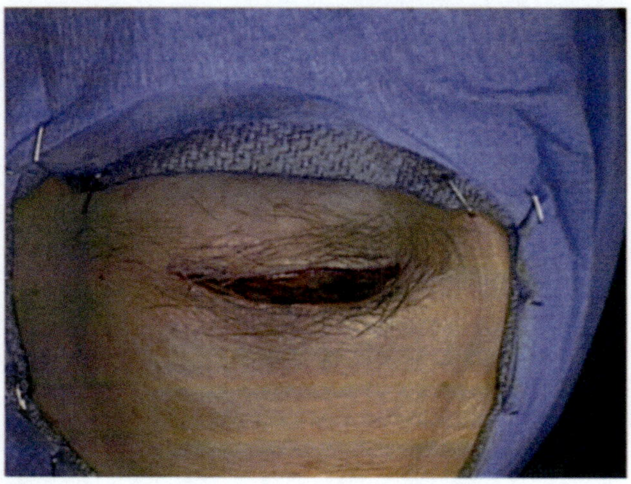

(B)

Fig. 3 (**A**)–(**C**) Draping and skin incision.

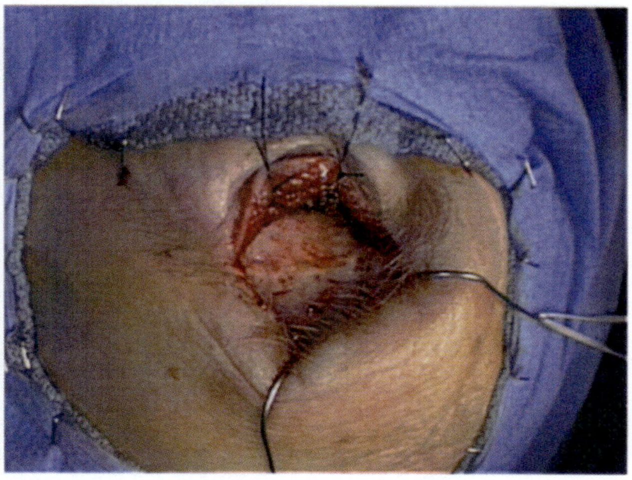

(**C**)

Fig. 3 (continued)

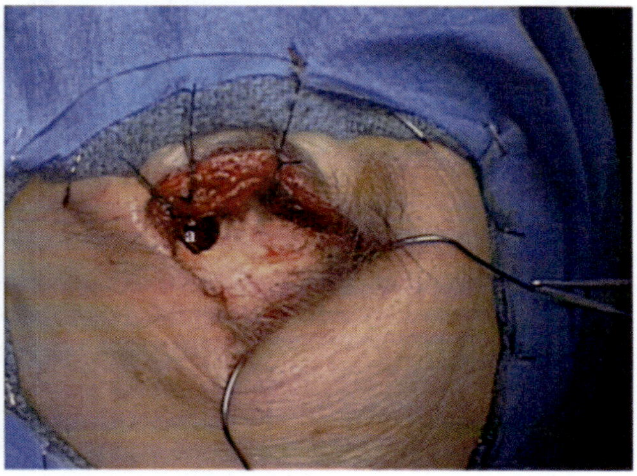

(A)

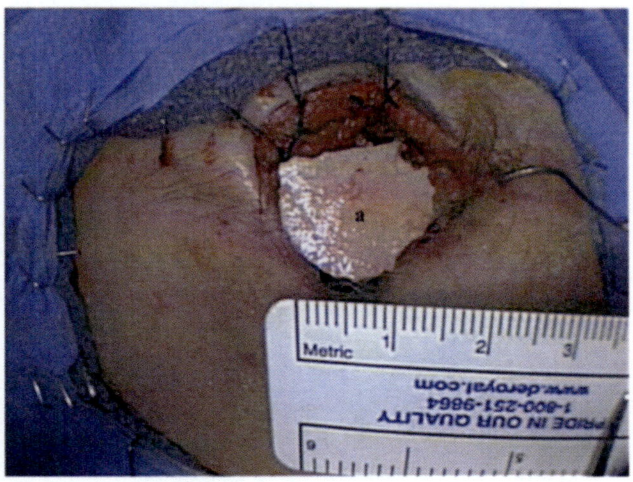

(B)

Fig. 4 (**A**)–(**D**) Burr hole and keyhole craniotomy. (**A**) *a* Burr hole. (**B**) *a* Keyhole bone flap. (**C**) *a* Frontal dura. (**D**) *a* Frontal dura. *b* Orbital roof after partial drilling improve the exposure.

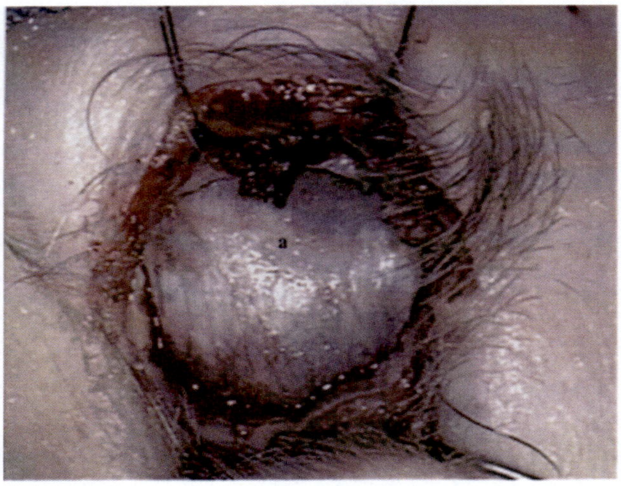

(C)

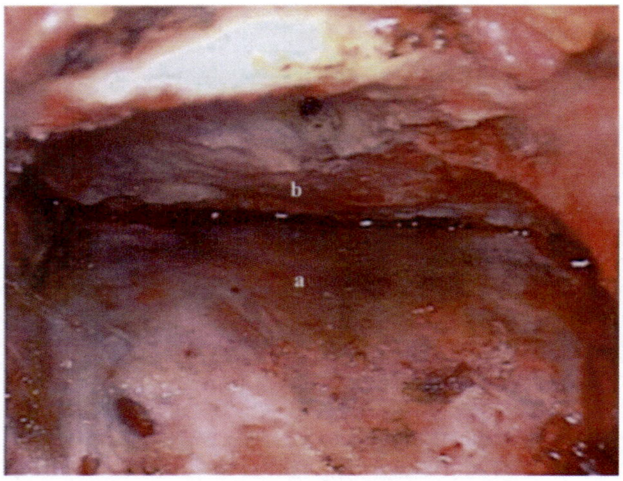

(D)

Fig. 4 (continued)

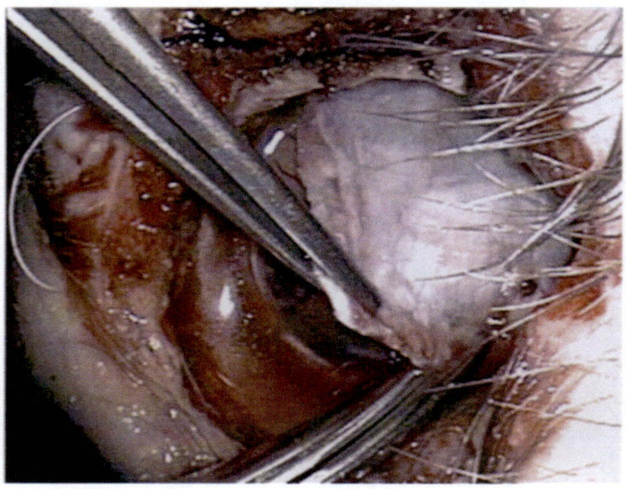

(A)

Fig. 5 (**A**) and (**B**) Dural opening. (**B**) *a* Reflected dura. *b* Lower surface of frontal lobe.

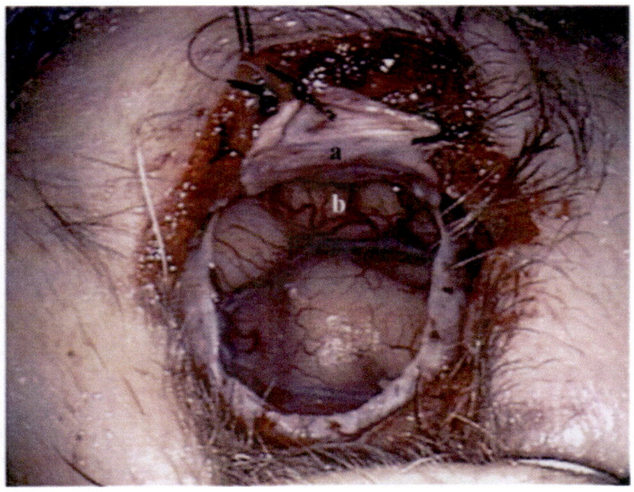

(B)

Fig. 5 (continued)

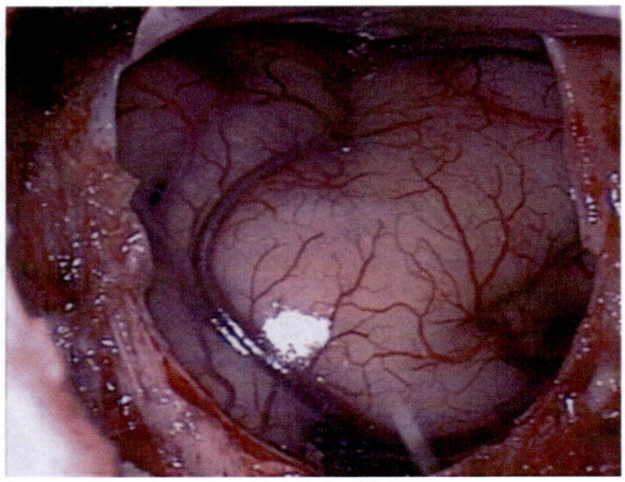

(A)

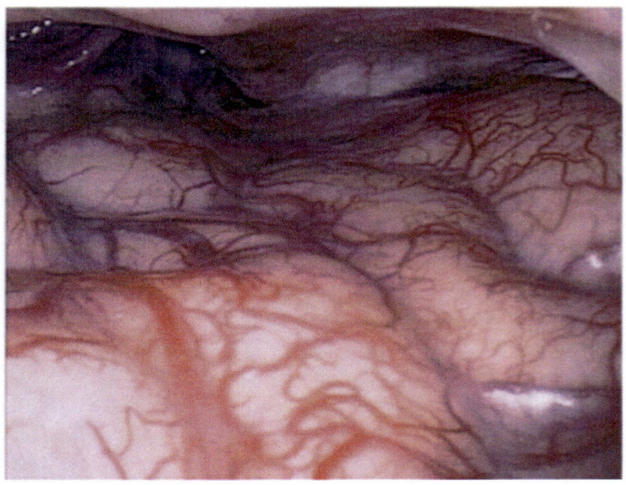

(B)

Fig. 6 (**A**)–(**C**) Regional endoscopic anatomy of the anterior cranial fossa. (**C**) *a* Left optic nerve.

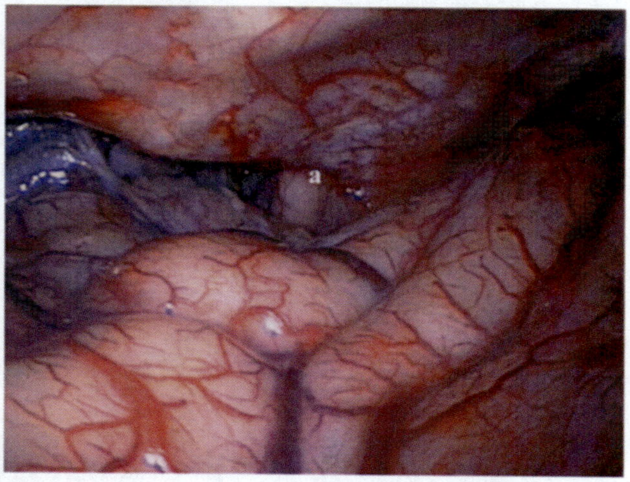

(C)

Fig. 6 (continued)

the frontal midline; the olfactory and optic nerves provide useful landmarks when accessing this region.

Using a combination of custom-designed bipolar electrocoagulation, a micro-Cavitron ultrasonic surgical aspirator (microCUSA), microinstruments, and microdissection techniques, the tumor is gradually internally decompressed, followed by sharp resection of the capsule. Once the resection is completed, the 0° endoscope is withdrawn, and a 30° endoscope is introduced and rotated along its longitudinal axis, clockwise and anticlockwise, to survey the entire region for any residual tumor out of the straight view of the 0° endoscope. Any tumor remnants are further resected to ensure total tumor excision. In middle cranial fossa tumors, the sphenoid ridge or the superior orbital roof could be drilled away to give either a better basal view or better access to the tumor.

Following tumor removal, the whole area is copiously irrigated, and hemostasis is secured. The dura is then closed watertight and covered with a layer of collagen dural substitute membrane and a dural sealant to prevent any CSF leak (Fig. 7A–C). The keyhole bone flap is then repositioned and secured in place using absorbable microplates and screws, and an injectable hydroxyapatite bone substitute is used to fill the bone defect around the keyhole bone flap (Fig. 8A,B). The pericranium, soft tissue, and skin incision are then sutured in layers with careful attention to the aesthetic repair. Steri-Strips and a small adhesive bandage dressing are then applied to the suture line (Fig. 9A–C). If the frontal sinus has been opened during the bony work, its mucosa is stripped away; the nasofrontal duct is obliterated, and the sinus is cranialized.

The majority of patients undergoing this procedure are monitored in either the intensive care unit (ICU) or a step-down unit overnight and thereafter transferred to the ward until discharged home, typically 48 hrs after the operation.

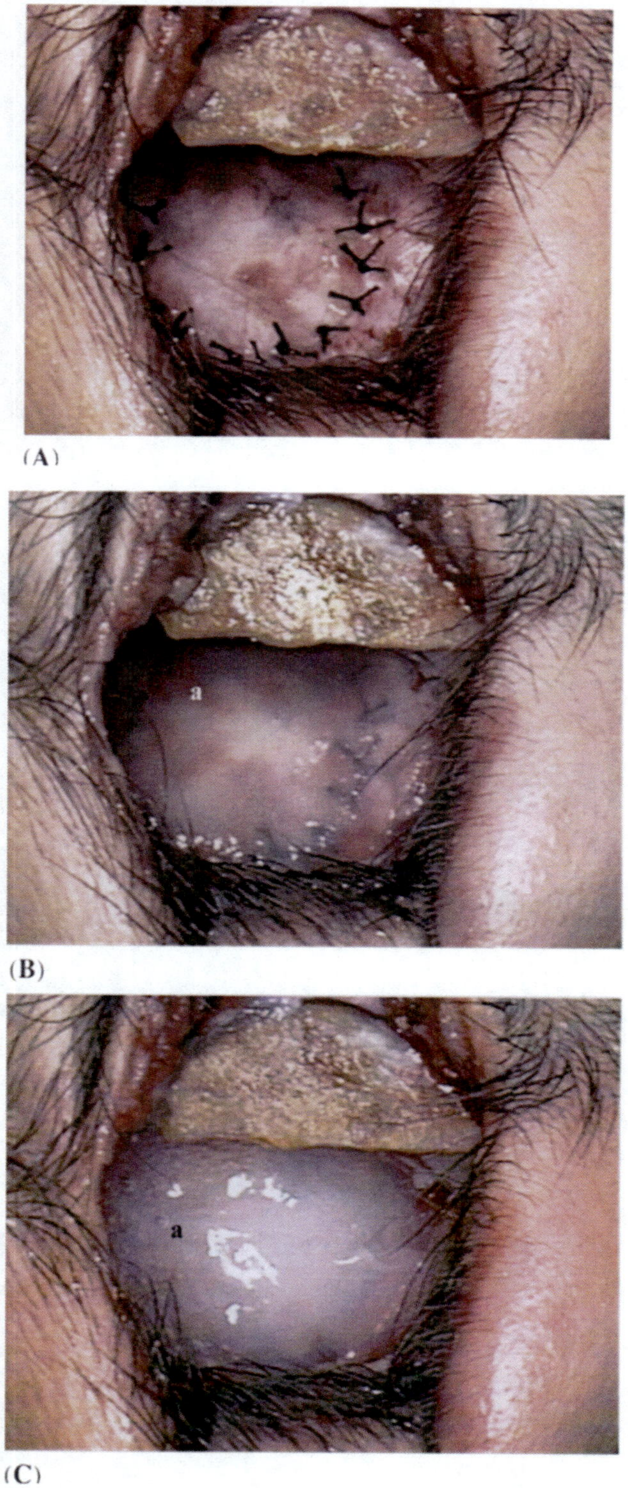

Fig. 7 (**A**)–(**C**) Closure of the dura. (**B**) *a* Collagen dural substitute (onlay graft). (**C**) *a* Fibrin glue.

7. ILLUSTRATIVE CASES

7.1. Anterior Cranial Fossa Tumors

7.1.1. Background (Fig. 10)

Midline or paramedian anterior skull base lesions, such as olfactory groove or planum sphenoidale meningiomas, esthesioneuroblastomas, and transcranial extensions of orbital or paranasal sinus tumors, have traditionally been approached through

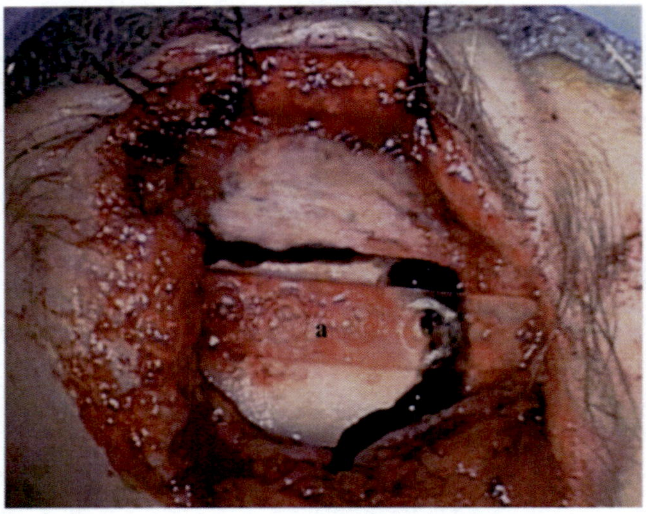

(**A**)

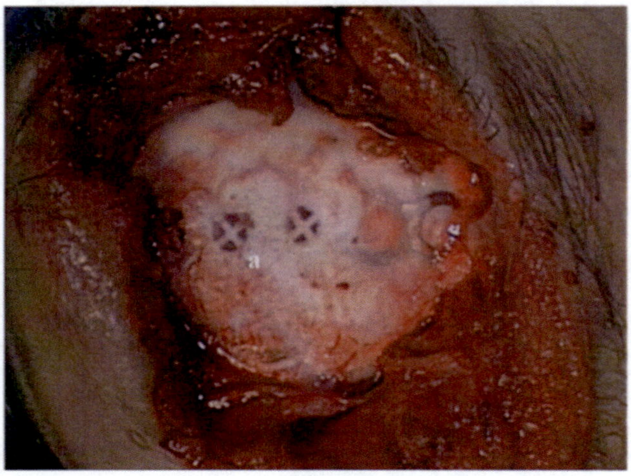

(**B**)

Fig. 8 (**A**) and (**B**) Cranioplasty. (**A**) *a* Absorbable microplate and screws. (**B**) *a* Hydroxyapatite bone substitute.

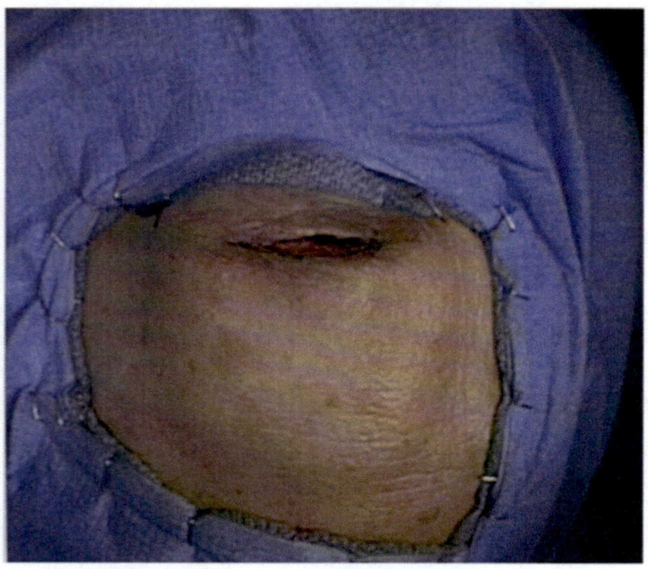

(**A**)

Fig. 9 (**A**)–(**C**) Skin closure. (**B**) *a* Close-up view of the eyebrow after complete skin closure.

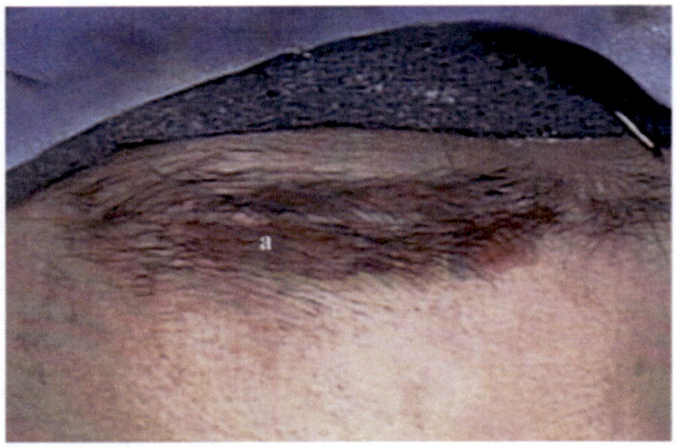

(**B**)

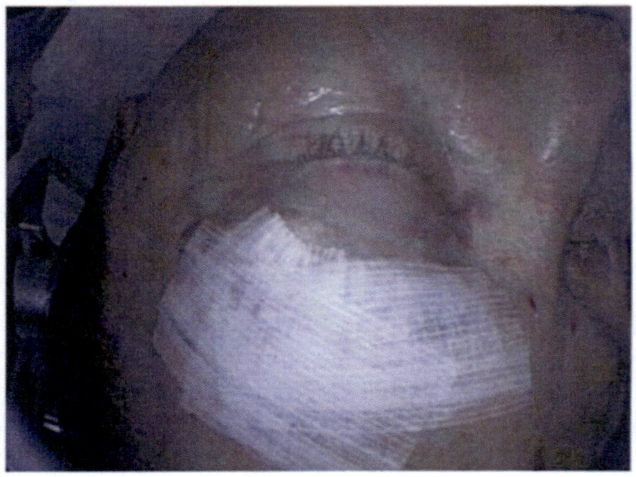

(**C**)

Fig. 9 (continued)

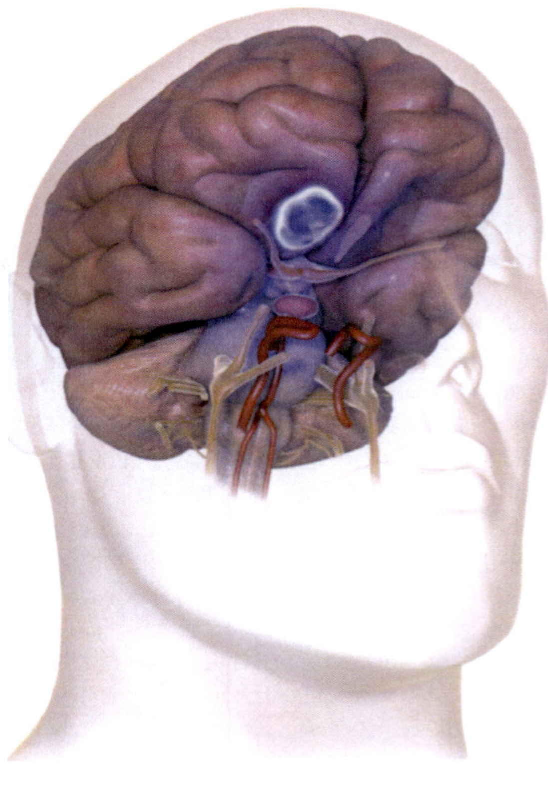

Fig. 10 Anterior cranial fossa tumors.

"craniofacial" unifrontal or bifrontal craniotomies with elevation of one or both frontal lobes and significant brain retraction. The most common surgical approaches have been variants of either the standard subfrontal or pterional approaches.

In our experience, despite the small size of the supraorbital keyhole craniotomy, the exploration followed by slow CSF drainage has proven to be large enough for safe intracranial microsurgical interventions, while the integrity of as much normal tissue as possible is preserved, and unnecessary manipulation or brain retraction is not required. The endoscopic supraorbital approach has allowed us excellent visualization of anterior cranial fossa tumors and vascular and neural structures in this region, while avoiding the deleterious effects of frontal lobe retraction without sacrificing exposure or final outcome.

7.1.2. Approach (Fig. 11) Under general anesthesia, after positioning, prepping, draping, and skin incision, a 1.5-cm supraorbital keyhole craniotomy is performed, the dura is incised open, and CSF is slowly drained. After adequate relaxation of the frontal lobe, a 0° endoscope is introduced and advanced along the floor of the anterior cranial fossa.

The operation then proceeds according to the exact pathology being addressed. For midfrontal skull base lesions, including meningiomas and esthesioneuroblastomas, following the initial exposure of the tumor, a small area of the surface is electrocoagulated and a biopsy obtained for intraoperative frozen section confirmation of the pathology. Dissection then proceeds along the floor of the anterior cranial fossa, and small feeding arteries from below are electrocoagulated and divided to devascularize the tumor. The tumor is then internally decompressed using a combination of a microCUSA, bipolar electrocautery, microinstruments, and microdissection techniques. Following internal debulking, the tumor capsule is identified, and a plane of dissection with the normal frontal lobes is started. The capsule is then gradually and circumferentially resected without undue pressure on the frontal lobes. In olfactory groove meningiomas (OGMs), the tumor is resected off the floor of the anterior cranial fossa and from both olfactory bulbs; the ipsilateral olfactory bulb is often circumferentially infiltrated by tumor, while the contralateral one may occasionally be preserved. The last portion of the tumor to be dealt with is typically the inferior posterior portion abutting the suprasellar area and the optic nerves and chiasm. Dissection off the optic nerves, chiasm, and anterior cerebral artery (ACA) complex is carried out using sharp dissection techniques.

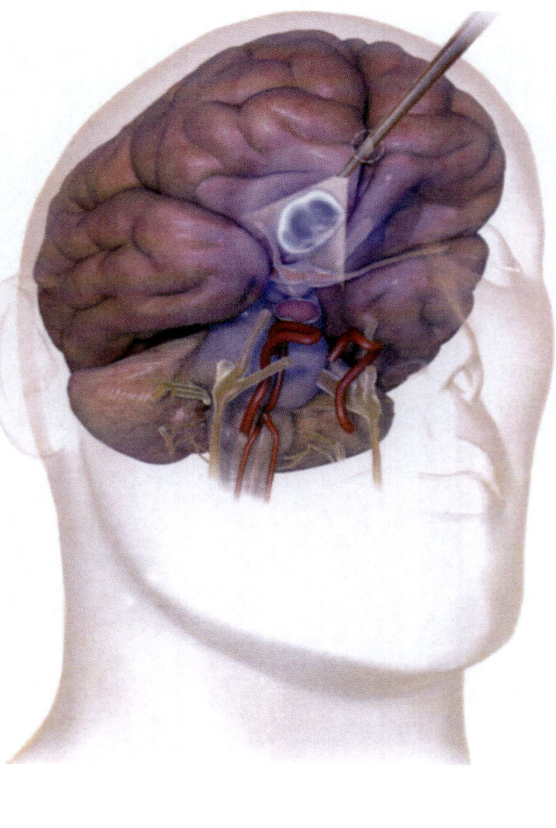

Fig. 11 Approach to anterior cranial fossa tumors.

Once the tumor is completely resected, hemostasis is secured, and the whole area is copiously irrigated. At this point, the endoscope is gradually withdrawn, and a second survey of the entire region is conducted using an angled endoscope to identify and remove any tumor remnants. The dura is then reapproximated, and cranioplasty is carried out, followed by layered suturing of the subcutaneous tissues and skin.

7.1.3. Cases

7.1.3.1. Olfactory Groove Meningioma (Fig. 12A–I)

7.1.3.2. Planum Sphenoidale Meningioma (Fig. 13A–T)

7.2. MIDDLE CRANIAL FOSSA TUMORS

7.2.1. Background Access to tumors of the middle cranial fossa has traditionally required aggressive transcranial approaches via open craniotomies, such as the frontotemporal, pterional, and extended orbitozygomatic approaches. These wide exposures, however, often involve significant frontal or temporal lobe brain retraction, unnecessary surgical dissection, and potentially disfiguring skin incisions, thus resulting in undesirable perioperative morbidity.

While routinely using the endoscopic supraorbital approach to access tumors of the anterior cranial base, we found that the adaptation of rigid endoscopy to the supraorbital approach broadens the available surgical exposure, thus also providing extended access to the middle cranial fossa without the need for additional dissection or retraction. Utilizing the fully endoscopic supraorbital approach to access the middle cranial fossa and the sylvian fissure area, we have enhanced our ability to appreciate the anatomy of this area due to superior visibility and to perform a more complete resection of middle cranial base tumors, including meningiomas, archacnoid cysts, and other lesions.

7.2.2. Approach Under general anesthesia, after positioning, prepping, draping, and an eyebrow skin incision, a 1.5-cm keyhole supraorbital craniotomy is performed, the dura is opened, and CSF is slowly drained until adequate relaxation of the frontal lobe is obtained. A 0° endoscope is then introduced and advanced subfrontally along the floor of the anterior cranial fossa. The endoscope is then advanced either all the way to the middle cranial fossa (for medial sphenoid wing/cavernous sinus meningiomas and other middle cranial fossa tumors) or toward the sellar region (for parasellar region tumors or tumor extensions).

For middle cranial fossa tumors, including medial sphenoid wing/cavernous sinus meningiomas or schwannomas, a small area of the tumor surface is electrocoagulated, and a piece of

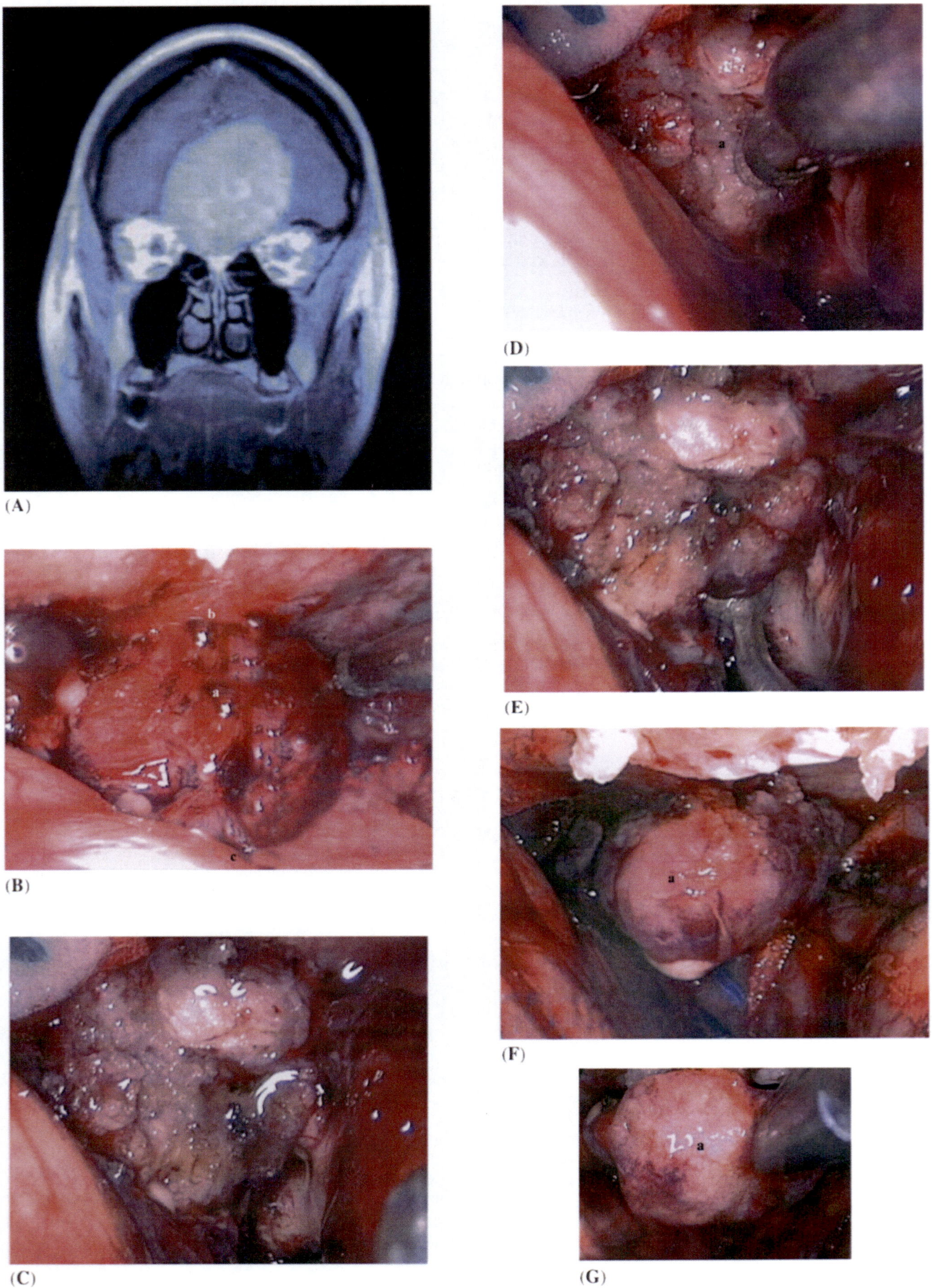

Fig. 12 (**A**) Contrast-enhanced, T_1-weighted coronal magnetic resonance image (MRI) showing an OGM. (**B**) Intraoperative endoscopic view showing

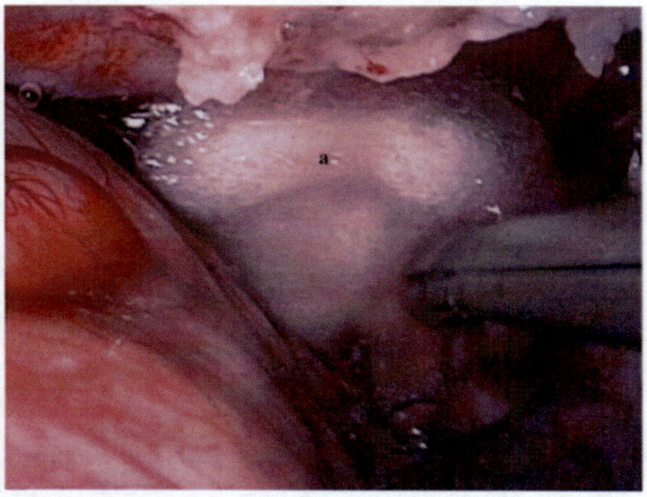

(H)

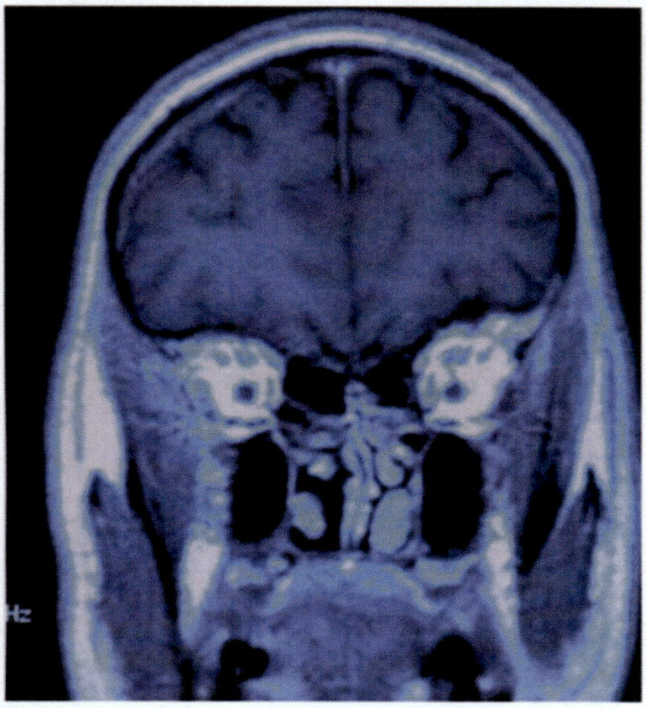

(I)

Fig. 12 (continued) the initial exposure of an olfactory groove meningioma (OGM). *a* Olfactory groove meningioma. *b* Cribriform plate and olfactory groove area. *c* Lower surface of frontal lobe. (**C**)–(**G**) Intraoperative endoscopic view showing the gradual resection of an OGM. (**D**) *a* Gradual debulking of OGM. (**F**) *a* Posterior capsule of OGM. (**G**) *a* Posterior capsule being removed. (**H**) *a* Gelfoam with dural graft underneath covering cribriform plate. (**I**) Postoperative contrast-enhanced, T_1-weighted coronal MRI

the tumor is sent for frozen section confirmation of the diagnosis. Following that and using a combination of custom-designed bipolar electrocautery, a microCUSA, microinstruments, and microdissecting techniques, the tumor is centrally decompressed and gradually resected. Attention is then shifted to the lateral and inferior aspects of the tumor, which usually extend down to the floor of the middle cranial fossa. Therefore, the superior orbital roof or the sphenoid ridge is drilled off for better access to the floor of the middle cranial fossa. Once this step is completed, excellent visualization of the floor of the middle cranial fossa is achieved, and the inferiormost aspect of the tumor is resected. The remaining tumor capsule is then dissected circumferentially and gradually resected off of the medial temporal and frontal lobes. The medial/inferior aspect of the tumor is usually the most hazardous to resect as it is closely related to the ipsilateral carotid artery and cavernous sinus; therefore, it is dealt with last. Using a combination of a bipolar electrocautery and sharp dissection with angled microscissors, this final portion of the tumor is gradually shaved off the internal carotid artery (ICA) and lateral cavernous sinus from anterior to posterior starting with the most medial anterior and inferior aspect of the tumor until the ICA is cleared.

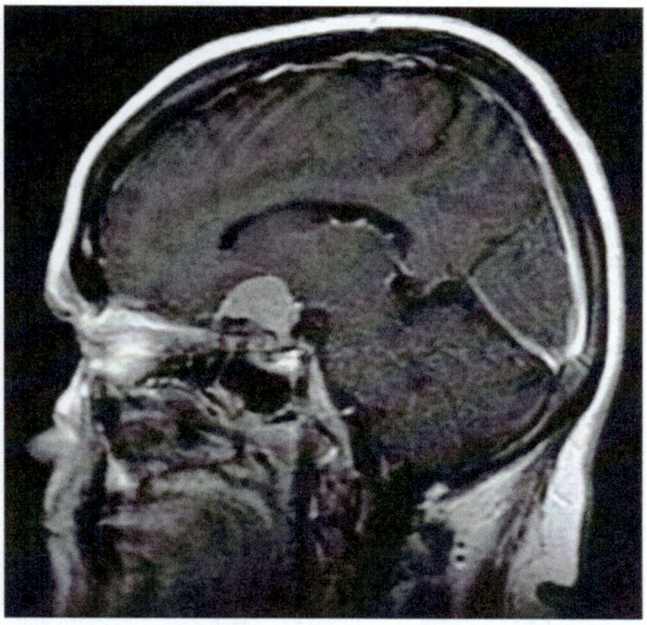

(A)

Fig. 13 (**A**) Contrast-enhanced, T_1-weighted sagittal MRI showing a planum sphenoidale meningioma. (**B**) Contrast-enhanced, T_1-weighted coronal MRI showing a planum sphenoidale meningioma. (**C**) and (**D**) Intraoperative endoscopic view showing the initial exposure of a planum sphenoidale meningioma. (**C**) *a* Meningioma. *b* Planum sphenoidale. (**E**)–(**P**) Intraoperative endoscopic view showing the decompression of a planum sphenoidale meningioma using a combination of blunt and sharp dissection. (**H**) *a* Close-up view during gradual decompression of meningioma. (**K**) *a* First appearance of ipsilateral optic nerve behind tumor. (**L**) *a* Sharp dissection of last remnants of meningioma from ipsilateral optic nerve. (**N**) *a* Ipsilateral optic nerve (II). *b* Contralateral optic nerve (II). (**P**) *a* Last remnant of meningioma adherent to ipsilateral optic nerve. (**Q**) and (**R**) Intraoperative endoscopic view following complete tumor removal and gradual withdrawal of the endoscope. (**R**) *a* Gelfoam. *b* Clean bone of planum sphenoidale. (**S**) Postoperative contrast-enhanced sagittal MRI. (**T**) Postoperative contrast-enhanced coronal MRI.

For parasellar region tumors or tumor extensions, such as in giant pituitary macroadenomas, the tumor is first exposed, and a biopsy is obtained and sent for frozen section confirmation. Following that and using a combination of custom-designed bipolar electrocautery, a microCUSA, microinstruments, and microdissection techniques, the tumor is gradually internally decompressed and resected. The parts of the tumor closest to the carotid artery, the cavernous sinuses, and the optic nerves and chiasm

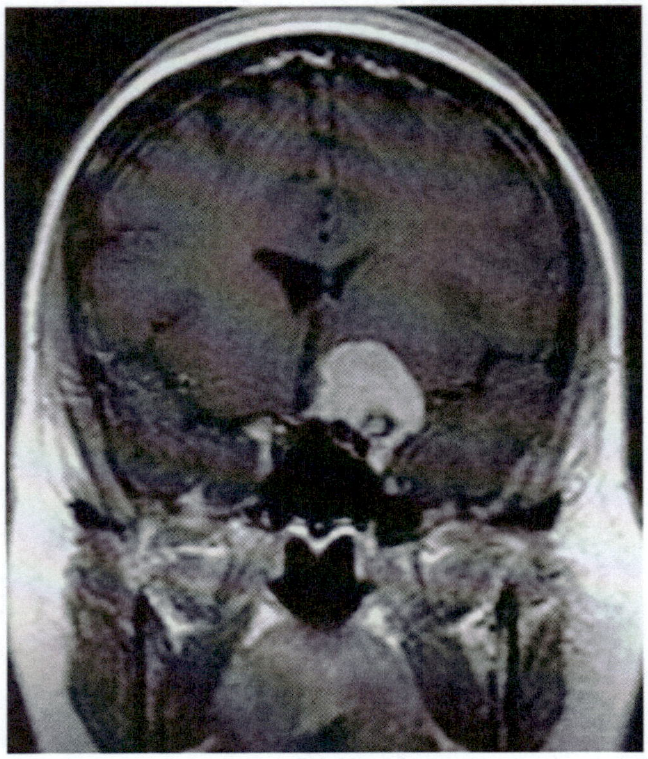

(B)

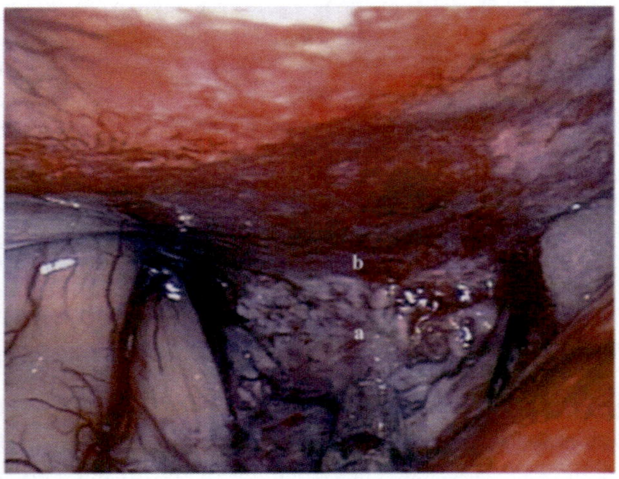

(C)

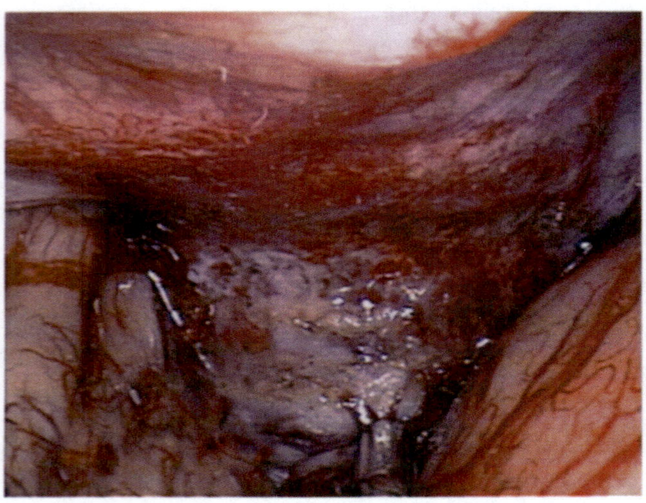

(D)

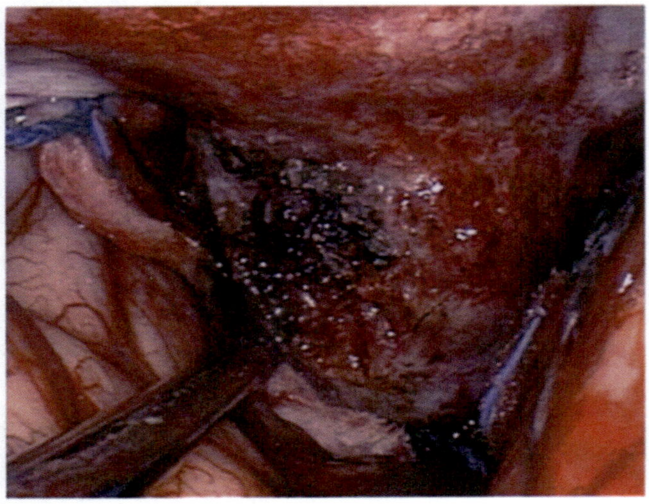

(E)

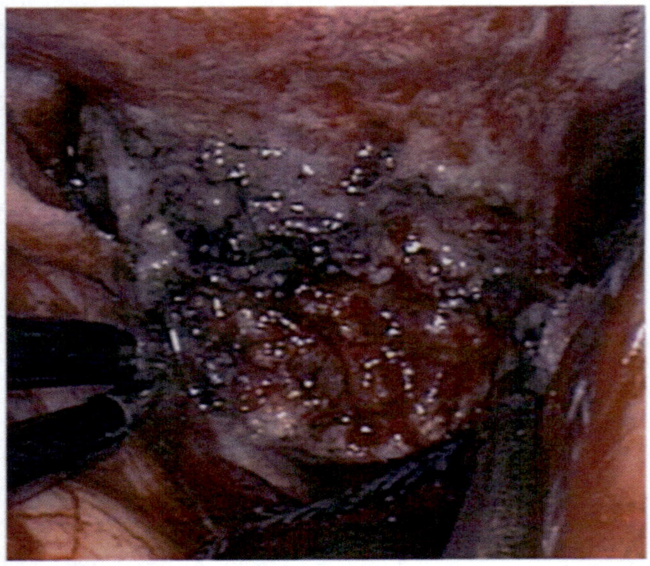

(F)

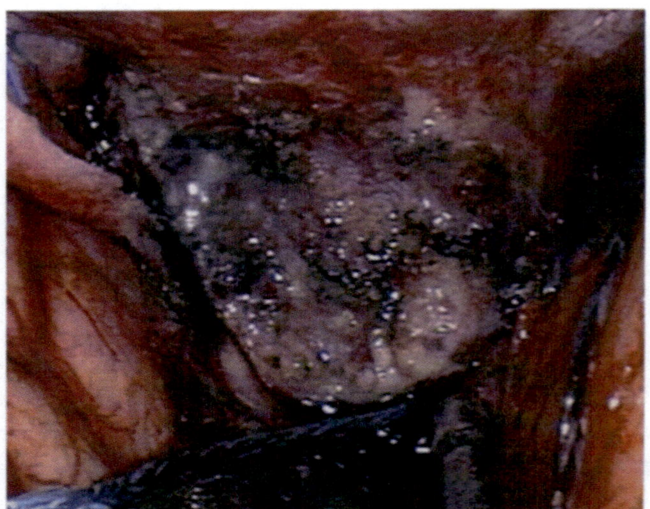

(G)

Fig. 13 (continued)

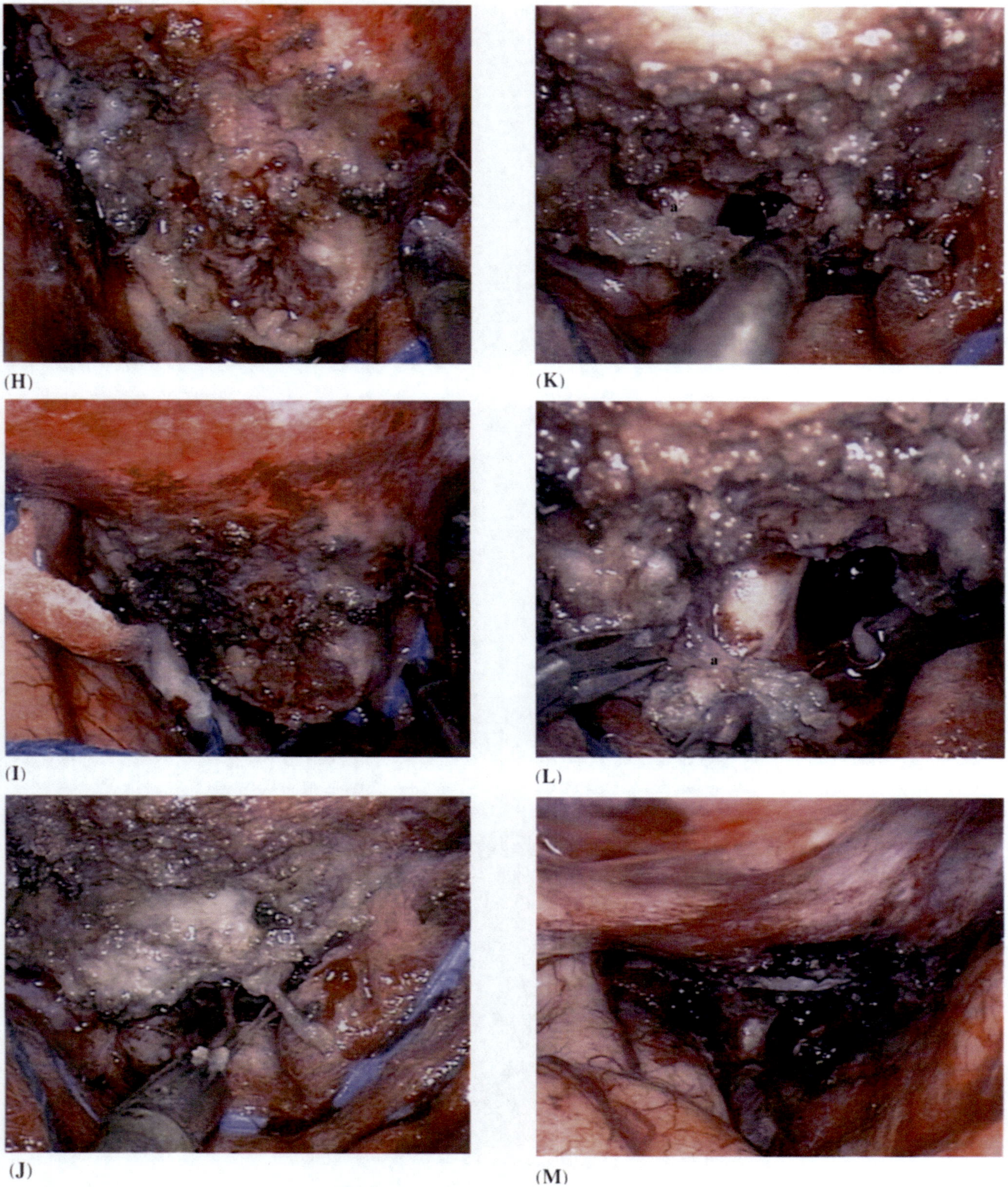

Fig. 13 (continued)

are dealt with last. Again using microdissection techniques and microinstruments, the medial and inferior portions of the tumor are gradually shaved off the critical neurovascular structures in this area using sharp dissection techniques. For suprasellar extensions of giant sellar lesions, a Teflon sponge may be left in the suprasellar cistern as a marker of the extent of suprasellar tumor resection if a second-stage operation is being planned.

After tumor resection is achieved, the 0° endoscope is slowly withdrawn, and a 30° or 70° endoscope is used to conduct a second survey of the entire region; any remaining tumor is further dissected and removed. Following that, hemostasis is secured, and the entire region is copiously irrigated. The dura is then closed, followed by cranioplasty and layered suturing of the subcutaneous tissue and skin.

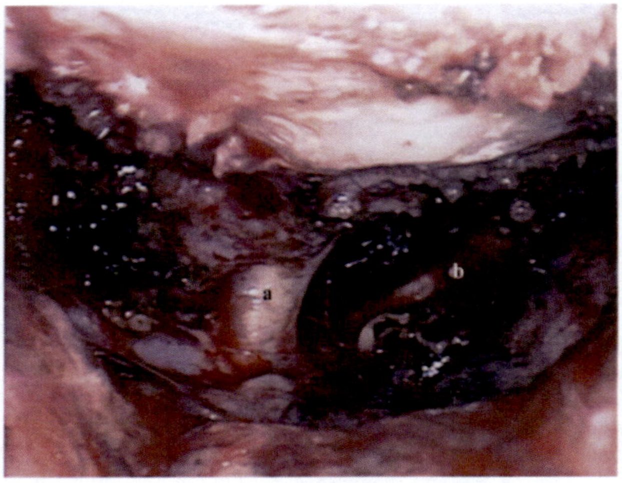

(N)

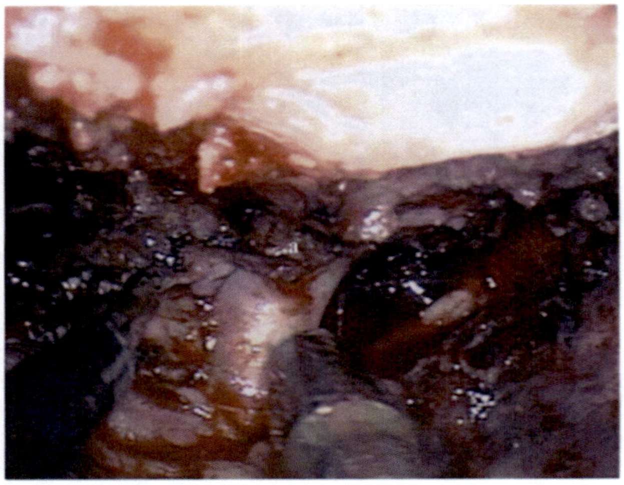

(P)

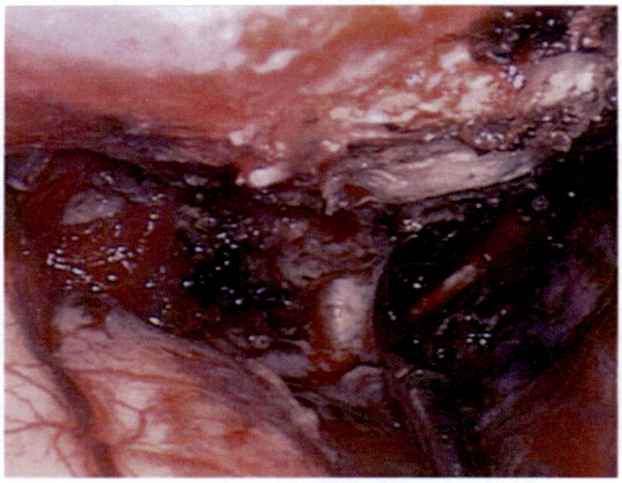

(O)

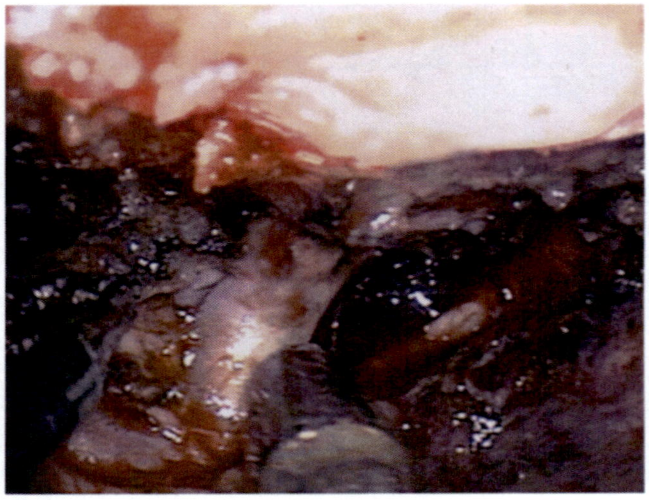

(Q)

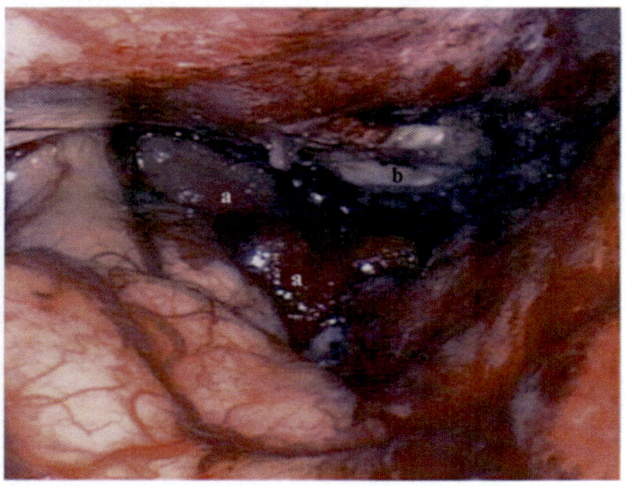

(R)

Fig. 13 (continued)

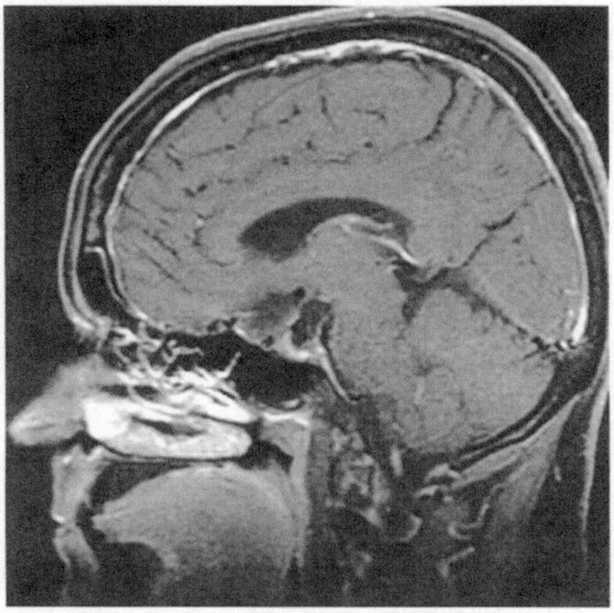

(S)

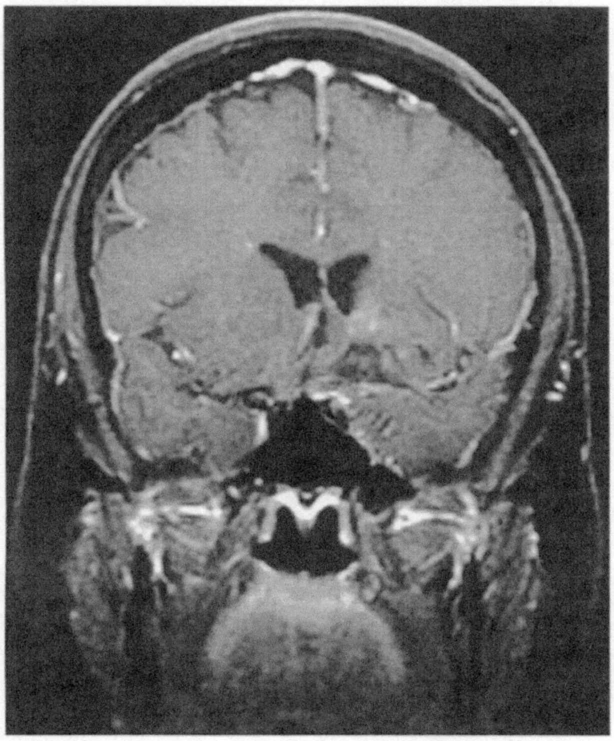

(T)

Fig. 13 (continued)

7.2.3. Cases

7.2.3.1. Medial Sphenoid Wing Meningioma (Right Sided) (Fig. 14A–O)

7.2.3.2. Suprasellar Epidermoid Tumor (Left Sided) (Fig. 15A–L)

8. POTENTIAL COMPLICATIONS

Potential complications of the fully endoscopic supraorbital approach include the following:

- Bleeding, infection, meningitis, cerebrovascular accident, CSF leak, and death, as well as the potential risk for endocrinological

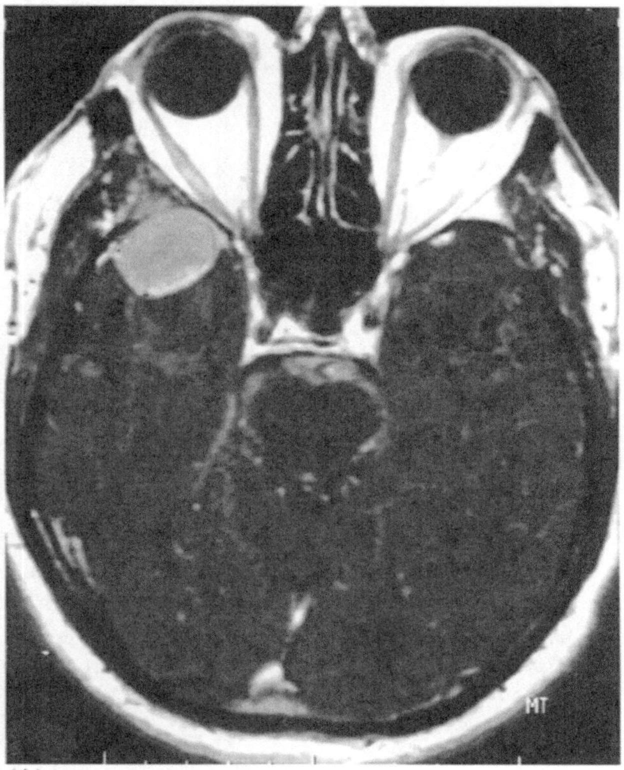

(A)

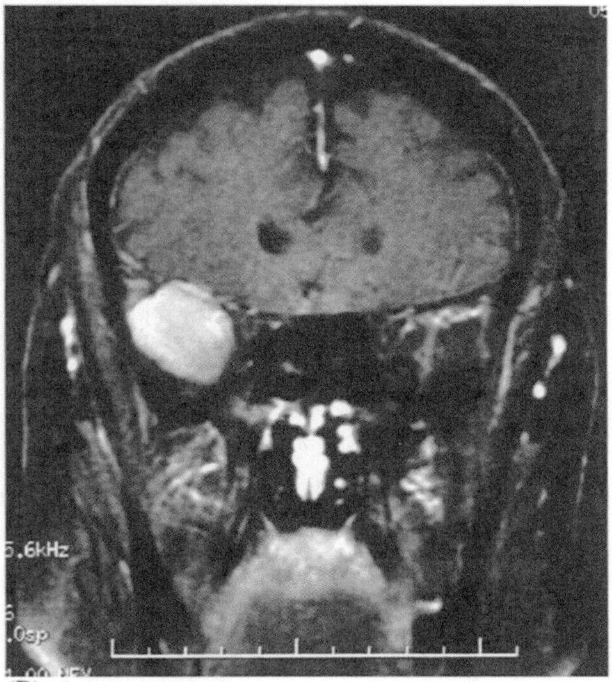

(B)

Fig. 14 (**A**) Contrast-enhanced, T_1-weighted axial MRI showing a medial sphenoid wing meningioma. (**B**) Contrast-enhanced, T_1-weighted coronal MRI showing a medial sphenoid wing meningioma. (**C**) and (**D**) Intraoperative endoscopic view showing the initial exposure of a medial sphenoid wing meningioma. (**C**) *a* Ipsilateral sphenoid ridge. *b* Meningioma. *c* Lower surface of ipsilateral frontal lobe. (**D**) *a* Ipsilateral sphenoid ridge. *b* Meningioma. *c* Lower surface of ipsilateral frontal lobe. *d* Arachnoid. (**E**)–(**K**) Intraoperative endoscopic view showing the resection of a medial sphenoid wing meningioma. (**F**) *a* Meningioma. *b* Lower surface of ipsilateral frontal lobe. *c* Medial

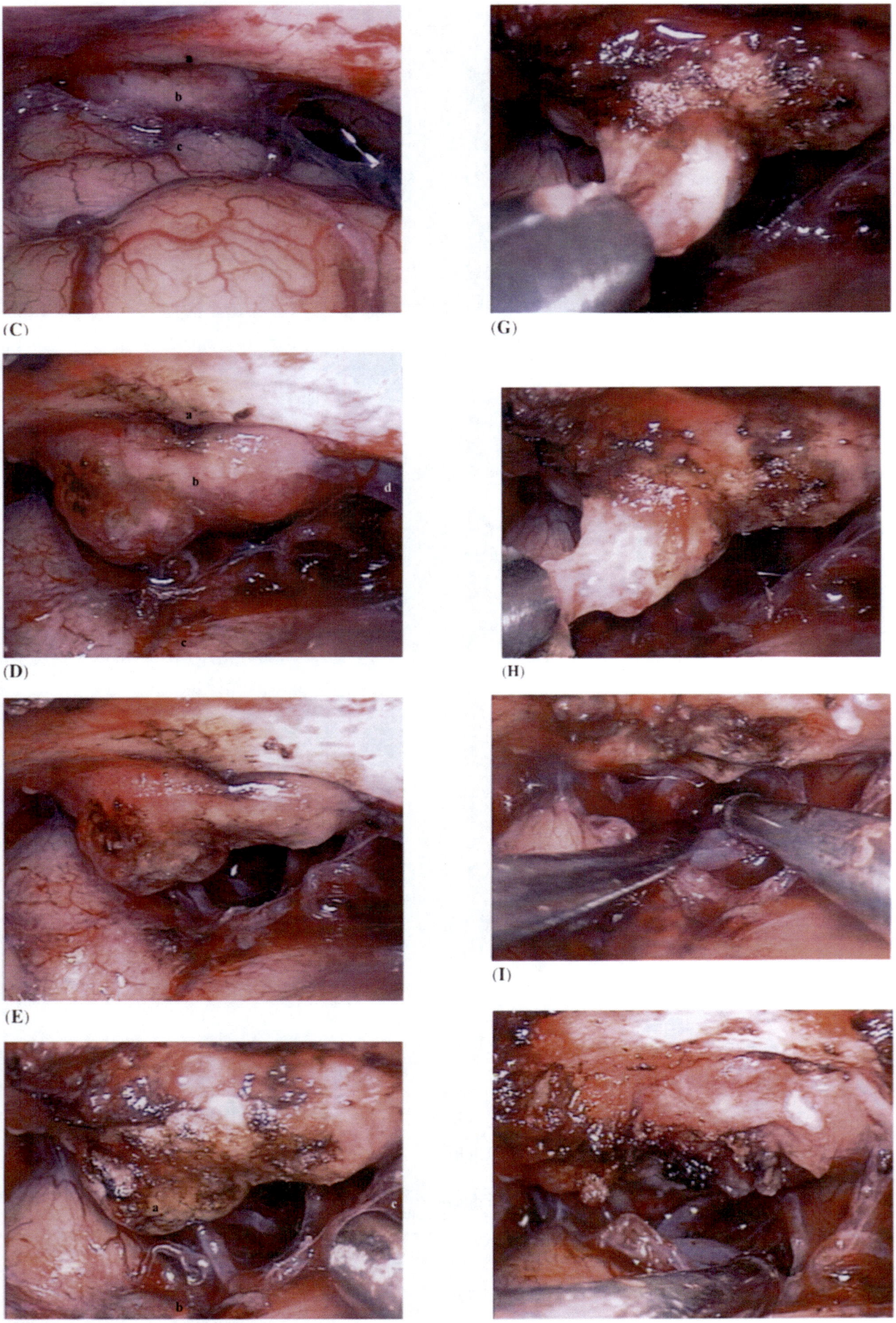

Fig. 14 (continued)

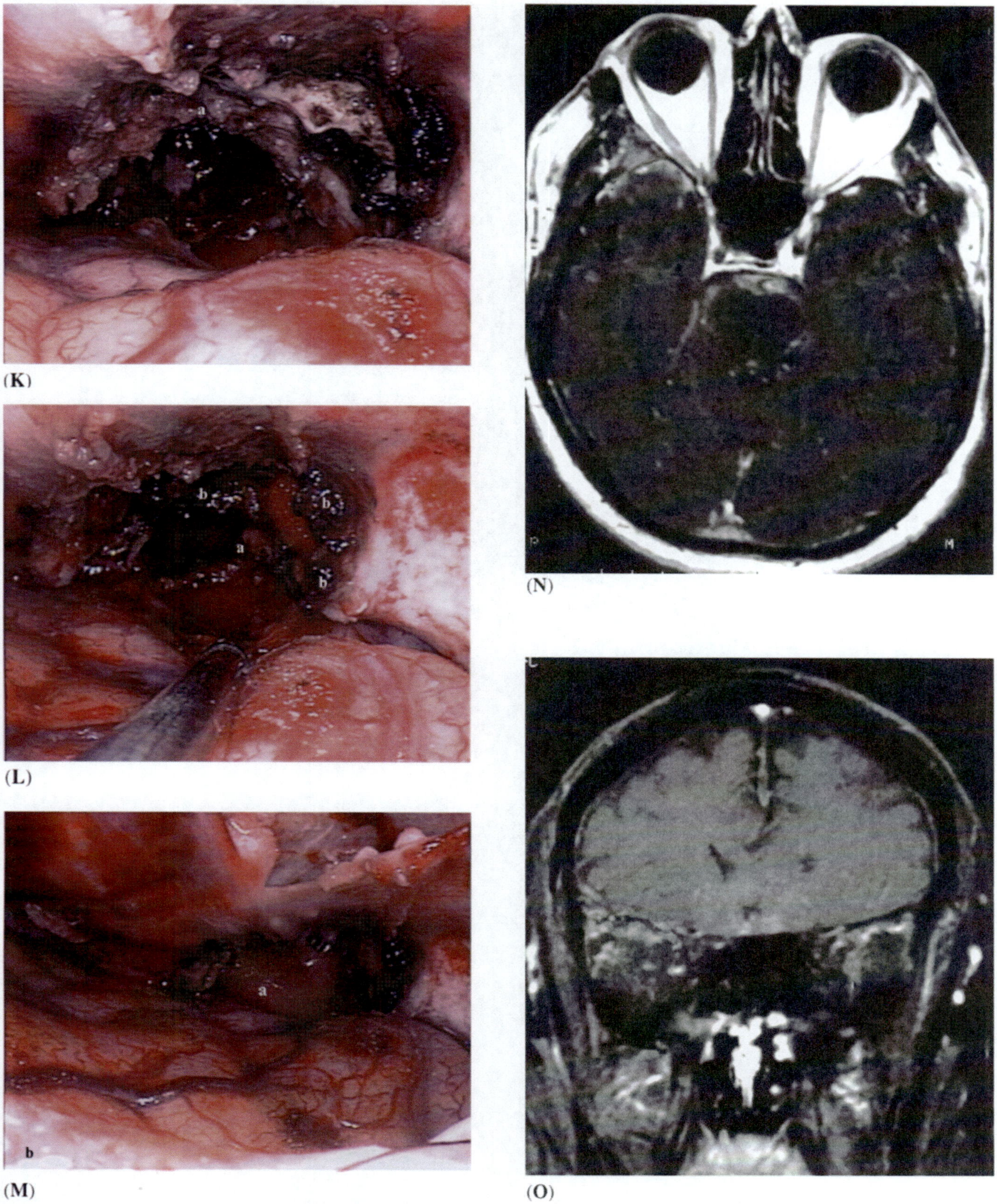

Fig. 14 (continued) surface of ipsilateral temporal lobe. (**K**) *a* Sphenoid ridge is partly drilled for better exposure of the middle skull base and its floor. (**L**) and (**M**) Intraoperative endoscopic view following complete tumor removal and gradual endoscope withdrawal. (**L**) *a* Tumor cavity following complete removal. *b* Dural attachments are cauterized or resected. (**M**) *a* Endoscopic view following complete tumor removal with Gelfoam in cavity. *b* Outer surface of eyebrow. (**N**) Postoperative contrast-enhanced, T_1-weighted axial MRI. (**O**) Postoperative contrast-enhanced, T_1-weighted coronal MRI.

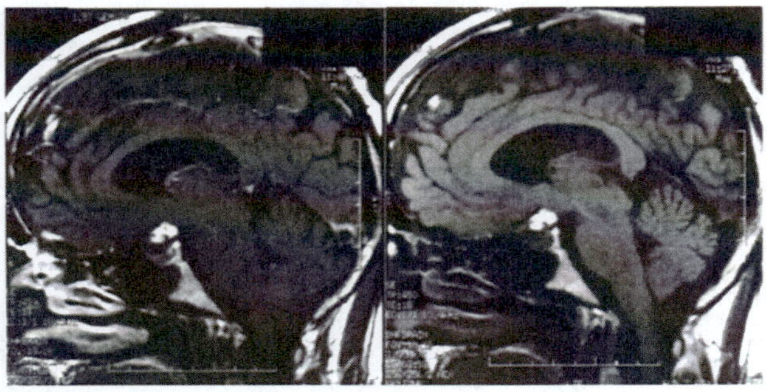

(A)

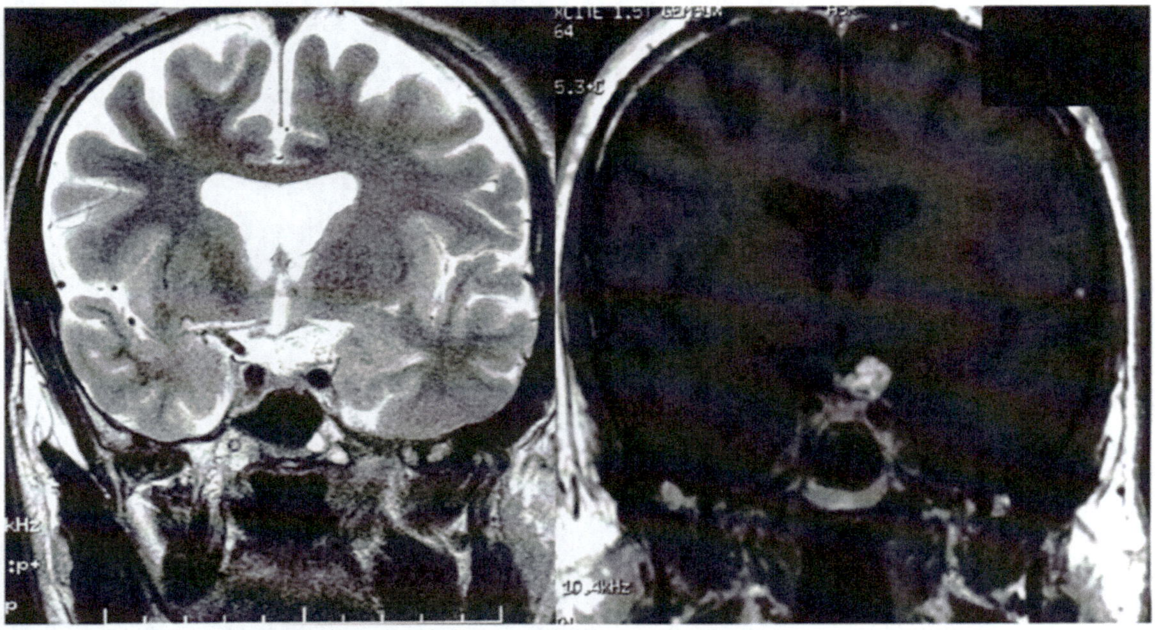

(B)

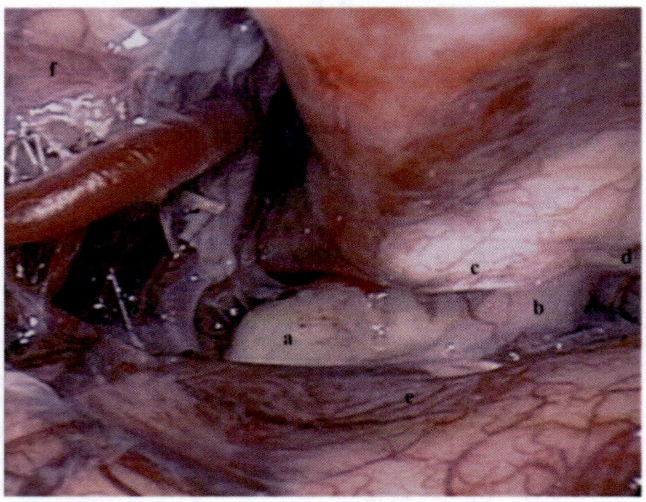

(C)

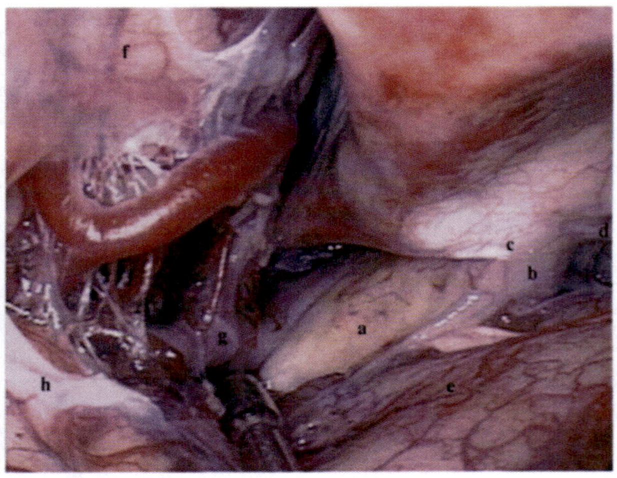

(D)

Fig. 15 (**A**) Contrast-enhanced and noncontrasted, T_1-weighted sagittal MRIs showing a suprasellar epidermoid tumor. (**B**) T_2-weighted and contrast-enhanced T_1-weighted coronal MRIs showing a suprasellar epidermoid tumor. (**C**) and (**D**) Intraoperative endoscopic view showing the initial exposure of a suprasellar epidermoid. *a* Epidermoid tumor. *b* Ipsilateral optic nerve (II). *c* Dura overlying ipsilateral anterior clinoid process. *d* Planum sphenoidale. *e* Lower surface of frontal lobe. *f* Temporal lobe. *g* Middle cerebral artery bifurcation *h* Arachnoid. (**E**) and (**F**) Intraoperative endoscopic view showing the gradual resection of a suprasellar epidermoid. (**E**) *a* Epidermoid tumor partially debulked. *b* Ipsilateral optic nerve (II). *c* Ipsilateral internal carotid artery. *d* Middle cerebral artery bifurcation. (**F**) *a* Ipsilateral internal carotid artery bifurcation. *b* Ipsilateral anterior cerebral artery. *c* Ipsilateral internal carotid artery. *d* Ipsilateral middle cerebral artery. *e* Middle cerebral artery bifurcation. *f* Tumor cavity. *g* Last remnants of epidermoid. (**G**)–(**J**) Intraoperative endoscopic view and close-up views following complete tumor removal and endoscope withdrawal. (**I**) *a* Ipsilateral internal carotid artery bifurcation. *b* Ipsilateral anterior cerebral artery. *c* Ipsilateral internal carotid artery. *d* Ipsilateral middle cerebral artery. *e* Tumor cavity following complete tumor removal. (**K**) Postoperative contrast-enhanced, T_1-weighted sagittal MRIs. (**L**) Postoperative contrast-enhanced, T_1-weighted coronal MRIs.

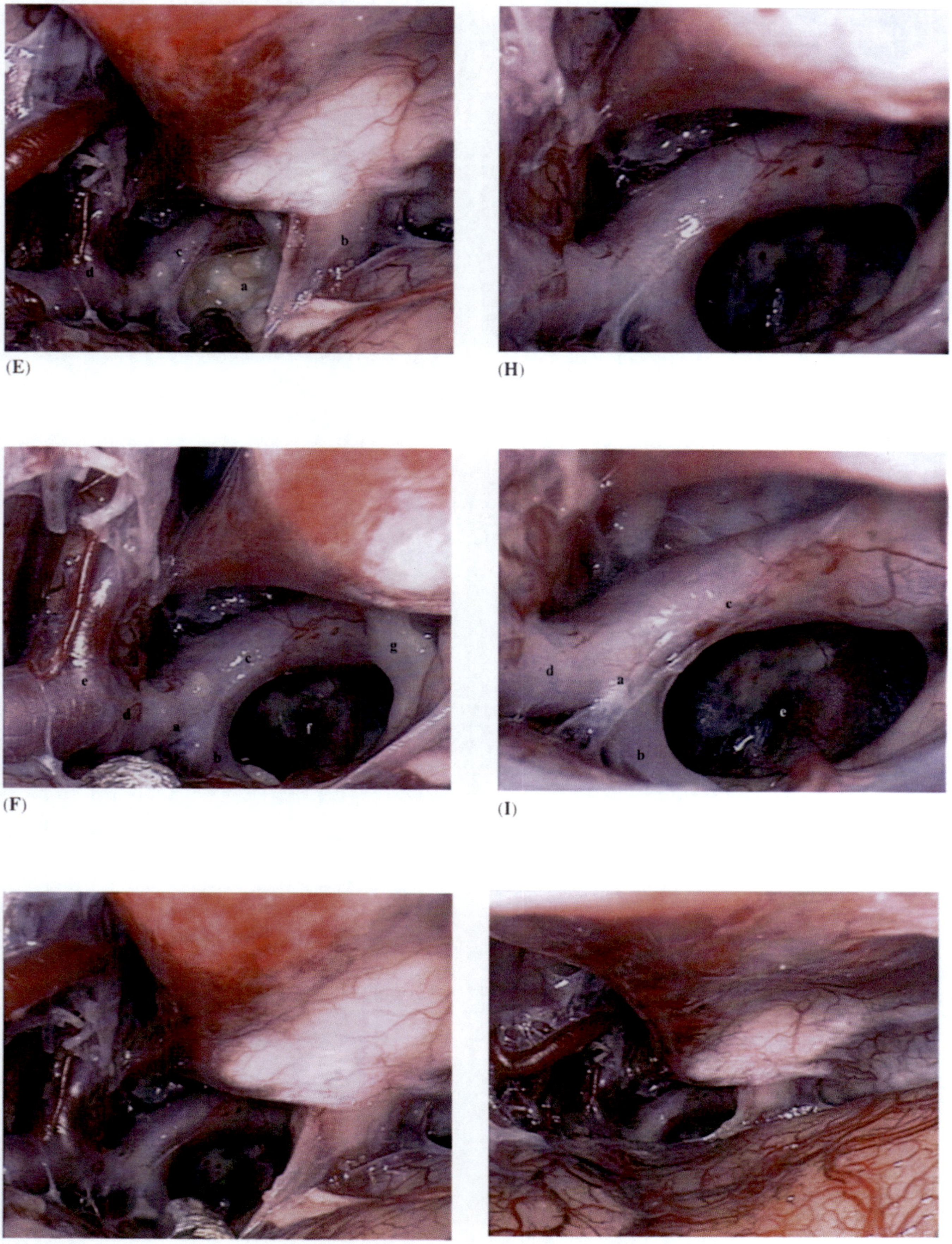

Fig. 15 (continued)

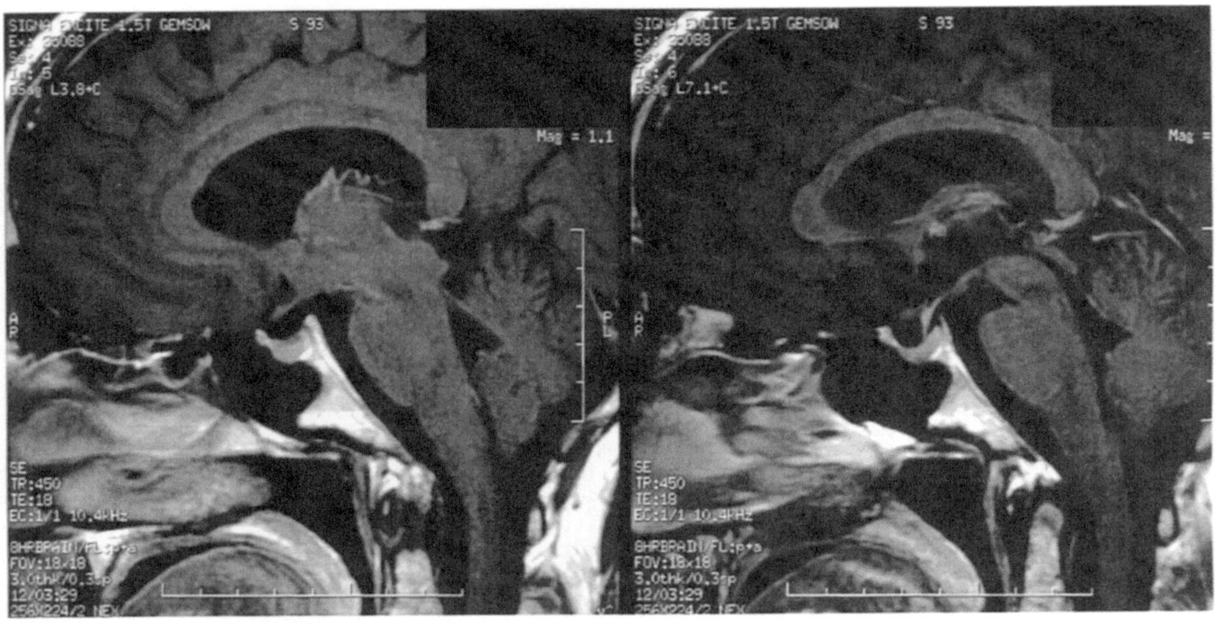

(K)

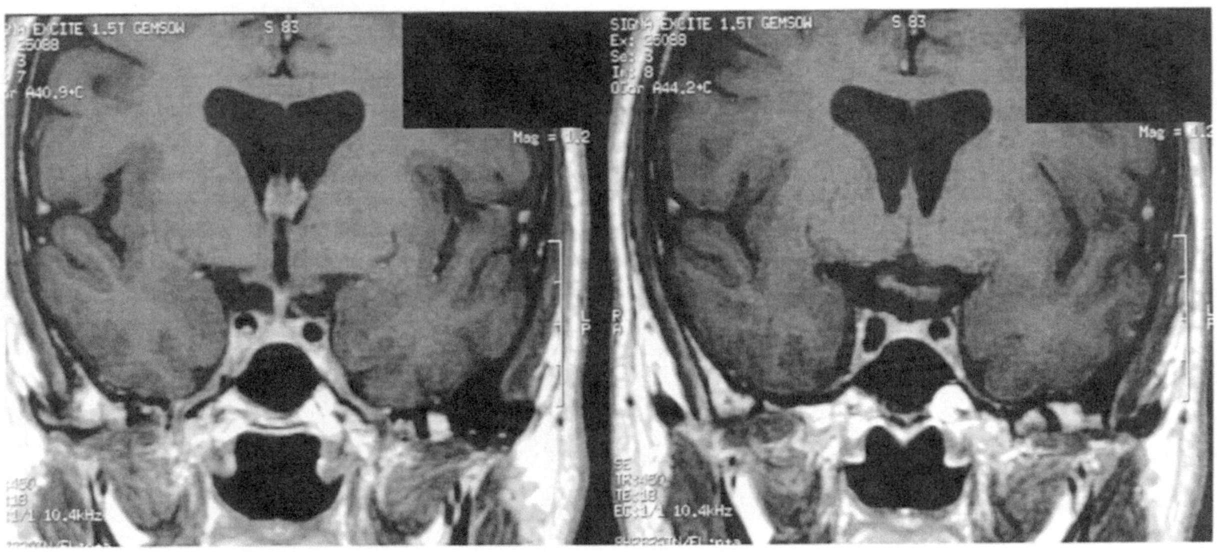

(L)

Fig. 15 (continued)

morbidity, vascular complications, neuropsychological and behavioral disorders, and neurocognitive disorders (these are also potential complications associated with open approaches with more extensive dissection).

- Postoperative severe headaches, lethargy, confusion, or slow mentation can occur due to pneumocephalus.
- A long postoperative course of recovery or a generally obtunded patient with no focal signs of neurological deficit is probably due to postoperative frontal lobe edema or contusion.
- CSF rhinorrhea can occur via an internal fistula through an occult frontal sinus opening.
- Transient or permanent anesthesia of the frontal scalp may occur due to stretching or sectioning of the supraorbital and supratrochlear nerves during the eyebrow incision.
- Transient swelling or cellulitis of the periorbital area may occur.
- Transient frontalis muscle palsy due to transmitted stretch on the frontal branch of the facial nerve.
- Orbital complications may be due to direct injuries such as globe perforation; postoperative diplopia is usually caused by extensive dissection, cerebral edema, or extensive removal of the orbital walls; enophthalmos may result from expansion of the volume of the orbital cavity due to resection of the orbital walls; pulsatile exophthalmos may result from extensive drilling of the orbital roof.
- Direct injuries to neural or vascular structures include direct cavernous sinus, cranial nerve, or carotid artery injuries (especially in patients with ICA encasement or displacement by the tumor or with tumor extending into the cavernous sinuses), which present with symptoms such as opthalmoplegia or cerebrovascular stroke (CVS); unilateral or bilateral loss of vision from injury to the optic nerves or their blood supply; loss of the

sense of smell (anosmia) from damage to the olfactory nerves; endocrinopathies such as temporary or permanent diabetes insipidus (DI) or various degrees of hypopituitarism resulting from direct injury to the pituitary stalk or gland, respectively.

9. AVOIDING COMPLICATIONS IN AUTHOR'S EXPERIENCE

To avoid these complications, the keyhole craniotomy should be far enough from the frontal sinus, the nasofrontal ducts should be obliterated, and the sinus cranialized in case of accidental opening. The medial limit of the incision should always be kept lateral to the supraorbital notch, bearing in mind that palsy of the supraorbital and supratrochlear nerves may be avoided. Pneumocephalus resulting in severe postoperative headache as well as meningitis, CSF leak, and osteomyelitis are usually complications of inadequate separation of the cranial cavity from the sinonasal tract during cranioplasty. Postoperative frontal edema or contusion is usually the result of prolonged traction; this is not required with the supraorbital approach and should be avoided. The frontal branch of the facial nerve virtually never crosses in this area when the eyebrow skin incision is performed correctly; therefore, it is not likely to be directly injured. However, overstretching of the skin is unnecessary and should be avoided as transient palsy of the frontalis muscle may occur due to transmitted stretch from the skin. As with open approaches, direct neurovascular injuries are avoided with careful use of microinstruments. Orbital complications, such as postoperative diplopia, are self-limited, but they may last for a few weeks and are managed conservatively. Enophthalmos and pulsatile exophthalmos are prevented by avoiding extensive removal of the superior orbital wall (not more than one half of the superior orbital roof should be drilled); however, reconstructing the orbital walls with autogenous bone or titanium mesh is another option in case of extensive orbital roof drilling. Diabetes insipidus is an infrequent occurrence and is usually temporary.

In planning the operation, it is important to consider the individual characteristics of each of the anterior cranial fossa tumors. For instance, in OGMs the blood supply comes into the tumor through the bone in the midline of the anterior fossa from branches of the ethmoidal, middle meningeal, and ophthalmic arteries, and the posterior capsule of the tumor may be densely attached to the optic nerves, chiasm, and anterior cerebral arteries. There may be small feeding vessels from the ACoA complex and from the A_2 segments of the ACAs; although these small feeding vessels can be sacrificed, it is critical to follow them carefully to ensure they are not perforating vessels. Preservation of these perforators, which supply the optic nerve, chiasm, and hypothalamus, is vital. If dissection of the tumor off of these perforators is difficult, or if the tumor has infiltrated the optic nerves, it is better to leave a small amount of tumor behind rather than create major deficits due to operative injury. Following complete tumor excision, the dural attachment of the tumor is totally excised, and any bone hyperostosis is removed. The region of the cribriform plate is covered with a graft of pericranial tissue and Gelfoam to prevent a CSF leak.

In some cases, massive nonfunctioning pituitary macroadenomas may enlarge to completely occupy the suprasellar cistern and the third ventricle up to the level of the foramen of Monro or even beyond. They may also extend laterally through the medial wall of the cavernous sinus, lateral to the carotid artery and into the middle cranial fossa, or anteriorly onto the planum sphenoidale and anterior skull base. These are frequent causes of the inability to completely resect these tumors from an endonasal approach. Therefore, in our practice we have adopted two-stage endoscopic approaches and found them ideal for complete resection of massive pituitary macroadenomas. The two-stage surgical approach involves an endoscopic endonasal approach for resection of the intrasellar/suprasellar components of the tumor, followed by a supraorbital (or transglabellar) resection of the extrasellar/parasellar components. This can be done either simultaneously or as two separate procedures. The approach (supraorbital versus transglabellar) is tailored depending on the extension and configuration of the tumor.

9 The Fully Endoscopic Retrosigmoid Approach

This chapter discusses the application of the fully endoscopic retrosigmoid approach to access the cerebellopontine angle (CPA) and petroclival and foramen magnum regions for surgical management of tumors such as schwannomas or meningiomas and neurovascular conflicts involving cranial nerves V through XII that occur in this region of the skull base. The limitations to viewing angles imposed on the surgeon by the operating microscope contrasts with the ability for broad panoramic surveys and different angles of view when endoscopes are used. In our experience, the improved exposure of the entire tumor with virtually no cerebellar retraction has reduced the risk of injury to the brainstem and the surrounding cranial nerves, resulted in more complete tumor removal, decreased the time required to access the CPA, allowed rapid recovery of the patients, and resulted in minimal postoperative discomfort. The chapter provides a thorough description of the fully endoscopic retrosigmoid approach, including indications, operating room setup, patient positioning, operative technique, state-of-the-art illustrative cases, potential complications, and ways to avoid these complications (in the authors' experience).

Keywords: Acoustic neuroma; Cerebellopontine angle (CPA); Endoscopic; Foramen magnum; Glossopharyngeal neuralgia; Hemifacial spasm; Intracanalicular; Meningioma; Minimally invasive; Posterior fossa; Retrosigmoid; Skull base; Surgery; Keyhole; Trigeminal neuralgia; Vestibular schwannoma.

1. INTRODUCTION

The neurovascular anatomy of the posterior cranial fossa is quite intricate. The limitations to viewing angles imposed on the surgeon by the operating microscope contrasts with the ability for broad panoramic surveys and different angles of view when endoscopes are used. The endoscope is particularly well suited to application at the cerebellopontine angle (CPA), where neurovascular structures are often obscured by the protrusion of the petrous portion of the temporal bone and where mass lesions, including meningiomas and vestibular schwannomas (VSs) that include portions within the internal auditory canal (IAC), are not always completely exposed microscopically. The endoscopic approach to the CPA, especially when angled endoscopes are used, allows the surgeon to visualize areas that were often hidden from the direct line of view of the operating microscope. Moreover, endoscopic procedures pose no additional risk to the patient and add no additional time to the total duration of surgery.

We have routinely used the endoscopic retrosigmoid approach for cranial nerve microvascular decompressions for trigeminal neuralgia, glossopharyngeal neuralgia, and hemifacial spasm, as well as for resection of CPA tumors, such as vestibular schwannomas, meningiomas, and others. The improved exposure of the entire tumor with virtually no cerebellar retraction has reduced the risk of injury to the brainstem and the surrounding cranial nerves, resulted in more complete tumor removal, decreased the time required to access the CPA, allowed rapid recovery of the patients, and resulted in minimal postoperative discomfort.

2. INDICATIONS

The fully endoscopic retrosigmoid approach provides minimally invasive access to the CPA, petroclival, and foramen magnum regions for surgical management of tumors such as schwannomas or meningiomas and neurovascular conflicts involving cranial nerves V through XII that occur in this region of the skull base.

3. INSTRUMENTATION

The instrumentation needed to execute this technique successfully include an endoscopic tower, a high-definition digital camera, a xenon or halogen light source, 0° and 30° rigid endoscopes, an endoscope irrigation sheath, two endoscope holding arms, and precision microinstruments.

4. OPERATING ROOM SETUP (FIG. 1)

Once the patient is anesthetized, the operating room table is turned 180°, and corrugated extension tubing is used to lengthen

From: *Endoscopic Skull Base Surgery: A Comprehensive Guide with Illustrative Cases.*
Edited by H. K. Shahinian © Humana Press, Totowa, NJ.

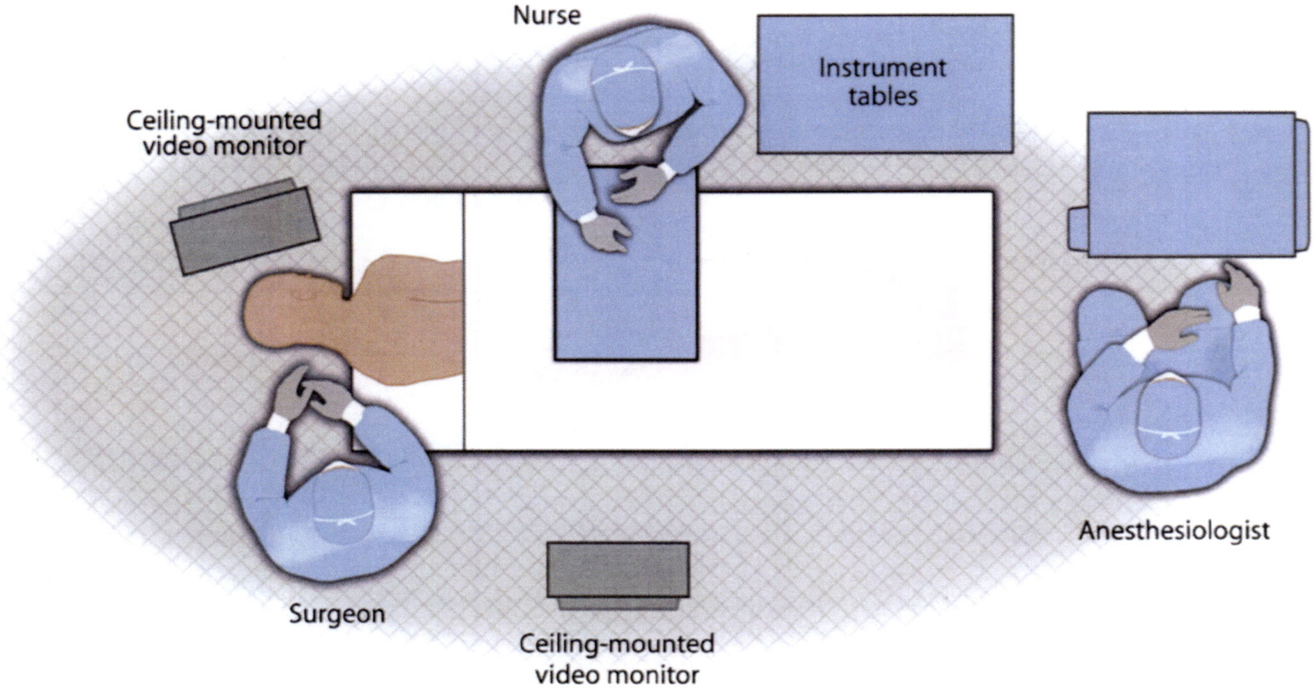

Fig. 1 Operating room setup.

the airway circuit. The patient is put in the lateral oblique (park bench) position, and the surgeon stands on the side to be operated on. Next, the endoscopic tower is placed directly opposite the surgeon. Two separate, pneumatically powered holding arms are affixed to the table, one on each side of the patient, and wrapped in sterile drapes. One holding arm is dedicated to holding the endoscope, and the second is used to hold other microinstruments in place. A second monitor placed behind the surgeon allows the scrub technician or assistant, who stands facing the surgeon, to monitor the operation.

5. PATIENT POSITIONING (FIG. 2)

A three-pin Mayfield clamp is applied to the patient's head, and the patient is rolled into the lateral oblique position while the surgeon controls the patient's head. A beanbag is placed under the patient to conform to the patient's body. The Mayfield head clamp is positioned so that the side with two pins is supporting the dependent side of the head. With the head of the bed raised 30° to facilitate venous drainage, the neck is flexed, rotated away from the surgeon, and fixed in position. The hip and knee joints are flexed, and a pillow is placed between both knees. The patient's body is then secured to the table with adhesive tape, and an axillary roll is placed beneath the axilla of the dependent arm to protect the brachial plexus. The ipsilateral arm is retracted caudad and tucked under the bedsheet.

6. OPERATIVE TECHNIQUE

Following the administration of general anesthesia (without paralysis), a color marker is used to draw the landmarks of the skin incision, and the retroauricular area is prepared with an antibacterial surgical scrub (Fig. 3A,B). Intraoperative cranial nerve and brainstem monitoring is performed in all cases. A longitudinal 3-cm retroauricular skin incision is performed, and small hooks are used to retract the skin and soft tissues. Dissection is then carried out down to the cranium in a subperiosteal plane (Fig. 4A–C). Using a microdrill and the asterion as a bony anatomical landmark, a 1.5-cm keyhole craniotomy is made at the confluence of the transverse and sigmoid sinuses; the bone flap is removed in one piece to be returned in place during cranioplasty at the end of the operation (Fig. 5A,B). Bone wax is used to fill any mastoid air cells entered during the bone drilling.

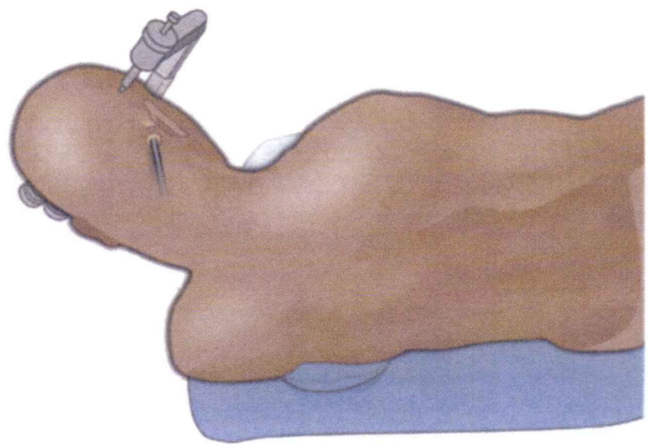

Fig. 2 Patient Positioning.

The dura is then incised in a curvilinear fashion and reflected laterally (Fig. 6). Cerebrospinal fluid (CSF) is then slowly drained

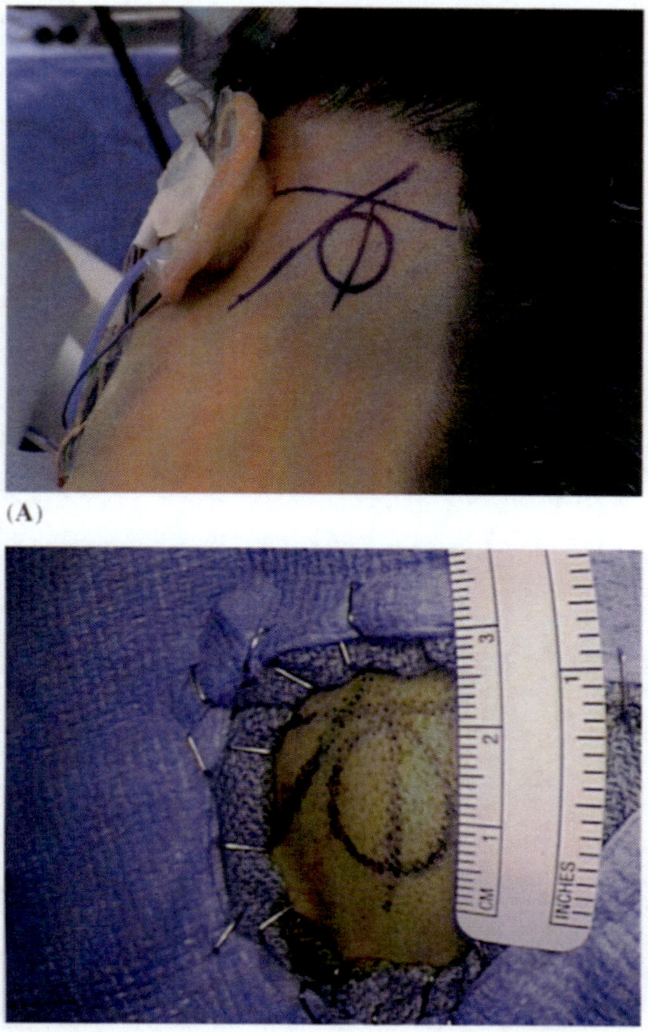

(A)

(B)

Fig. 3 (**A**) and (**B**). Marking and draping.

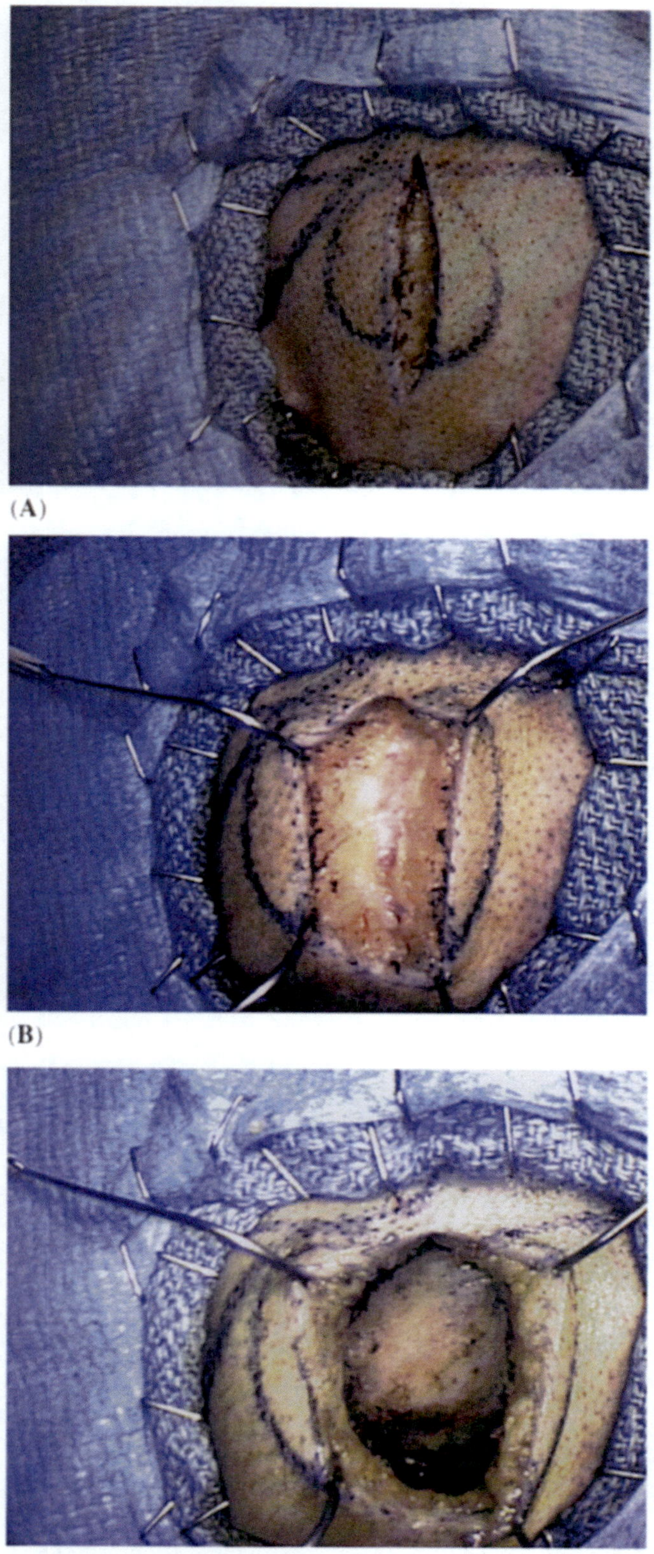

(A)

(B)

(C)

Fig. 4 (**A**)–(**C**) Skin incision.

from the paracerebellar cisterns. The combination of positioning, mild hyperventilation, and intravenous administration of mannitol allows the cerebellum to retract spontaneously, opening a narrow path between the posterior aspect of the petrous bone and the cerebellum through which a 2.7- or 4.0-mm 0° endoscope is introduced and then advanced slowly to the CPA (Fig. 7A–C). On entering the CPA, the surgeon conducts a preliminary survey of the surrounding structures, including tentorial and emissary veins, the petrous temporal bone, the lower cranial nerves and jugular foramen, the acousticofacial bundle and the internal auditory meatus, the trigeminal nerve and Meckel's cave, the trochlear nerve along the tentorium, as well as the regional vascular anatomy (Fig. 8A–E). The irrigation sheath clears blood and debris from the lens of the endoscope, eliminating the time-consuming and dangerous practice of removing and reinserting the endoscope. The holding arm secures the endoscope in place, allowing bimanual surgical dexterity.

From this point, the procedure will vary according to the pathological condition being addressed (i.e., microvascular decompression vs. tumor extirpation). Once the intracranial portion of the procedure is completed and hemostasis is obtained, the dura is then closed in a watertight fashion and covered with a collagen dural substitute membrane followed by a dural sealant to prevent any CSF leak (Fig. 9A–C). The bone plug is then replaced and secured in place by resorbable microplates and screws, and an injectable hydroxyapatite bone substitute is applied to fill the bone defect (Fig. 10A,B). The incision is then closed in ana-

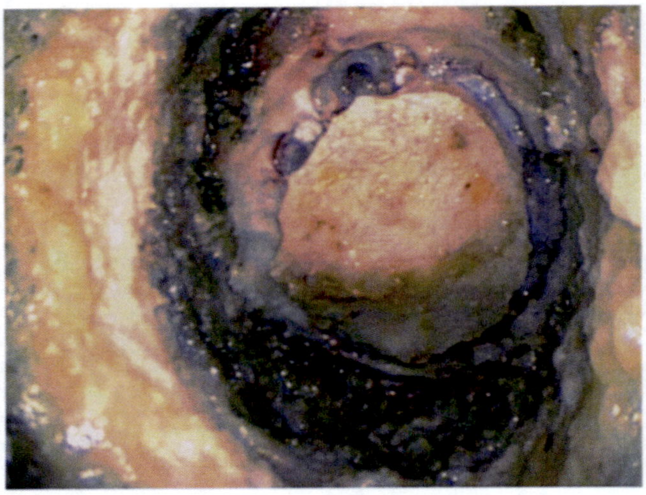

(A)

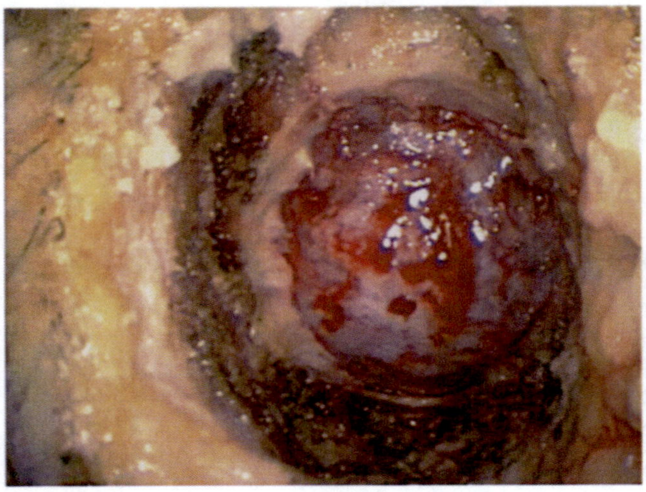

(B)

Fig. 5 (**A**) and (**B**) Keyhole craniotomy.

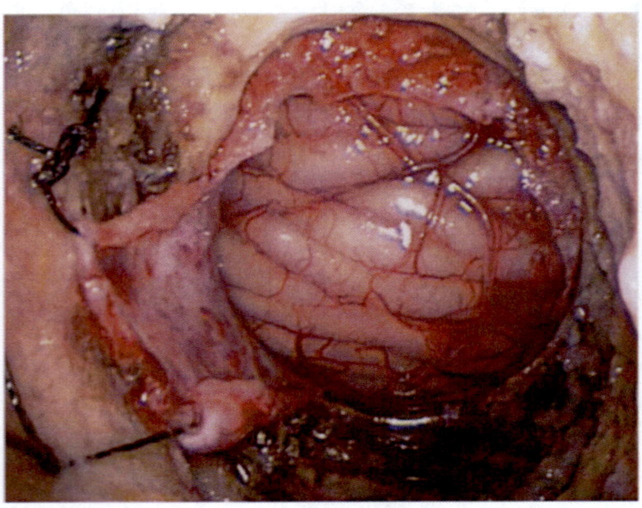

Fig. 6 Dural opening.

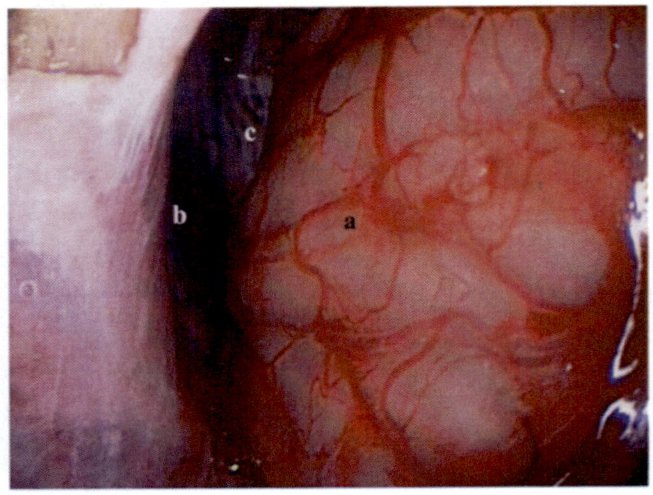

(A)

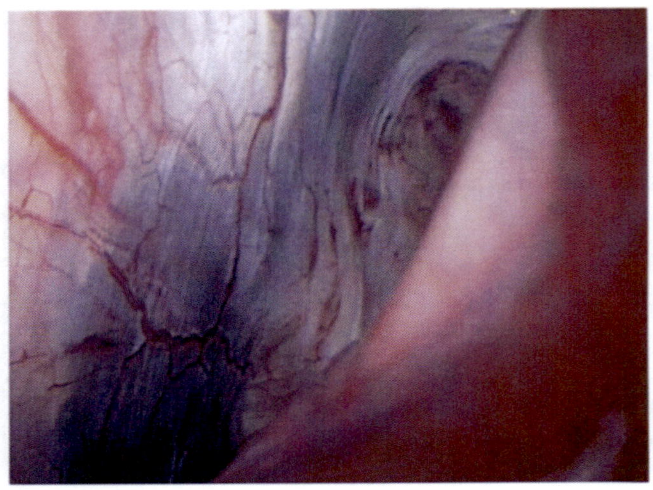

(B)

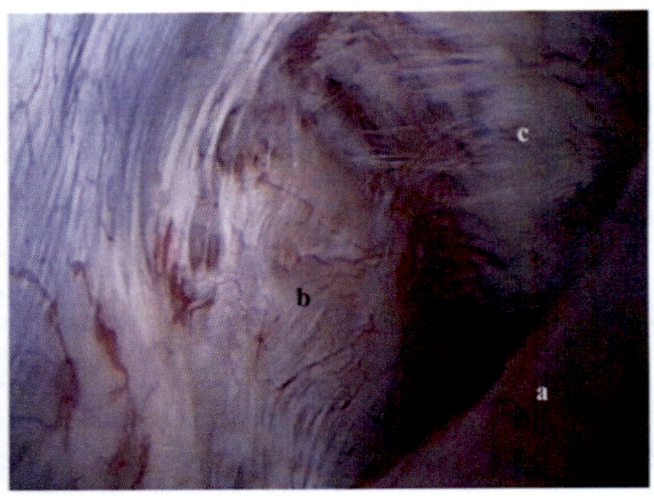

(C)

Fig. 7 (**A**)–(**C**) Endoscope advancement to the cerebellopontine angle (CPA). (**A**) *a* Lateral aspect of cerebellar hemisphere (left side). *b* Petrous temporal bone. *c* Endoscope trajectory. (**C**) *a* Lateral aspect of cerebellar hemisphere. *b* Petrous temporal bone. *c* Tentorium.

tomical layers without the use of any subcutaneous drains, and an adhesive bandage dressing is applied to the suture line (Fig. 11A,B). Following extubation, the patient is typically transferred to either a step-down unit or the intensive care unit (ICU) for overnight monitoring. The vast majority of patients are discharged 48 h after the operation.

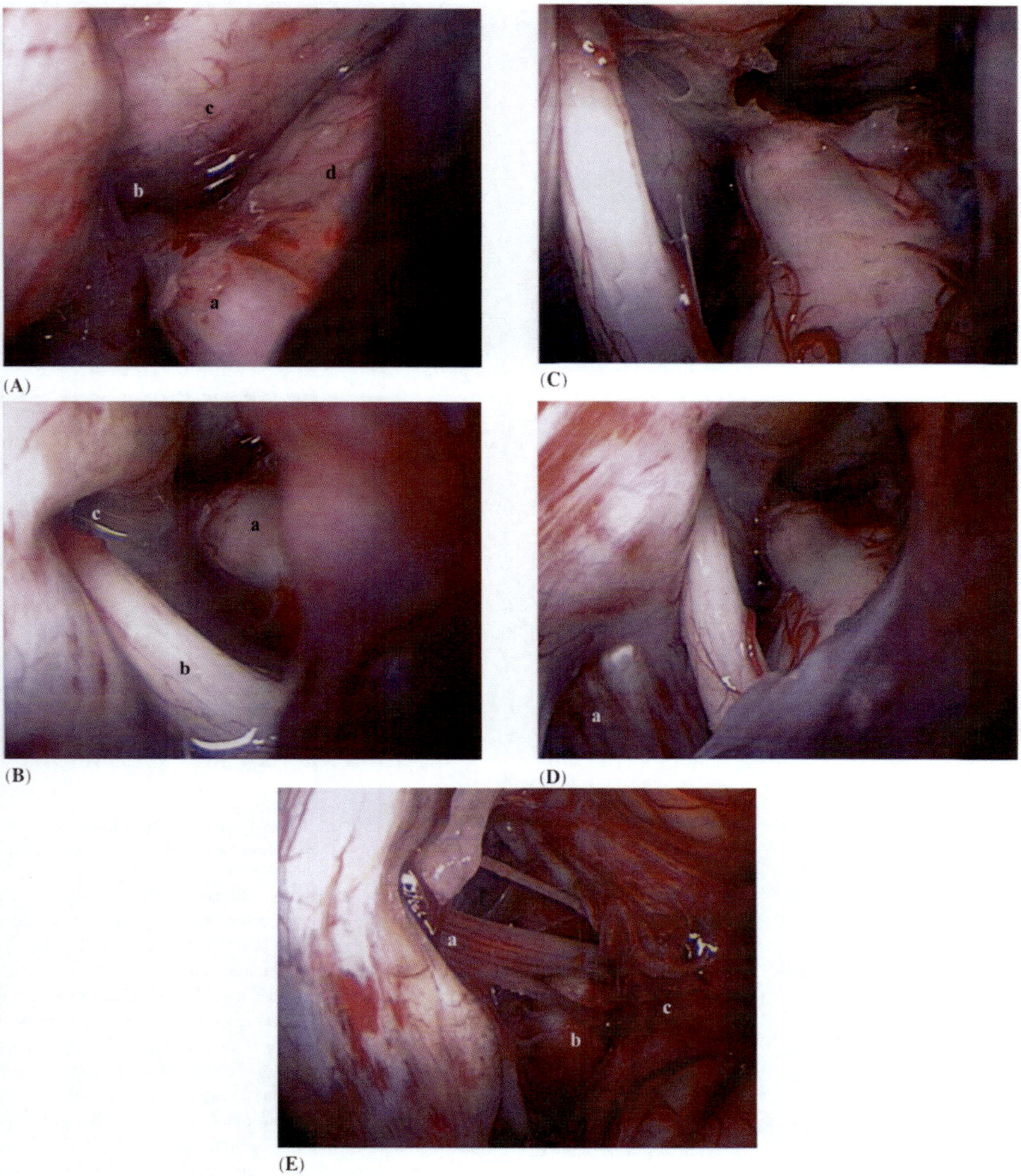

Fig. 8 (**A**)–(**E**) Endoscopic anatomy of the cerebellopontine angle (CPA). (**A**) *a* Ipsilateral trigeminal nerve (V). *b* Meckel's cave. *c* Tentorium. *d* Brainstem. (**B**) *a* Ipsilateral trigeminal nerve (V). *b* Ipsilateral acousticofacial nerve bundle (VII, VIII). *c* Internal auditory meatus (IAM). (**D**) *a* Ipsilateral lower cranial nerves (IX–XI). (**E**) *a* Ipsilateral lower cranial nerves (IX–XI). *b* Brainstem. *c* Inferior lateral aspect of cerebellum.

7. ILLUSTRATIVE CASES

7.1. TRIGEMINAL NEURALGIA

7.1.1. Background (Fig. 12) Trigeminal neuralgia is a disease characterized by severe and often debilitating facial pain that occurs along the distribution of any of the three branches of the trigeminal nerve. As classically defined, attacks are intermittent, and the quality of the pain is sharp or stabbing or mimics an electric shock. The mainstay of treatment for patients with trigeminal neuralgia prior to the modern surgical era was confined to medical treatment of episodic symptoms, ablative procedures, or sectioning

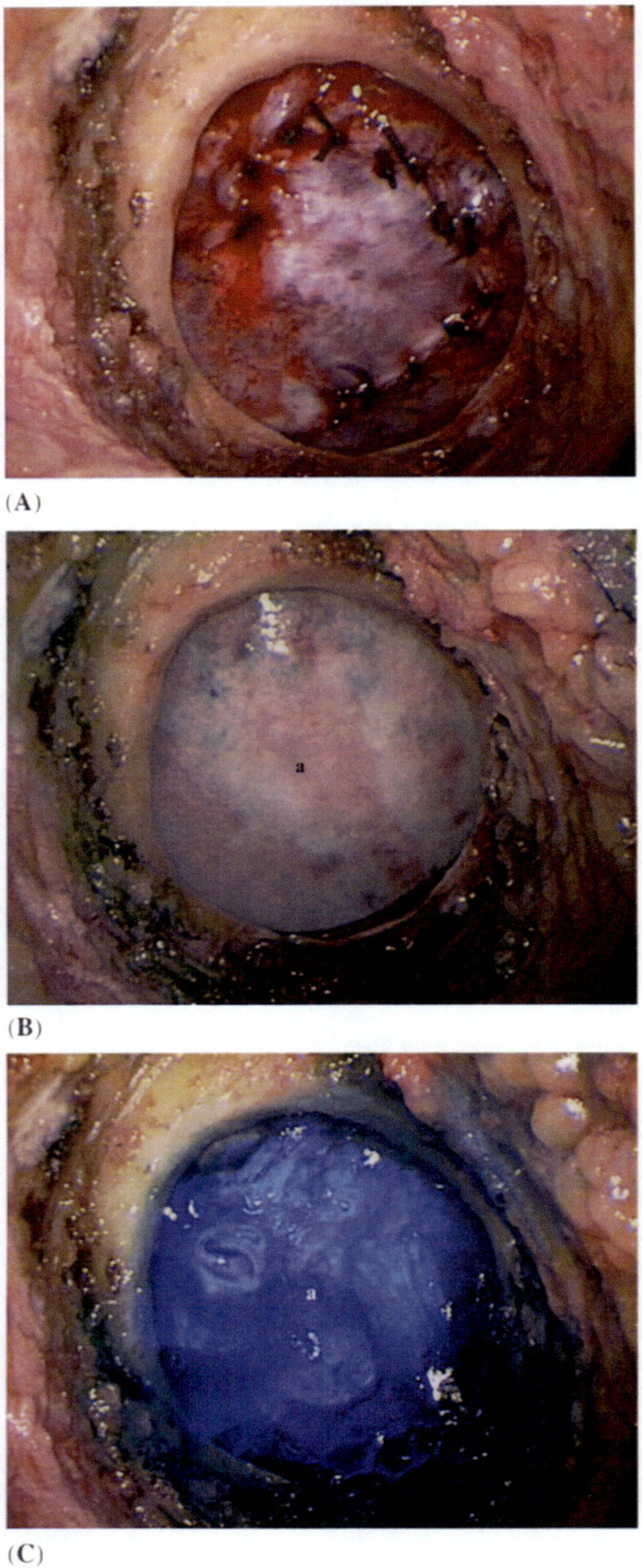

Fig. 9 (**A**)–(**C**) Closure of dura. (**B**) *a* Collagen dural substitute (onlay graft). (**C**) *a* Dural sealant.

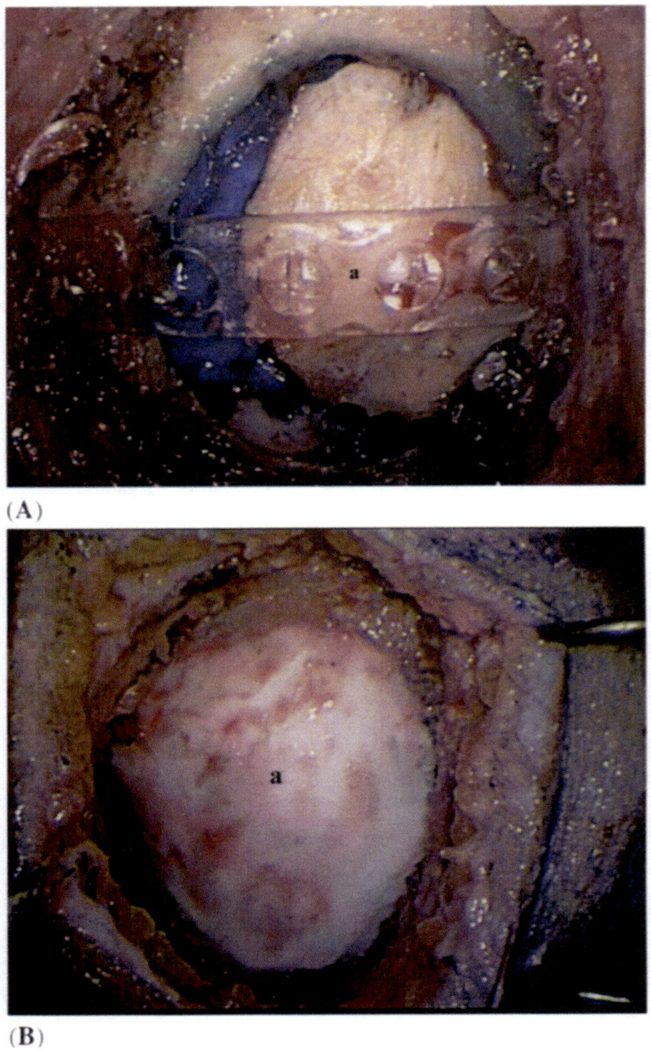

Fig. 10 (**A**) and (**B**) Cranioplasty. (**A**) *a* Absorbable microplate and screws. (**B**) *a* Hydroxyapatite bone substitute.

of the trigeminal nerve. According to our current understanding of the pathogenesis of trigeminal neuralgia, the most common cause is compression and distortion of the root entry zone (REZ) of the trigeminal nerve by aberrant arterial or venous structures (often the superior cerebellar artery), and thus removal of these traumatic insults results in alleviation of the neuropathic pain experienced by patients. Microvascular decompression (the Janetta procedure) rarely results in the numbness commonly associated with other destructive and ablative procedures.

Although trigeminal neuralgia is clinically diagnosed without the need for any additional investigations in the majority of cases, all suspected patients should have a magnetic resonance imaging/magnetic resonance angiographic (MRI/MRA) scan of the brain. These are reviewed by the surgeon and an experienced neuroradiologist to look for vessels abutting the trigeminal nerve, especially areas suspicious for compression of the trigeminal nerve at the REZ. In some cases, no discrete offending vessel is identified, but the suggestion of abnormal vascular anatomy within the prepontine and CPA cisterns coupled with the patient's clinical presentation are enough to merit surgical exploration. The MRI/MRA is also pertinent in ruling out other pathologies, such as tumors or aneurysms.

7.1.2. Approach Following the initial exposure and once the cerebellum has fallen away from the petrous portion of the temporal bone, a 0° rigid endoscope is inserted through the craniotomy, and a panoramic inspection of the CPA region is conducted. The trigeminal nerve is identified, and contiguous vessels are viewed. Particular attention is given to the parts

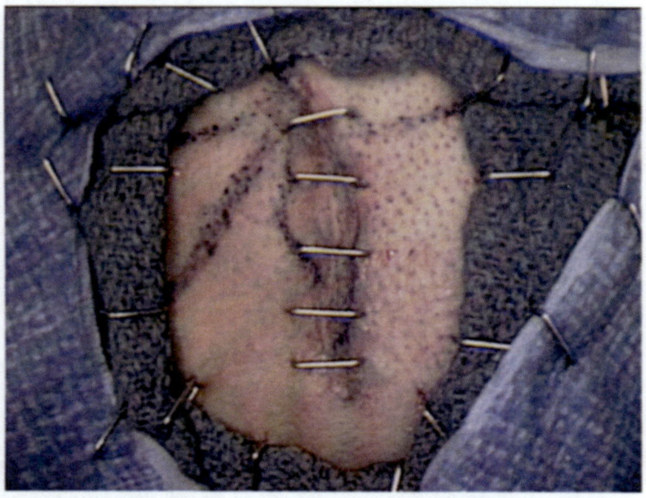

(A)

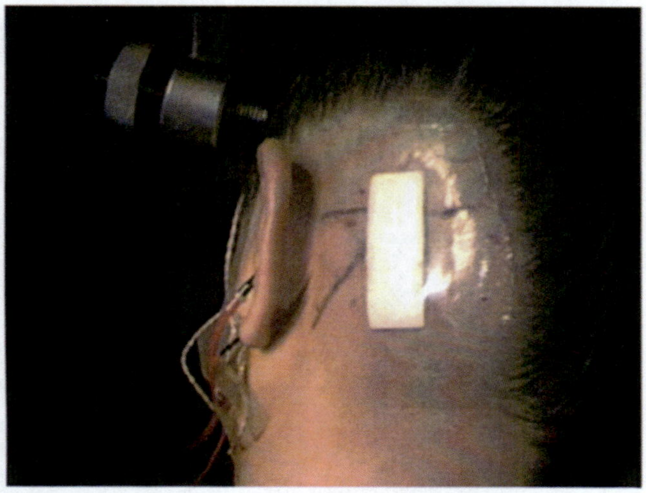

(B)

Fig. 11 (**A**) and (**B**) Skin closure and dressing.

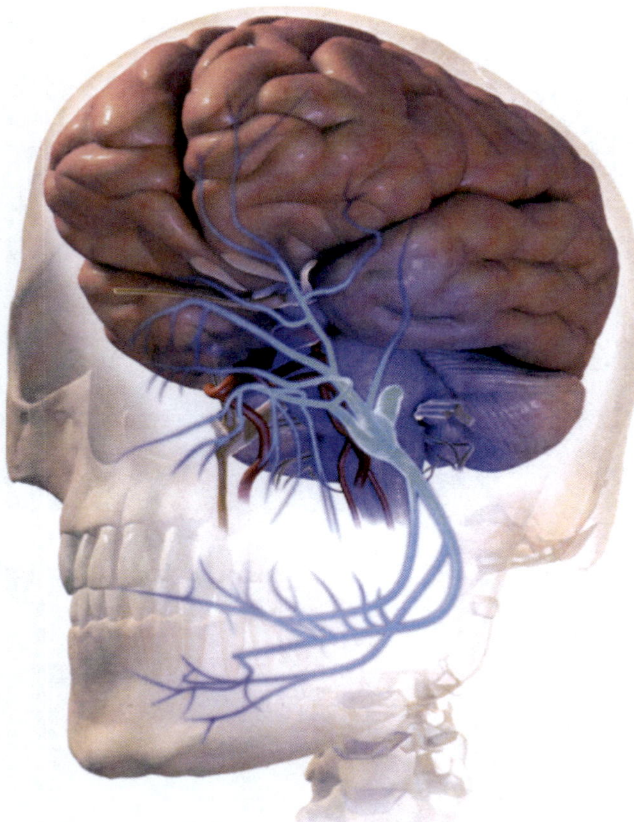

Fig. 12 Neurovascular Anatomy of Trigeminal Nerve.

of the nerve that are more obscure, including the medial and inferior aspects of the nerve at the REZ; the superior, inferior, and medial aspects of the cisternal portion of the nerve; and the site of entry of the nerve into Meckel's cave. The offending vascular structures are identified and mapped proximally and distally. A *site of compression* is defined as an area of contact between the nerve and a vessel that results in a grossly appreciable change in the appearance of the nerve, including indentation, discoloration, or other evidence of trauma to the nerve.

Once a thorough examination of the nerve is completed and the conflict is satisfactorily identified, the 0° endoscope is replaced with the 30° endoscope, and the examination is repeated. This secondary survey is critical in confirming that all neurovascular conflicts are identified because sites of compression can be multiple and complex. Dissecting instruments are then used to gently liberate the nerve from the compressing vessel. Teflon pads are interposed between the nerve and vessel to maintain the separation and to "cushion" the nerve. A final survey, utilizing the 30° endoscope, is then conducted, and further decompression is carried out if necessary. The entire area is then copiously irrigated and bathed with fibrin-based tissue glue to secure the Teflon pledgets in place; the dura is closed, followed by cranioplasty and layered closure of the soft tissues and skin.

7.1.3. Cases

7.1.3.1. Trigeminal Neuralgia (Left Sided) (Fig. 13A–F)

7.1.3.2. Trigeminal Neuralgia (Left Sided) (Fig. 14A–I)

7.1.3.3. Trigeminal Neuralgia (Right Sided) (Fig. 15A–I)

7.1.3.4. Trigeminal Neuralgia (Right Sided, Post-Gamma Knife twice) (Fig. 16A–K)

7.2. HEMIFACIAL SPASM AND GLOSSOPHARYNGEAL NEURALGIA

7.2.1. Background (Fig. 17) Hemifacial spasm is an uncommon disorder manifesting as a unilateral, involuntary, sporadic contraction of the musculature innervated by the facial nerve. The disorder almost always presents unilaterally, although bilateral involvement may occur rarely. In essentially all cases, primary hemifacial spasm is caused by an ectatic blood vessel (often the anterior inferior cerebellar artery [AICA]) that irritates, compresses, or forms a loop around the facial nerve as it exits the brainstem.

The complex anatomy of the posterior cranial fossa, as well as the limited size of the craniotomy, makes adequate visualization of the facial nerve using an operating microscope difficult. Use of an operating microscope has several limitations. The

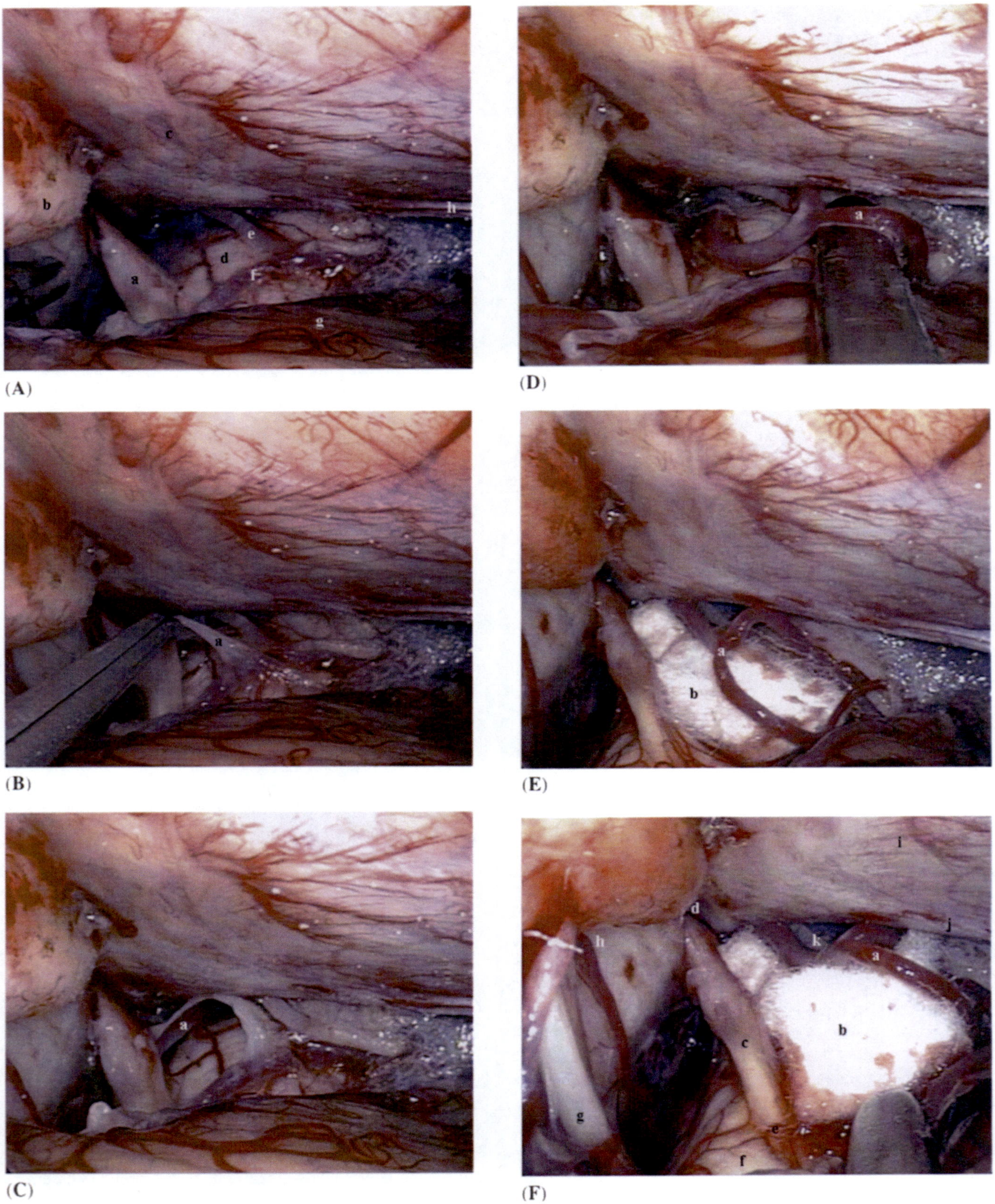

Fig. 13 (**A**) Intraoperative endoscopic close-up view showing initial exposure of trigeminal nerve and the related offending artery. *a* Trigeminal nerve (V). *b* Petrous apex. *c* Tentorium. *d* Brainstem. *e* Trochlear nerve (IV). *f* Offending artery. *g* Superior aspect of cerebellum *h* Tentorial incisura. (**B**)–(**D**) Intraoperative endoscopic view showing dissection of offending artery from the trigeminal nerve. (**B**) *a* Arachnoid. (**C**) *a* Main offending artery identified (loop of superior cerebellar artery [SCA]). (**D**) *a* Lifting of offending artery away from the trigeminal nerve REZ. (**E**) and (**F**) Intraoperative endoscopic view showing Teflon placement. (**E**) *a* Offending artery separated from the trigeminal nerve. *b* Teflon. (**F**) *a* Offending artery following complete decompression. *b* Teflon. *c* Trigeminal nerve (V). *d* Meckel's cave. *e* REZ. *f* Brainstem. *g* Acousticofacial nerve bundle. *h* Internal auditory meatus (IAM). *i* Tentorium. *j* Tentorial incisura. *k* Trochlear nerve (IV).

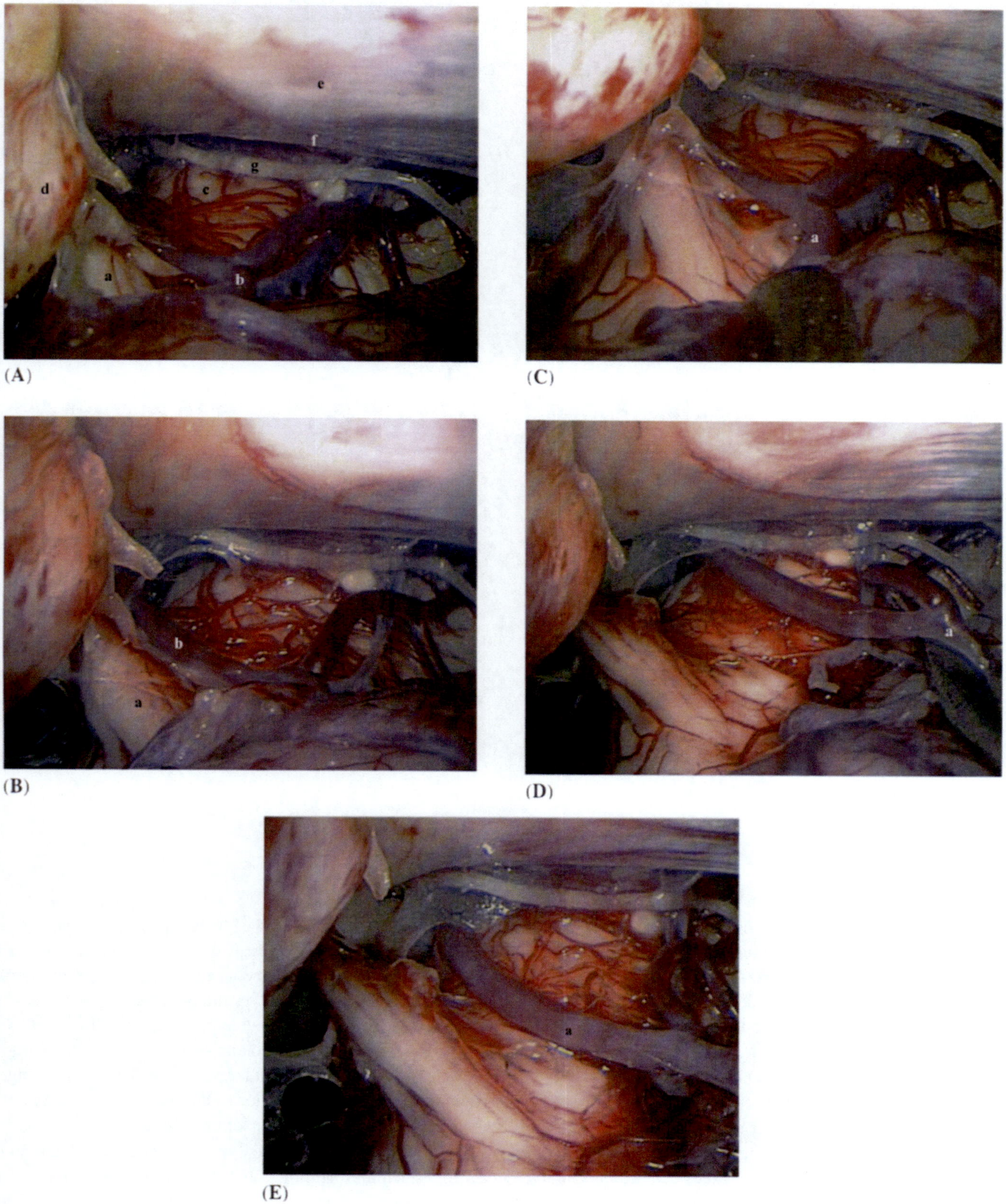

Fig. 14 (**A**) and (**B**) Intraoperative endoscopic close-up view showing the trigeminal nerve and related offending artery. (**A**) *a* Trigeminal nerve (V). *b* Offending artery. *c* Brainstem. *d* Petrous apex. *e* Tentorium. *f* Tentorial incisura. *g* Trochlear nerve (IV). (**B**) *a* Close-up view of trigeminal nerve (V). *b* Offending artery. (**C**)–(**E**) Intraoperative endoscopic view showing dissection of offending artery from trigeminal nerve. (**C**) *a* Decompression of the trigeminal nerve. (**D**) *a* Lifting of offending artery away from trigeminal nerve. (**E**) *a* Offending artery completely separated from trigeminal nerve. (**F**)–(**H**) Intraoperative endoscopic view showing Teflon placement. (**F**) *a* Trigeminal nerve (V). *b* Offending artery separated from trigeminal nerve. *c* Teflon. *d* Trochlear nerve (IV). (**G**) *a* Trigeminal nerve (V). *b* Offending artery separated from trigeminal nerve. *c* Teflon. (**H**) *a* Trigeminal nerve (V). *b* Offending artery following complete decompression. *c* Teflon. *d* Petrous apex. *e* Tentorium. *f* Trochlear nerve (IV). *g* Superior aspect of cerebellum. (**I**) Intraoperative endoscopic view showing the entire area bathed in fibrin glue. *a* Fibrin glue.

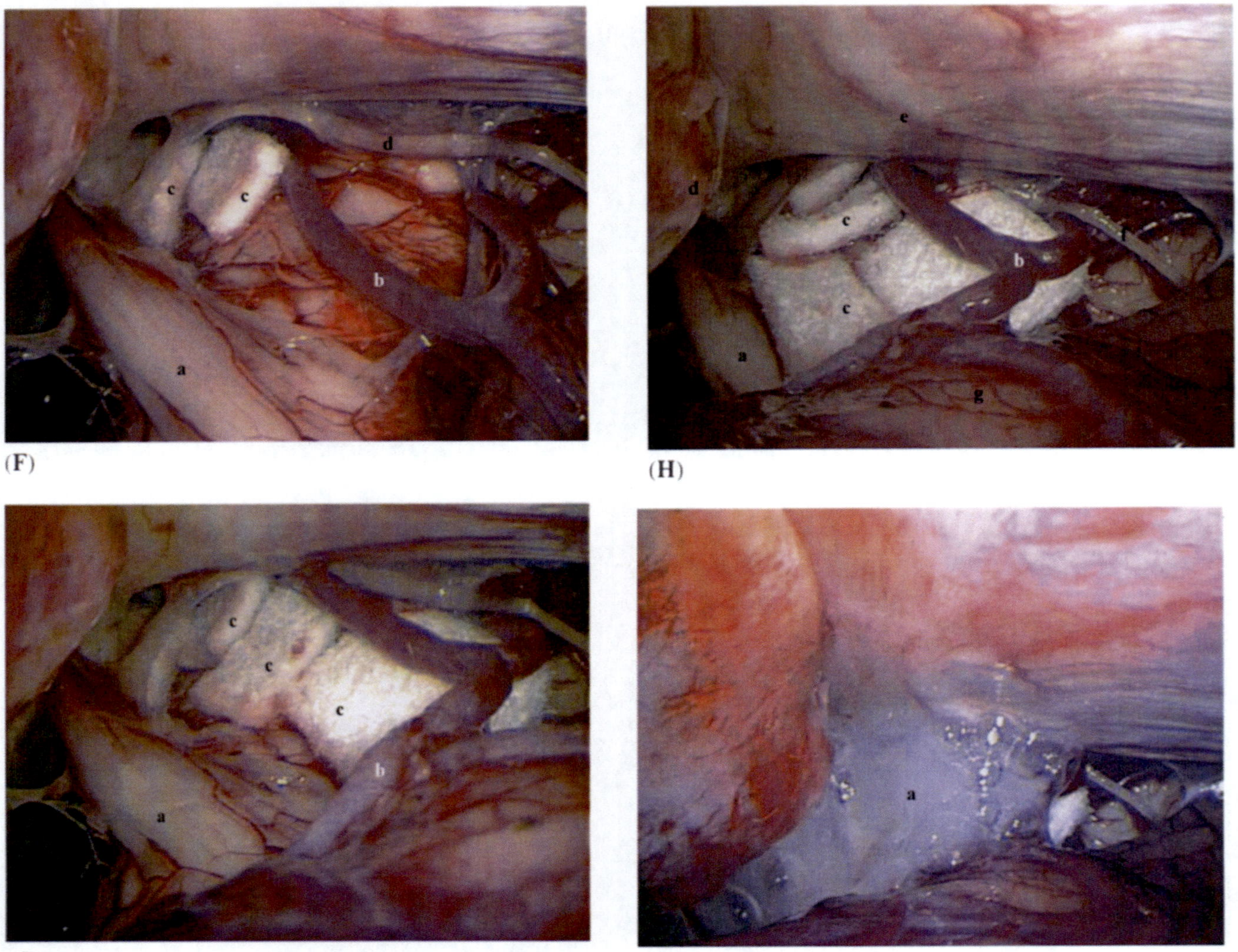

(F) (H) (G) (I)

Fig. 14 (continued)

facial nerve may not be clearly visualized medially because of an offending arterial loop, with the flocculonodular lobe of the cerebellum or the choroid plexus of the lateral recess in the way. Because the surgeon can only visualize objects directly ahead and is unable to see around objects or down narrow tortuous pathways, access to the site of disease may require wide exposure and retraction of adjacent structures. Retraction injury of the cerebellum or brainstem during decompressive surgery for hemifacial spasm can be a considerable source of morbidity. In contrast, the unimpeded view of the endoscope provides excellent panoramic views of the posterior fossa, CPA, and the root exit zone of the facial nerve and allows for identification of the nerve–vessel conflicts in all cases without the need for brain retraction. The improved visualization enhances the surgeon's ability to perform the surgical dissection and assess the adequacy of the decompression, both of which are often difficult to appreciate using the operating microscope.

Glossopharyngeal neuralgia is a rare clinical entity; it is characterized by severe paroxysmal attacks of sharp, lancinating pain affecting the sensory distribution of the glossopharyngeal nerve, including the base of the tongue, soft palate, tonsils, pharyngeal pillars, posterior pharyngeal wall, and the inner ear. Attacks may be associated with vagally mediated cardiovascular and hemodynamic compromise, such as bradycardia, hypotension, and cardiac syncope; rarely, asystole may occur with episodes of neuralgia. Microvascular decompression of the glossopharyngeal nerve is an effective treatment for patients with glossopharyngeal neuralgia in whom compression of the nerve by a blood vessel is implicated in the pathogenesis of the disease.

In the surgical management of glossopharyngeal neuralgia, as for trigeminal neuralgia and hemifacial spasm, the use of endoscopes of varying angles is ideal because all neurovascular conflicts can be identified, and decompression of the nerve can be successfully performed with minimal disturbance to the surrounding structures.

7.2.2. Approach Following entry into the CPA, the acousticofacial bundle is visualized, and the facial nerve is stimulated and positively identified. Once identified, the surrounding vascular structures are surveyed to identify the nerve–vessel conflict compressing the facial nerve. The 0° endoscope is replaced

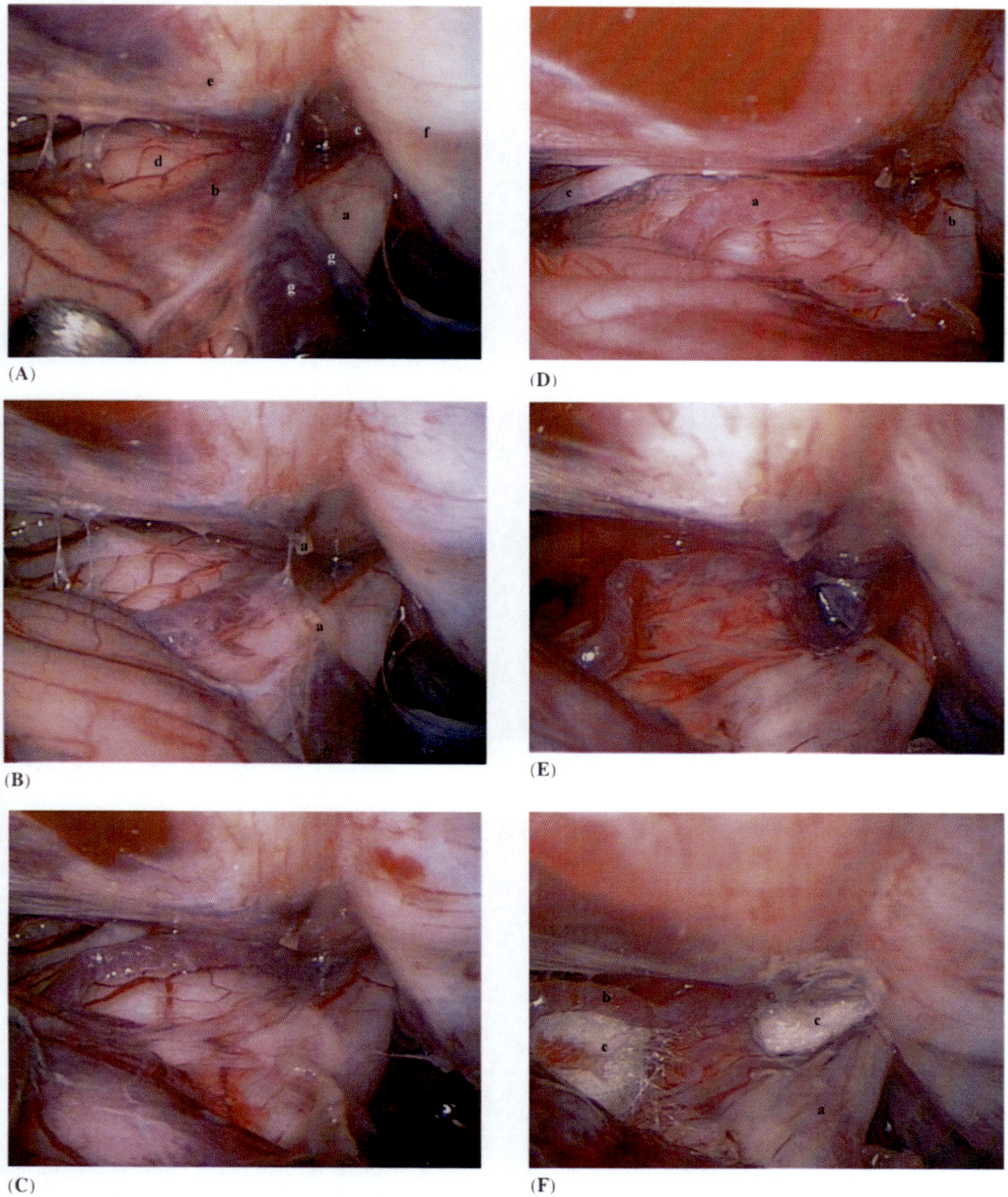

Fig. 15 (**A**) Intraoperative endoscopic close-up view showing the trigeminal nerve and related offending vessels. *a* Trigeminal nerve (V). *b* Offending artery. *c* Meckel's cave. *d* Brainstem. *e* Tentorium. *f* Petrous apex. *g* Cross-compressing offending veins. (**B**)–(**E**) Intraoperative endoscopic view showing dissection of offending vessels from the trigeminal nerve. (**B**) *a* Cross-compressing veins are electrocoagulated and divided. (**D**) *a* Close-up view of offending artery after separation from trigeminal nerve. *b* Trigeminal nerve (V). *c* Trochlear nerve (IV). (**F**)–(**H**) Intraoperative endoscopic view showing Teflon Placement. (**F**) *a* Trigeminal nerve (V). *b* Offending artery separated from the trigeminal nerve. *c* Teflon. (**G**) *a* Close-up view of the trigeminal nerve. (**H**) *a* Trigeminal nerve (V). *b* Teflon pieces completely padding the trigeminal nerve. *c* Superior aspect of cerebellum. *d* Acousticofacial nerve bundle (VII, VIII). *e* Tentorium. *f* Petrous temporal bone. (**I**) Intraoperative endoscopic view showing the entire area bathed in fibrin glue. *a* Fibrin glue.

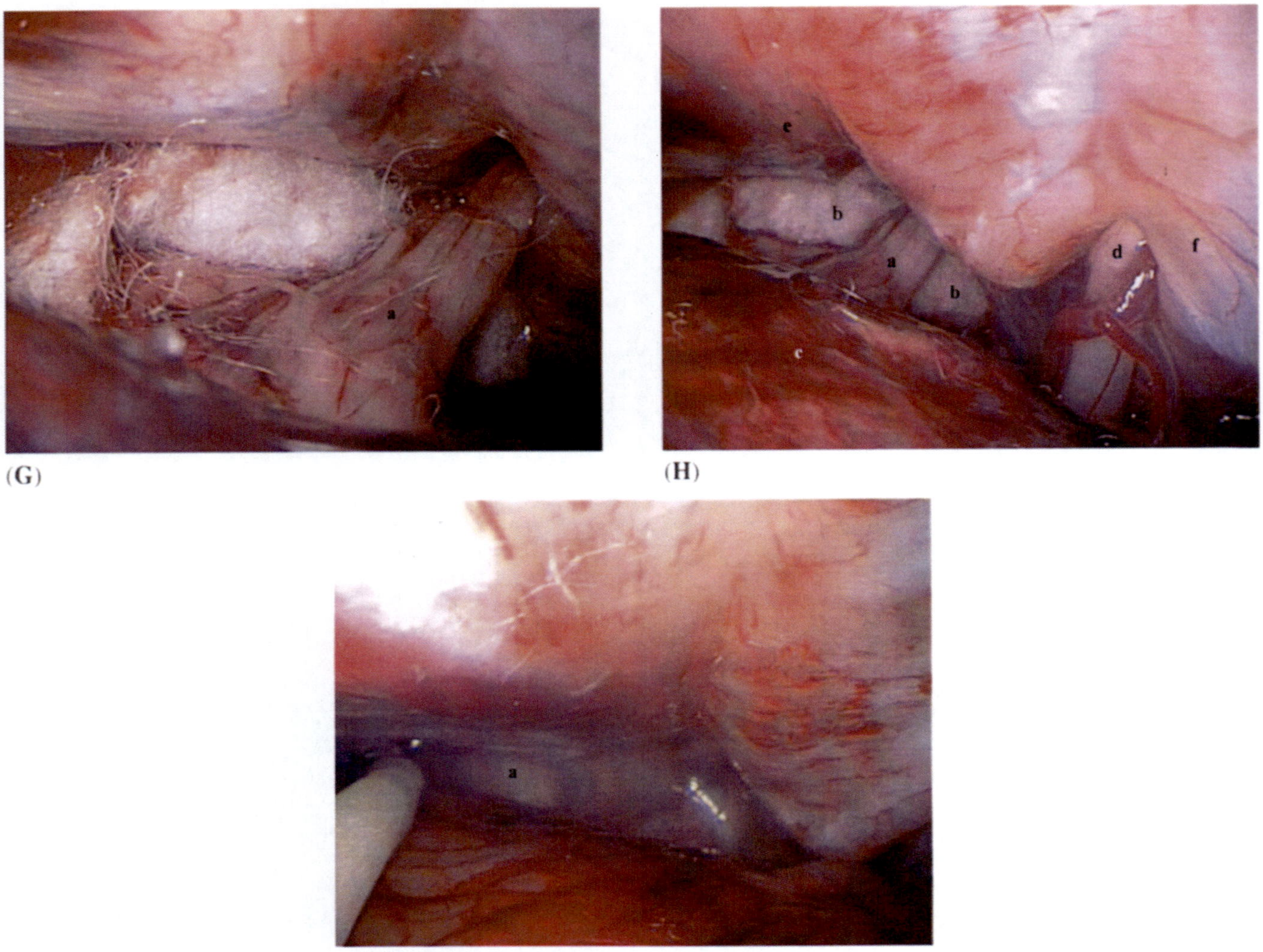

(G) (H)

(I)

Fig. 15 (continued)

with the 30° endoscope, and as in cases of trigeminal neuralgia, a secondary survey is conducted to confirm that all neurovascular conflicts are identified. Using microdissection and gentle manipulation, vascular compressions of the facial nerve are dissected free. Teflon pledgets are then placed between the nerve and compressing vessels to provide complete decompression; they are secured in place with fibrin glue. The dura is then reapproximated, providing a watertight closure, and layered suturing of the wound is carried out.

The surgical approach to the lower cranial nerves, as in glossopharyngeal neuralgia, is essentially identical to that described above. Once the endoscope is passed into the CPA cistern, cranial nerves IX to XI are located caudally in the surgical field. They are identified by their "guitar-string" appearance and are seen passing into the jugular foramen. Closure is then carried out in the usual fashion. Care must be taken while manipulating the endoscope and dissecting instruments so the neurovascular structures located immediately cranially but out of view of the lens are not damaged.

7.2.3. Cases

7.2.3.1. Hemifacial Spasm (Left Sided) (Fig. 18A–H)

7.2.3.2. Hemifacial Spasm (Right Sided) (Fig. 19A–F)

7.2.3.3. Hemifacial Spasm (Right Sided) (Fig. 20A–J)

7.2.3.4. Hemifacial Spasm (Left Sided) (Fig. 21A–H)

7.2.3.5. Glossopharyngeal Neuralgia (Left Sided) (Fig. 22A–D)

7.3. VESTIBULAR (ACOUSTIC) SCHWANNOMA AND POSTERIOR FOSSA MENINGIOMA

7.3.1. Background (Fig. 23) Vestibular schwannoma, also known as acoustic neuroma or neurinoma, is a benign overproliferation of the Schwann cells of the eighth cranial nerve sheath. MRI is the gold standard in assessing patients with this tumor. Acoustic neuromas are typically described as small (less than 1.5 cm), medium (1.5 to 2.5 cm), or large (greater than 2.5 cm). A small acoustic neuroma is also referred to as *intracanalicular* because it is confined within the bony IAC. A medium-size acoustic neuroma has extended from the bony canal into the brain cavity without producing pressure on

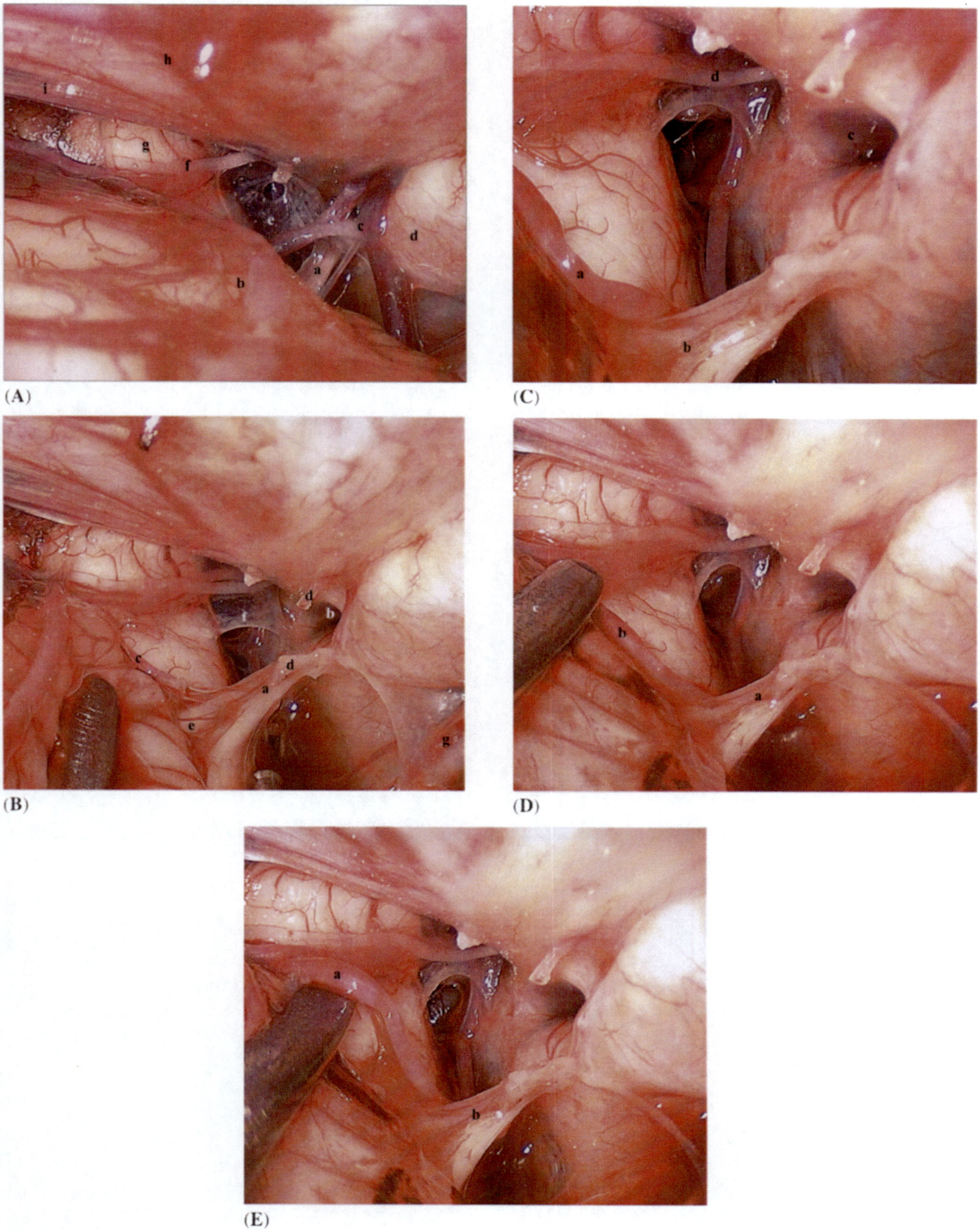

Fig. 16 (**A**) Intraoperative endoscopic close-up view showing the trigeminal nerve and the related neurovascular anatomy. *a* Trigeminal nerve (V). *b* Superior aspect of cerebellum. *c* Petrosal veins. *d* Petrous apex. *e* Dense arachnoid adhesions (post-Gamma KnifeX2). *f* Trochlear nerve (IV). *g* Brainstem. *h* Tentorium. *i* Tentorial incisura. (**B**)–(**F**) Intraoperative endoscopic view showing dissection of offending artery from trigeminal nerve. (**B**) *a* Trigeminal nerve (V). *b* Meckel's cave. *c* Offending artery (superior cerebellar artery [SCA]). *d* Petrosal veins electrocoagulated and divided. *e* REZ. *f* Arachnoid adhesions. *g* Acousticofacial nerve bundle (VII, VIII). (**C**) *a* Close-up view of offending artery. *b* Trigeminal nerve (V). *c* Meckel's cave. *d* Trochlear nerve (IV). *e* Contralateral trigeminal nerve (V). (**D**) *a* Close-up view of the trigeminal nerve. *b* Offending artery. *c* An elevator is introduced to separate the offending artery from the nerve. (**E**) *a* Elevation of offending artery away from trigeminal nerve. *b* Trigeminal nerve (V).

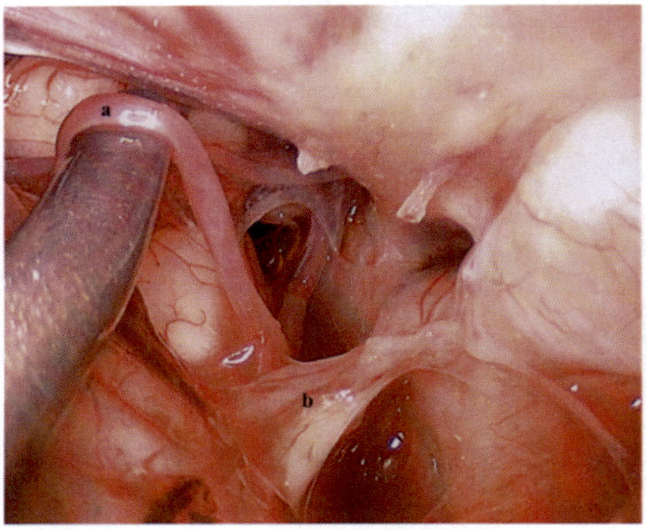

(F)

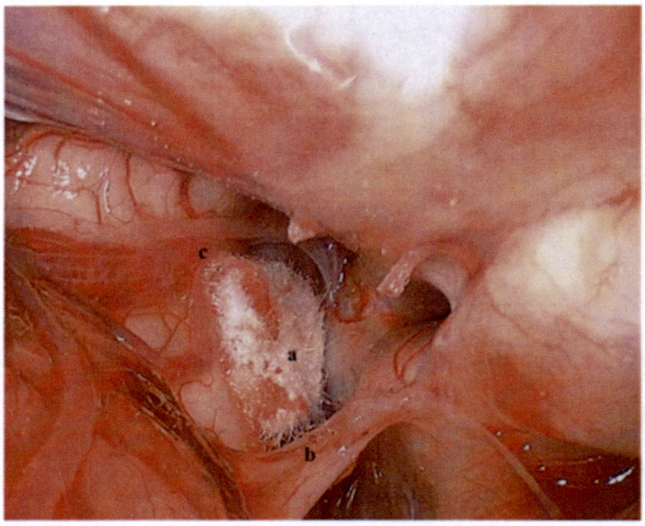

(G)

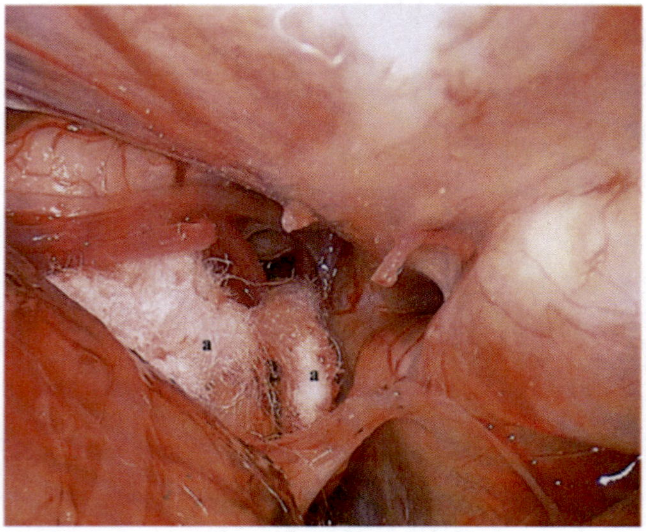

(H)

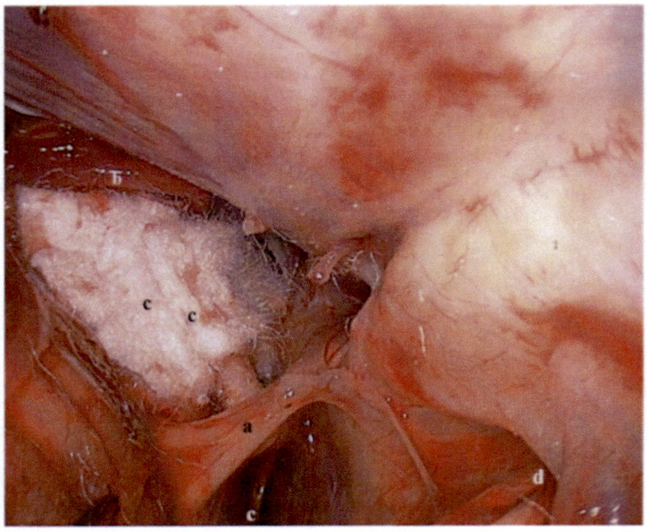

(I)

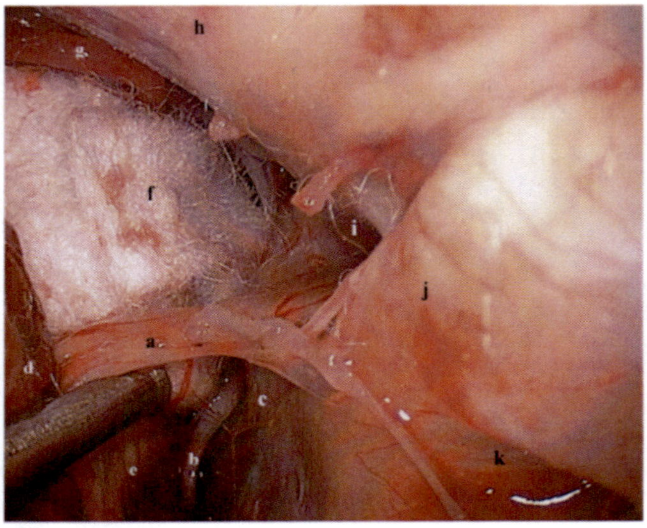

(J)

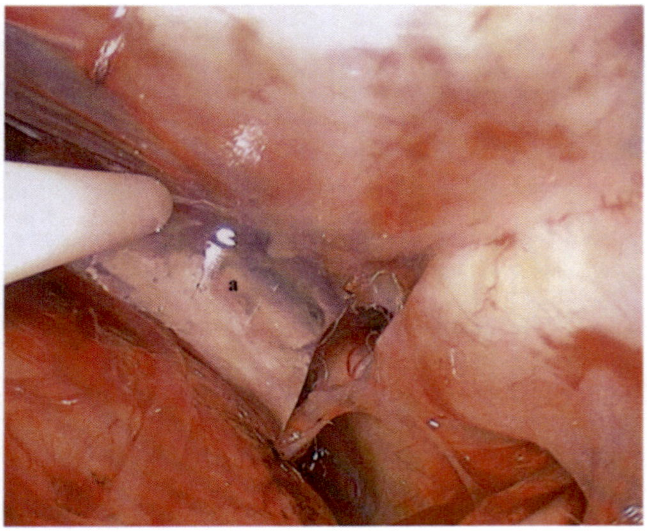

(K)

Fig. 16 (continued) (**F**) *a* Close-up view showing elevation of offending artery. *b* Trigeminal nerve (V). (**G**)–(**J**) Intraoperative endoscopic view showing the Teflon placement. (**G**) *a* Teflon. *b* Trigeminal nerve (V). *c* Offending artery. (**H**) *a* Teflon. (**I**) *a* Trigeminal nerve (V). *b* Offending artery completely separated from trigeminal nerve. *c* Teflon. (**J**) *a* Trigeminal nerve (V). *b* Abducent nerve. *c* Clivus. *d* Lateral aspect of cerebellum. *e* Brainstem. *f* Teflon. *g* Offending artery. *h* Tentorium. *i* Meckel's cave. *j* Petrous apex. *k* Internal auditory meatus (IAM). (**K**) Intraoperative endoscopic view showing the entire area bathed in fibrin glue. *a*. Fibrin glue.

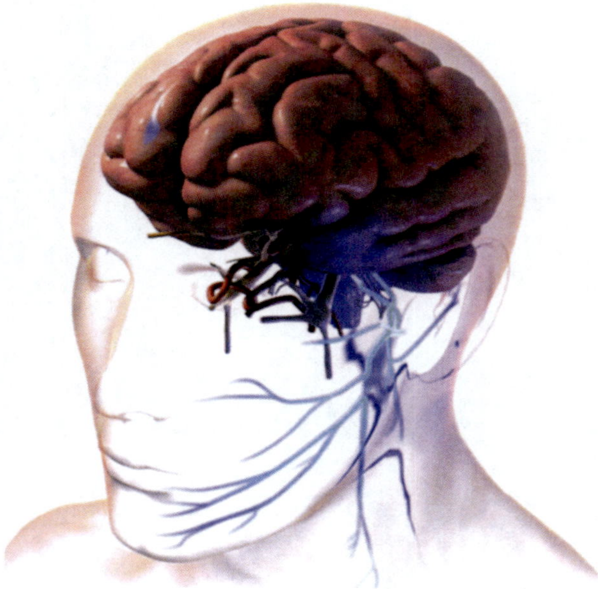

Fig. 17 Neurovascular Anatomy of Facial Nerve.

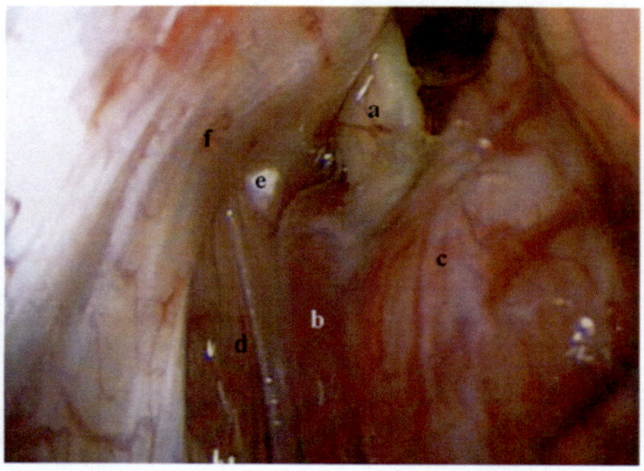

(A)

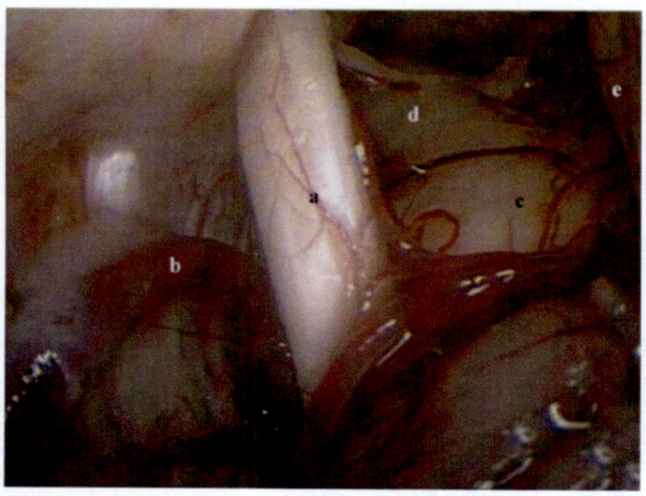

(B)

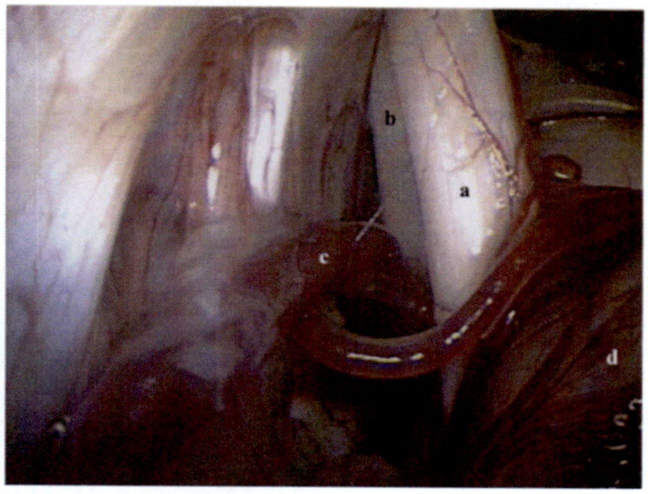

(C)

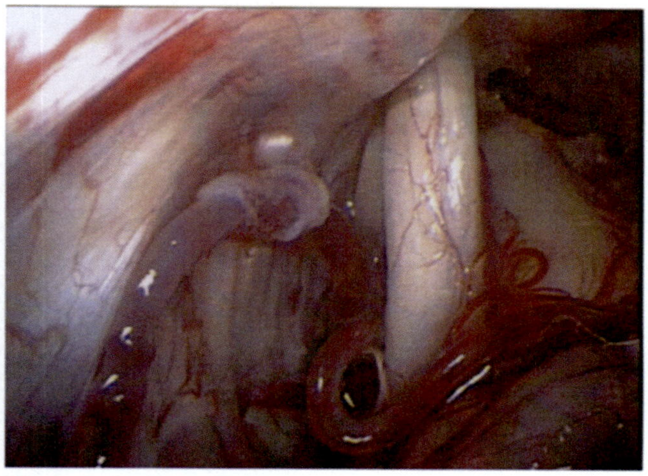

(D)

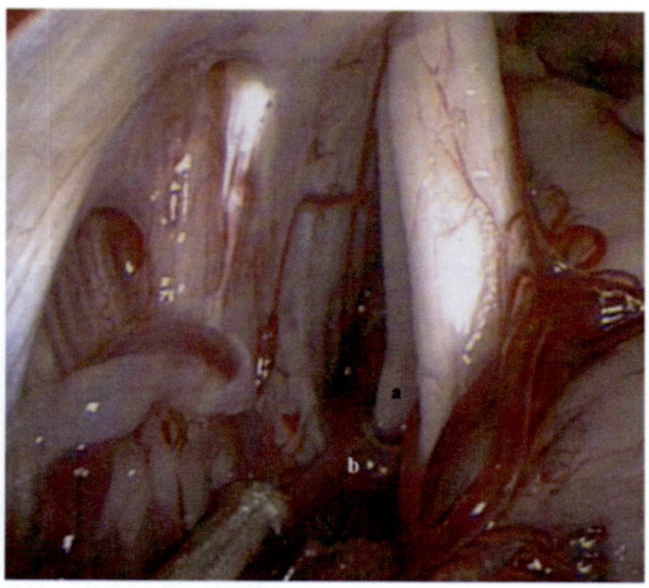

(E)

Fig. 18 (**A**) Intraoperative endoscopic close-up view showing acousticofacial nerve bundle and related offending artery. *a* Acousticofacial nerve bundle. *b* Offending artery covered with arachnoid layer (anterior inferior cerebellar artery [AICA]). *c* Lateral aspect of cerebellum. *d* Lower cranial nerves. *e* Jugular foramen. *f* Petrous temporal bone. (**B**)–(**E**) Intraoperative endoscopic view showing dissection of offending

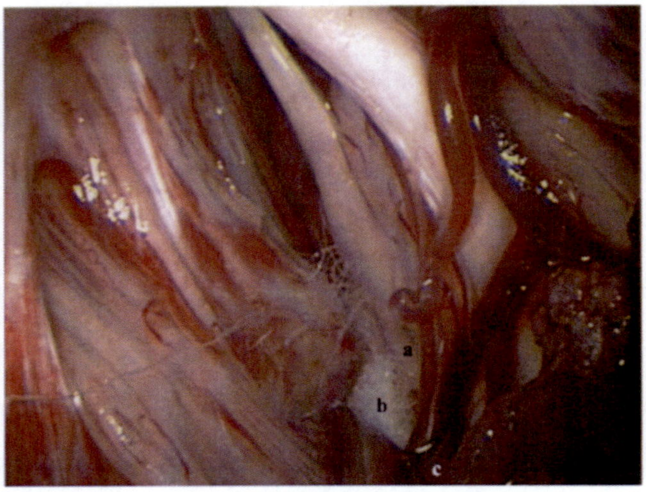

(F)

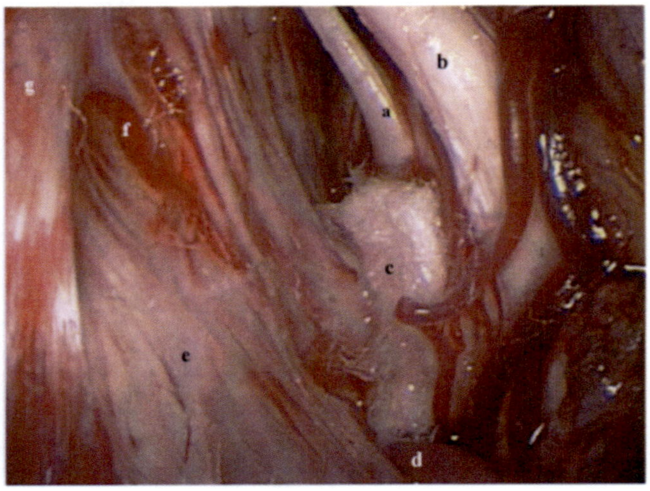

(G)

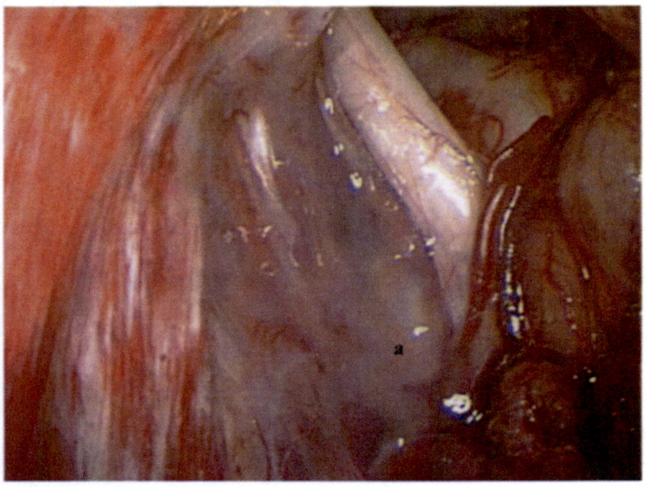

(H)

Fig. 18 (continued) artery from the facial nerve. (**B**) *a* Acousticofacial nerve bundle (VII, VIII). *b* Offending artery. *c* Brainstem. *d* Trigeminal nerve (V). *e* Lateral aspect of cerebellum. (**C**) *a* Vestibulocochlear nerve (VIII). *b* Facial nerve (VII). *c* Offending artery. *d* Brainstem. (**E**) *a* Close-up view of facial nerve (VII). *b* Site of contact between facial nerve and offending artery. (**F**) and (**G**) Intraoperative endoscopic view showing the Teflon pads separating the vessel from the facial nerve. (**F**) *a* Facial nerve (VII). *b* Teflon. *c* Offending artery. (**G**) *a* Facial nerve (VII). *b* Vestibulocochlear nerve (VIII). *c* Teflon. *d* Offending artery. *e* Lower cranial nerves. *f* Jugular foramen. *g* Petrous temporal bone. (**H**) Intraoperative endoscopic view showing entire area bathed in fibrin glue. (**H**) *a* Fibrin glue.

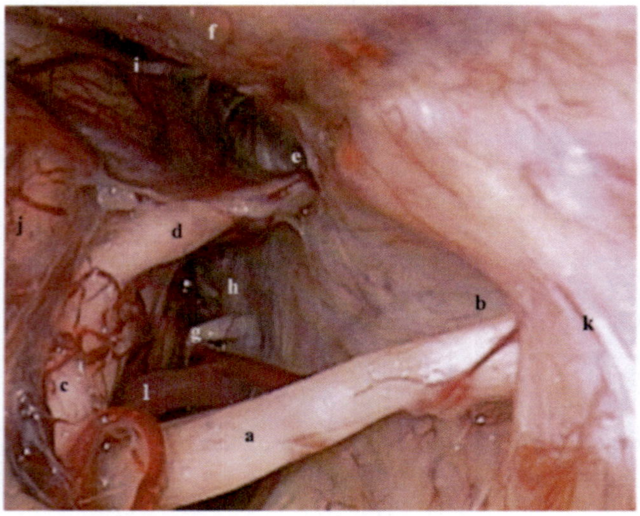

(A)

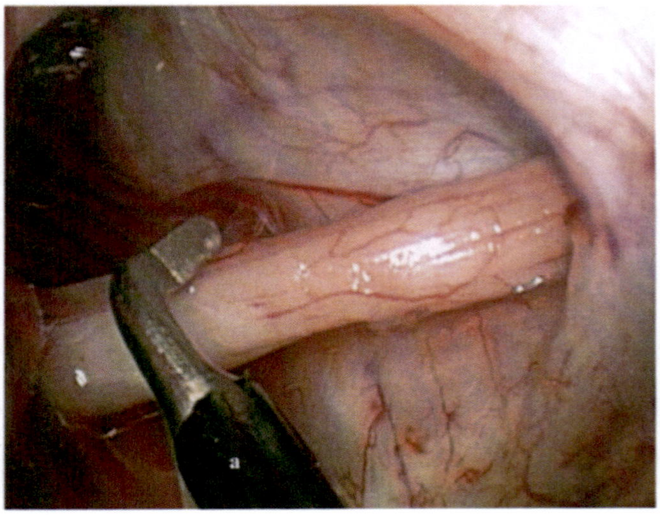

(B)

Fig. 19 (**A**) and (**B**) Intraoperative endoscopic view showing acousticofacial nerve bundle and offending arteries. (**A**) *a* Acousticofacial nerve bundle. *b* Internal auditory meatus (IAM). *c* Brainstem. *d* Trigeminal nerve (V). *e* Meckel's cave. *f* Tentorium. *g* Abducent Nerve. *h* Clivus. *i* Trochlear nerve (IV). *j* Lateral aspect of cerebellum. *k* Petrous temporal bone. *l* Offending artery (anterior inferior cerebellar artery [AICA]).

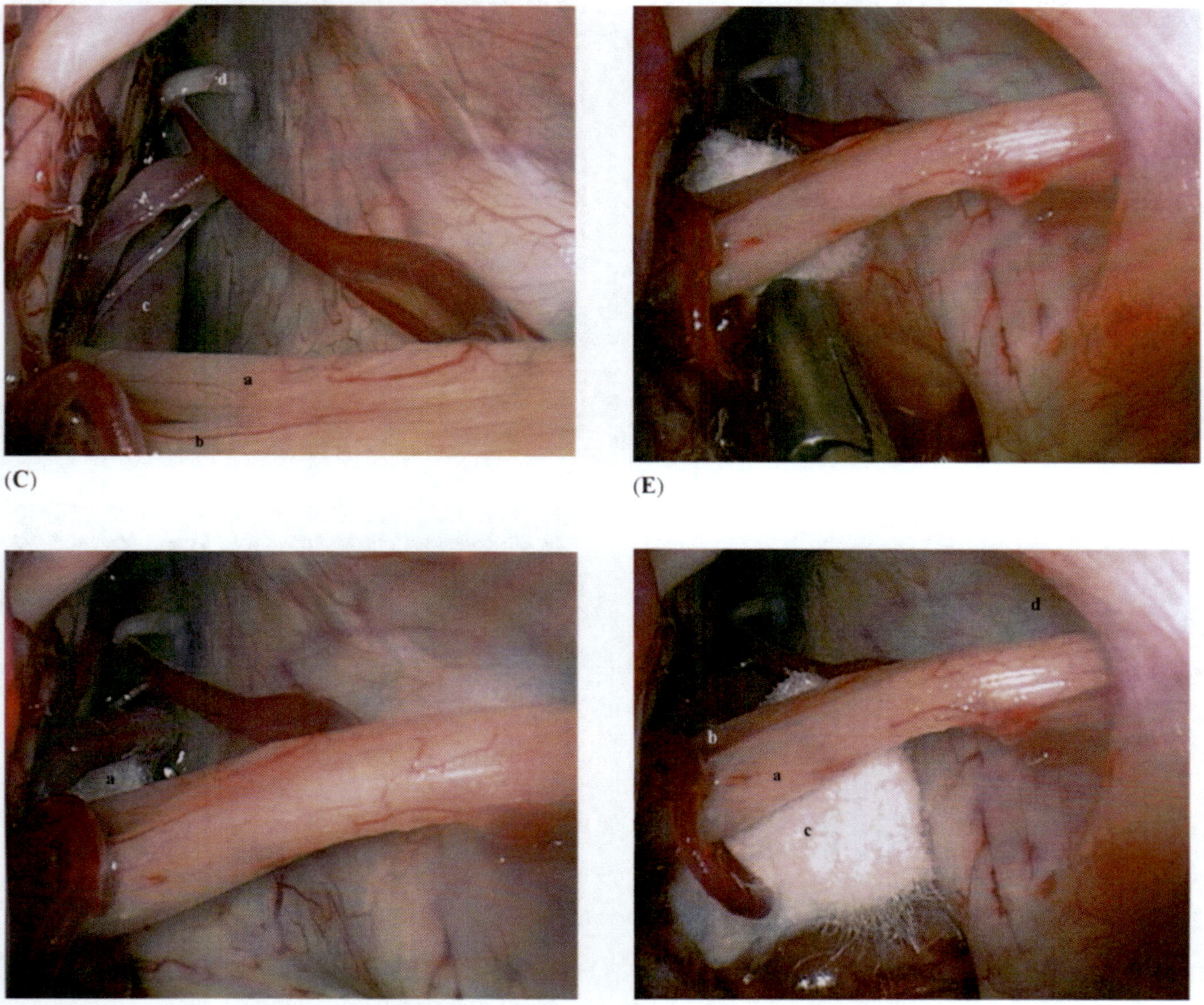

(C) (E)

(D) (F)

Fig. 19 (continued) (**B**) Close-up view of the acousticofacial nerve bundle and the regional anatomy. *a* Facial nerve stimulator (**C**) Intraoperative endoscopic view showing offending artery. (**C**) *a* Facial nerve (VII). *b* Vestibulocochlear nerve (VIII). *c* Main offending artery (vertebral artery). *d* Abducent nerve (VI) passing thru Dorello's canal. (**D**)–(**F**) Intraoperative endoscopic view showing Teflon placement. (**D**) *a* Teflon. (**F**) *a* Vestibulocochlear nerve (VIII). *b* Facial nerve (VII). *c* Teflon. *d* Internal auditory meatus (IAM).

the brain tissue itself. Large acoustic neuromas usually produce pressure manifestations.

Traditionally, either the translabyrinthine or the open suboccipital approach have been used to access and remove CPA tumors such as vestibular schwannomas. The traditional suboccipital approach suffers from the disadvantages of the operating microscope with its direct forward view, including the inability to completely visualize the lateral extent of the tumor within the IAC. Using the operating microscope, it is virtually impossible to "look around the corner" due to the oblique angle of the canal in relation to the trajectory of the dissection, as well as incomplete visualization of exposed air cells, which may lead to CSF rhinorrhea or otorrhea. The translabyrinthine approach allows wide exposure of the IAC and early identification of the facial nerve, which assists its preservation. However, this approach requires a wide disfiguring skin incision along with excessive drilling through the mastoid bone and inner ear, unfortunately resulting in complete hearing loss in all cases, as well as a significantly higher incidence of postoperative CSF leakage.

The endoscope, with its superior visualization and imaging, provides improved recognition of exposed air cells and allows for more complete tumor removal by direct visualization of the

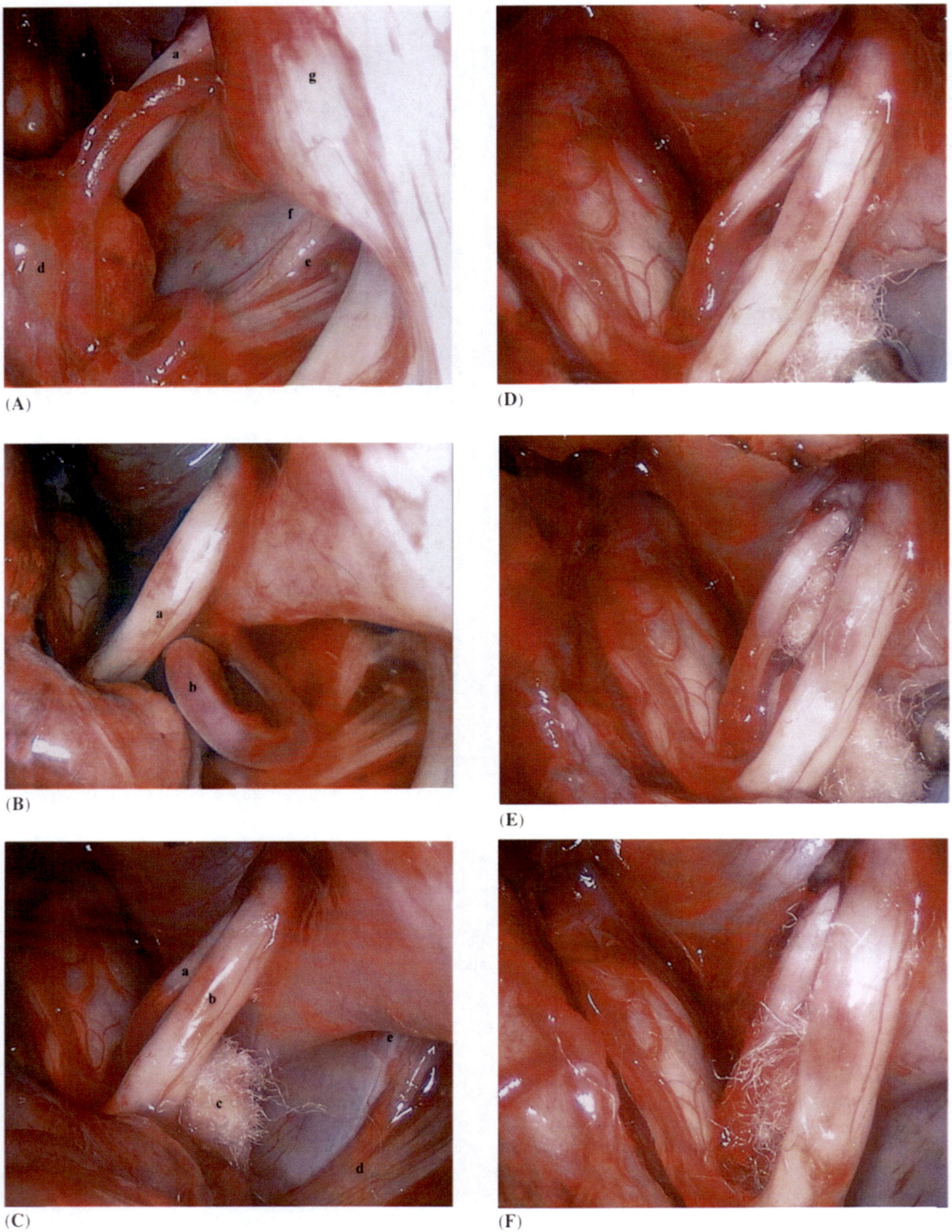

Fig. 20 (**A**) Intraoperative endoscopic close-up view showing acousticofacial bundle and offending arteries. *a* Acousticofacial nerve bundle (VII, VIII). *b* Offending artery. *c* Brainstem. *d*. Lateral aspect of cerebellum. *e* Lower cranial nerves (IX–XI). *f* Jugular foramen. *g* Petrous temporal bone. (**B**)–(**J**) Intraoperative endoscopic view showing dissection of offending arteries from facial nerve and Teflon placement. (**B**) *a* Acousticofacial nerve bundle (VII, VIII). *b* Offending artery. (**C**) *a* Facial nerve (VII). *b* Vestibulocochlear nerve (VIII). *c* Teflon. *d* Lower cranial nerves (IX–XI). *e* Jugular foramen. (**G**) *a* Facial nerve (VII). *b* Vestibulocochlear nerve (VIII). *c* Offending artery. *d* Teflon. (**H**) *a* Facial nerve (VII). *b* Vestibulocochlear nerve (VIII). *c* Offending artery. *d* Teflon. (**I**) *a* Facial nerve (VII). *b* Vestibulocochlear nerve (VIII). *c* Offending artery. *d* Teflon. *e* Brainstem. *f* Petrous temporal bone. *g* Lower cranial nerves (IX–XI). (**J**) *a* Fibrin glue.

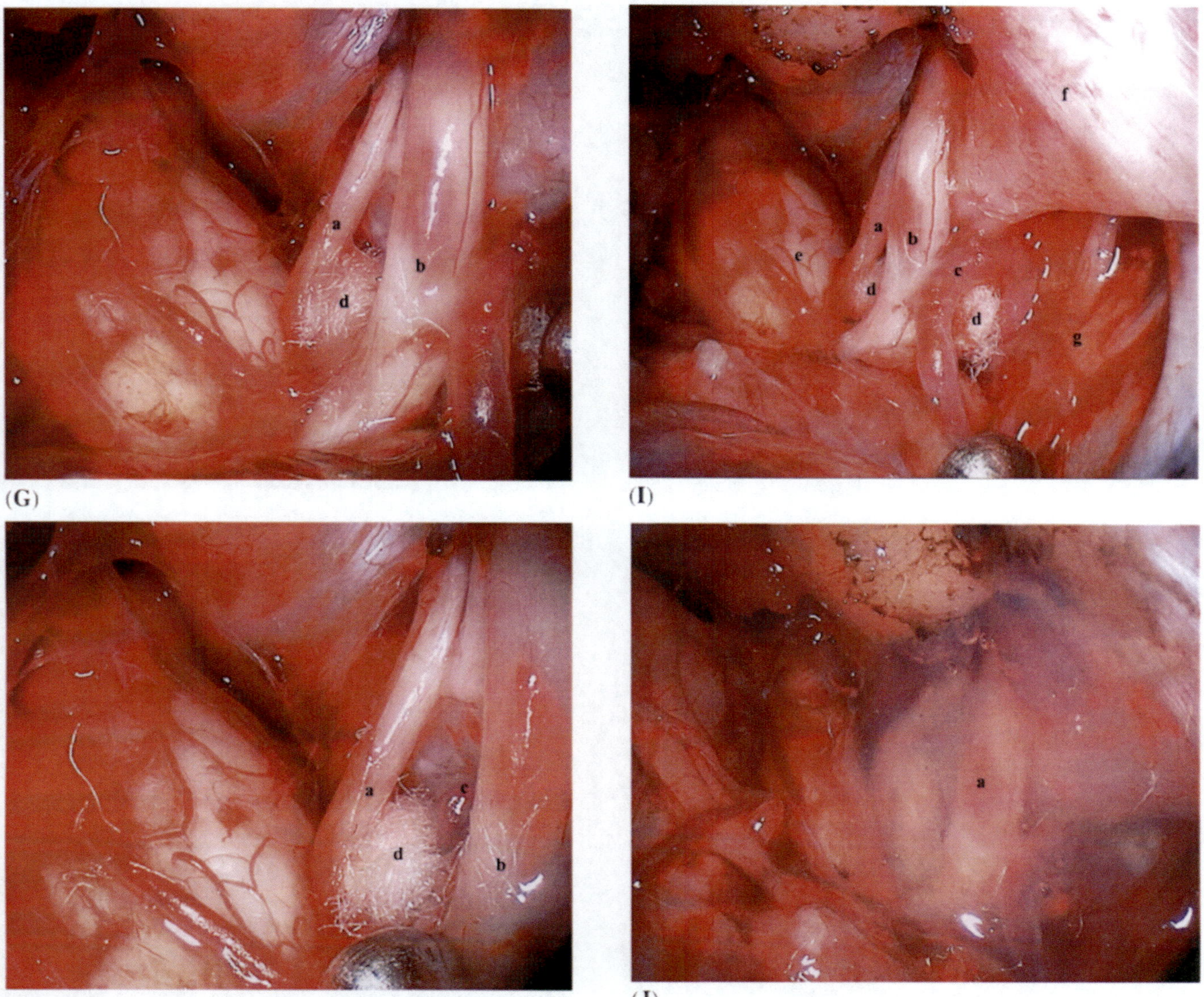

(G) (I) (H) (J)

Fig. 20 (continued)

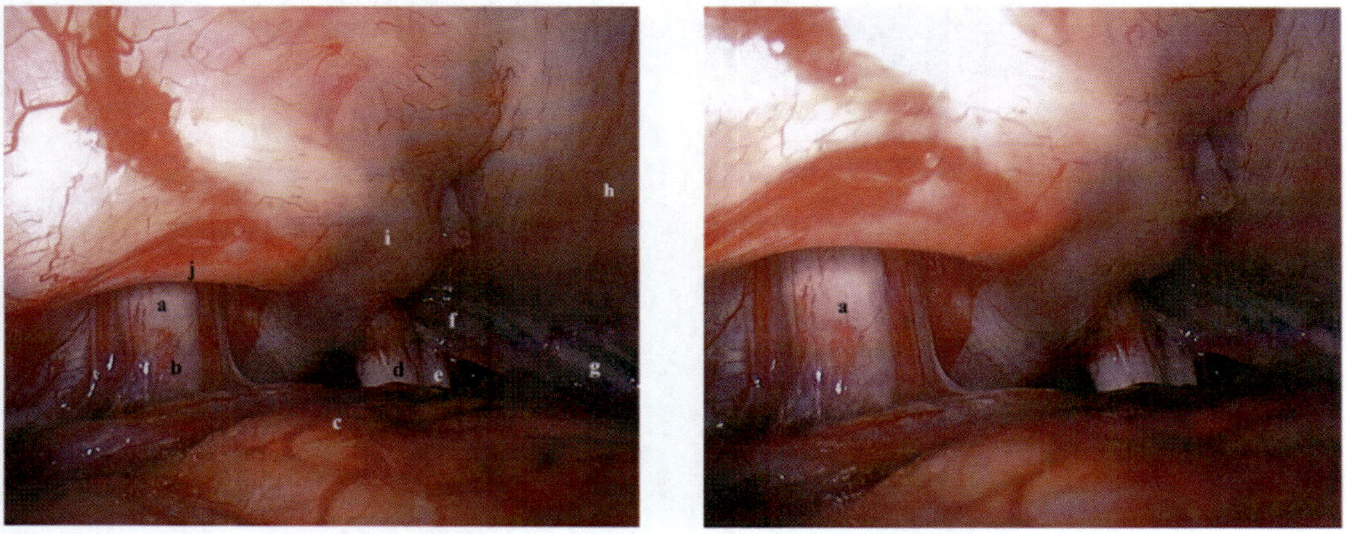

(A) (B)

Fig. 21 (**A**) Intraoperative endoscopic close-up view showing initial exposure of acousticofacial nerve bundle. *a* Facial nerve (VII). *b* Vestibulocochlear nerve (VIII). *c* Superior aspect of cerebellum. *d* Trigeminal nerve (V) sensory root. *e* Trigeminal nerve (V) motor root. *f* Superior cerebellar artery (SCA). *g* Trochlear nerve (IV). *h* Tentorium. *i* Petrous apex. *j* Internal auditory meatus (IAM). (**B**) *a* Close-up view of facial nerve (VII) and regional anatomy. (**C**)–(**H**) Intraoperative endoscopic view showing dissection of offending artery from facial nerve and Teflon placement. (**C**) *a* Facial nerve (VII). *b* Vestibulocochlear nerve (VIII). *c* Offending artery loop (anterior inferior cerebellar artery [AICA]). *d* Abducent nerve (VI). *e* brainstem (**D**) *a* Close-up view of offending artery loop and regional anatomy. (**E**) *a* Elevation of offending arterial loop away from facial nerve. *b* Acousticofacial nerve bundle (VII, VIII). *c* Lower cranial nerves (IX–XI). (**F**) *a* Close-up view using 30° endoscope showing offending arterial loop completely

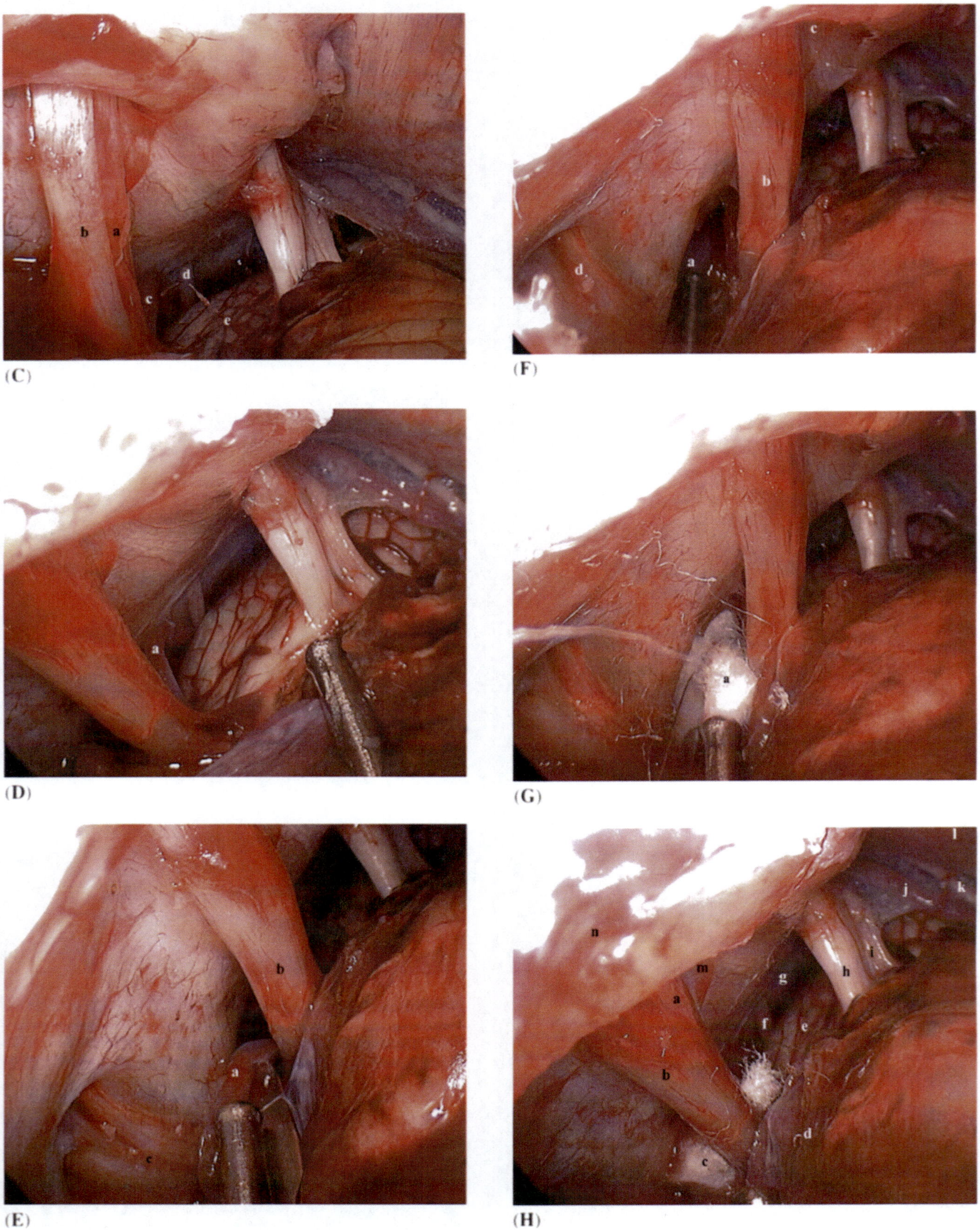

Fig. 21 (continued) separated from facial nerve. *b* Acousticofacial nerve bundle (VII, VIII). *c* Internal auditory meatus (IAM). *d* Lower cranial nerves (IX-XI). **(G)** *a* Teflon. **(H)** *a* Facial nerve (VII). *b* Vestibular nerve (VIII). *c* Teflon. *d* Lateral aspect of cerebellum. *e* Brainstem. *f* Abducent nerve (VI). *g* Clivus. *h* Trigeminal nerve (V) sensory root. *i* Trigeminal nerve (V) motor root. *j* Superior cerebellar artery (SCA). *k* Trochlear nerve (IV). *l* Tentorium. *m* Internal auditory meatus (IAM). *n* Petrous temporal bone.

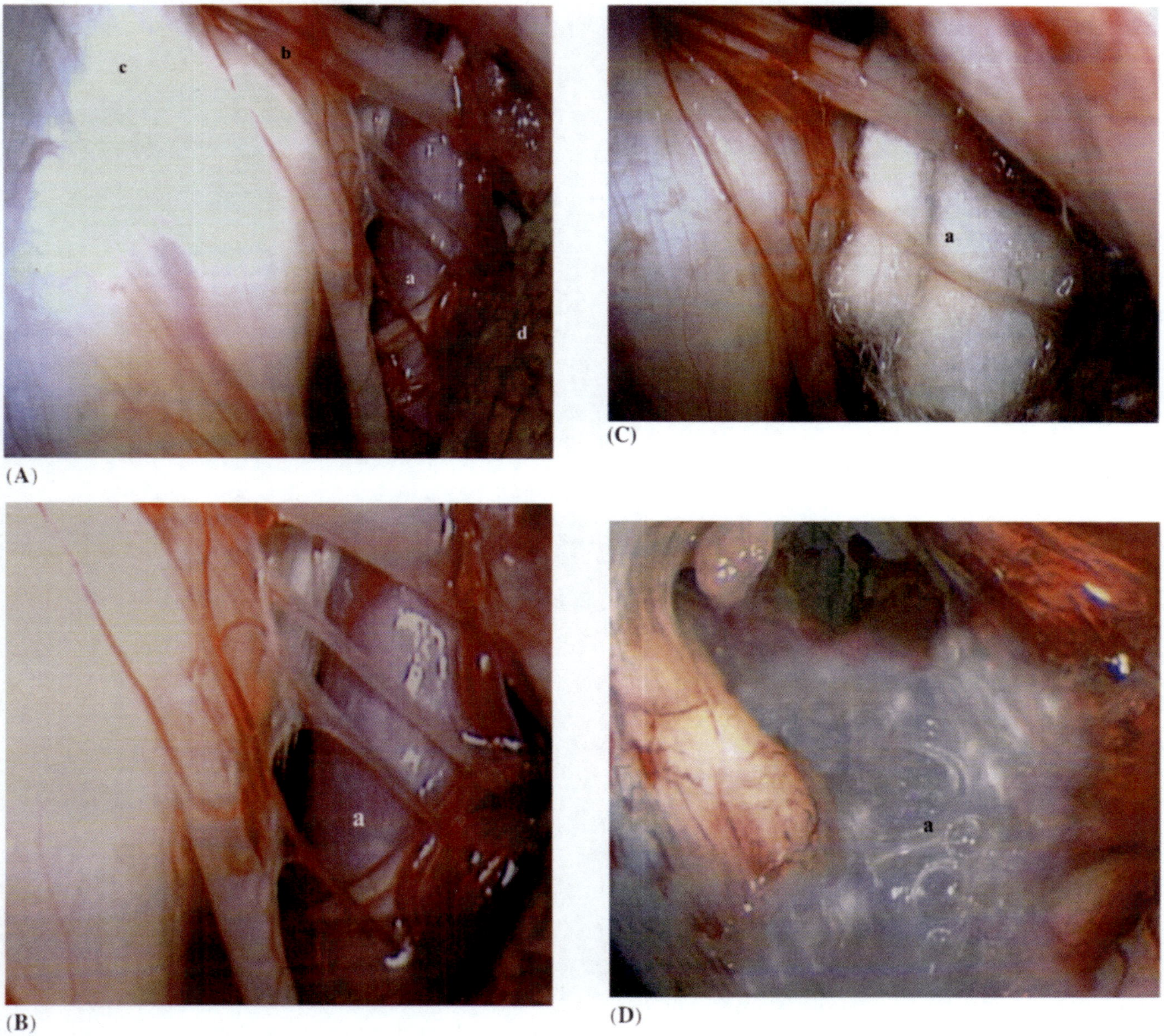

Fig. 22 (**A**) and (**B**) Intraoperative endoscopic view showing lower cranial nerves (IX–XI) and offending artery. (**A**) *a* Offending artery (vertebral artery). *b* Lower cranial nerves. *c* Petrous temporal bone. *d* Lower lateral aspect of cerebellum. (**B**) *a* Close-up view of the offending artery and regional anatomy. (**C**) and (**D**) Intraoperative endoscopic view showing separation of offending artery from lower cranial nerves by Teflon pads. (**C**) *a* Teflon. (**D**) *a* Fibrin glue.

IAC with direct view and angled endoscopes to remove any residual tumor that is out of the view of the operating microscope. In addition to the higher possibility of hearing preservation and avoidance of blind dissection behind the facial nerve, the endoscope provides improved visualization of the skull base—where narrow recesses and angled trajectories impair the direct forward view of the operating microscope—without the need for cerebellar retraction. Endoscopic surgery allows for smaller craniotomies, less dissection, and virtually no cerebellar retraction without compromising the goals of the operation.

7.3.2. Approach ***(Fig. 24)*** On entering the CPA, the surgeon conducts a preliminary survey of the surrounding structures, including the trigeminal and lower cranial nerves, as well as the regional vascular anatomy. The topography of the tumor and its relation to the surrounding structures are appreciated. The facial nerve is located and stimulated, and its response is measured with the facial nerve monitor. Once these relationships are identified, the tumor is gradually cored from its center using a combination of the micro-Cavitron ultrasonic surgical aspirator (microCUSA), bipolar electrocoagulation, suction–irrigation, and microinstruments. The capsule of the tumor is then gently dissected off the facial nerve. Attention is then directed to the IAC. A diamond burr is used to remove the posterior wall of the canal, and the dura overlying the IAC is cauterized and incised. IAC dissection proceeds until the lateral extent of the tumor is visualized and normal nerve is identified. In cases of smaller tumors in patients with "serviceable"

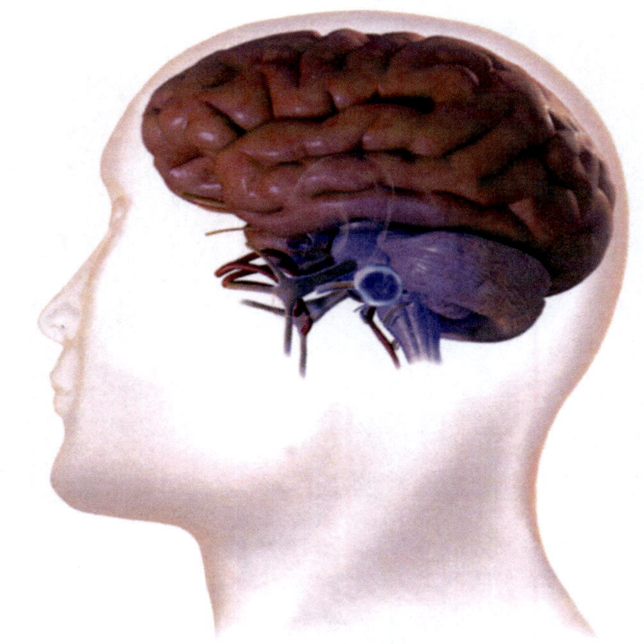

Fig. 23 Cerebellopontine (CPA) Angle Tumor.

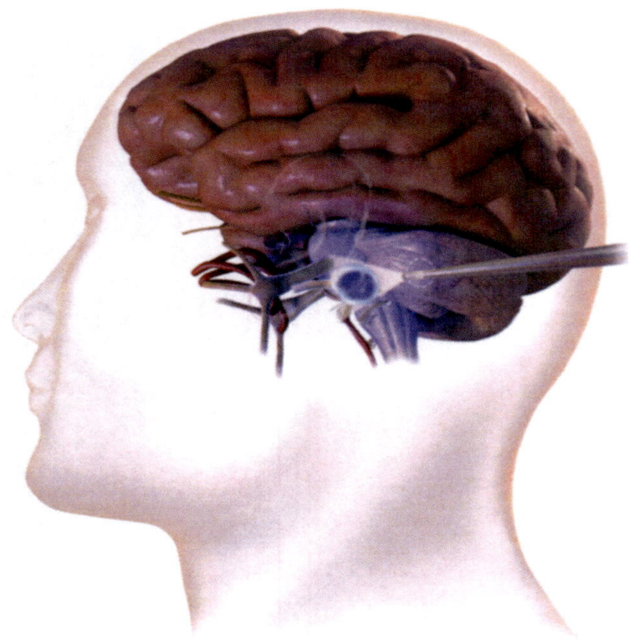

Fig. 24 Approach to Cerebellopontine (CPA) Angle Tumor.

hearing, this portion of the dissection is performed with hearing preservation in mind and extreme caution not to injure the cochlear nerve. Further tumor dissection within the IAC is guided by the 30° endoscope, allowing complete visualization of the lateral extent of the tumor as it is separated from the facial nerve. Once tumor resection is complete, the facial nerve is again stimulated to confirm its function. Complete hemostasis is then confirmed, followed by closure of the dura, cranioplasty, and layered suturing of the soft tissue and skin.

The dissection of CPA or cerebellar convexity meningiomas is essentially the same as for vestibular schwannomas. The tumor is often more dense, and the dissection can be more difficult, but extension into the IAC is rare. Because of the potentially adherent nature of the disease to nearby vessels and nerves in such a limited space, the chance of damage to surrounding critical structures is real; therefore, great care must be taken to identify and preserve these structures during tumor removal.

7.3.3. Cases

7.3.3.1. Large Acoustic Neuroma (Right Sided) (Fig. 25A–J)

7.3.3.2. Large Acoustic Neuroma (Right Sided) (Fig. 26A–R)

7.3.3.3. Large Acoustic Neuroma (Left Sided) (Fig. 27A–P)

7.3.3.4. Large Acoustic Neuroma (Right Sided) (Fig. 28A–V)

7.3.3.5. Medium Acoustic Neuroma (Right Sided) (Fig. 29A–N)

7.3.3.6. Medium Acoustic Neuroma (Left Sided) (Fig. 30A–T)

7.3.3.7. Medium Acoustic Neuroma (Left Sided) (Fig. 31A–O)

7.3.3.8. Small, Purely Intracanalicular Acoustic Neuroma (Left Sided) (Fig. 32A–L)

7.3.3.9. Small, Purely Intracanalicular Acoustic Neuroma (Right Sided) (Fig. 33A–I)

7.3.3.10. Small, Intracanalicular Acoustic Neuroma (Right Sided) (Fig. 34A–S)

7.3.3.11. Superior Cerebellar Convexity Meningioma Extending to CPA (Left Sided) (Fig. 35A–L)

7.3.3.12. Lateral CPA Meningioma (Left Sided) (Fig. 36A–L)

7.3.3.13. Medial CPA Meningioma (Left Sided) (Fig. 37A–T)

8. POTENTIAL COMPLICATIONS

Potential complications of the fully endoscopic retrosigmoid approach include the following:

- Brainstem and cerebellar injuries, quadriparesis, hemiparesis, infection, bacterial or aseptic meningitis, hemorrhage (subdural/epidural/intraaxial), and death (these are also potential complications associated with open approaches with more extensive dissection)
- Direct injuries include cerebellar injuries (cerebellar edema, hematoma, or infarction and direct injury to the cerebellar hemisphere); vascular injuries (to the AICA or its branches, e.g., labyrinthine artery, or less commonly to the posterior inferior cerebellar artery [PICA]); and venous injuries (sigmoid sinus, petrosal vein, or vein of Labbé)
- Early or delayed CSF leakage from the wound, ear (otorrhea), or nose (rhinorrhea)
- Facial weakness or paralysis, which may be transient or permanent or may partially improve with some residual facial weakness
- Eye complications such as dryness or redness secondary to facial paralysis
- Hearing loss or tinnitus (VIII)
- Other cranial nerve deficits (V, VI, IX–XII)

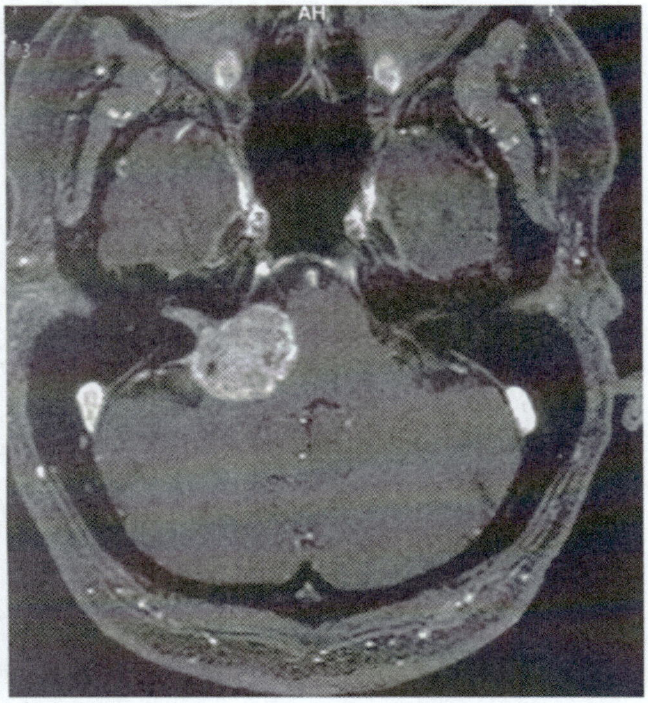

(A)

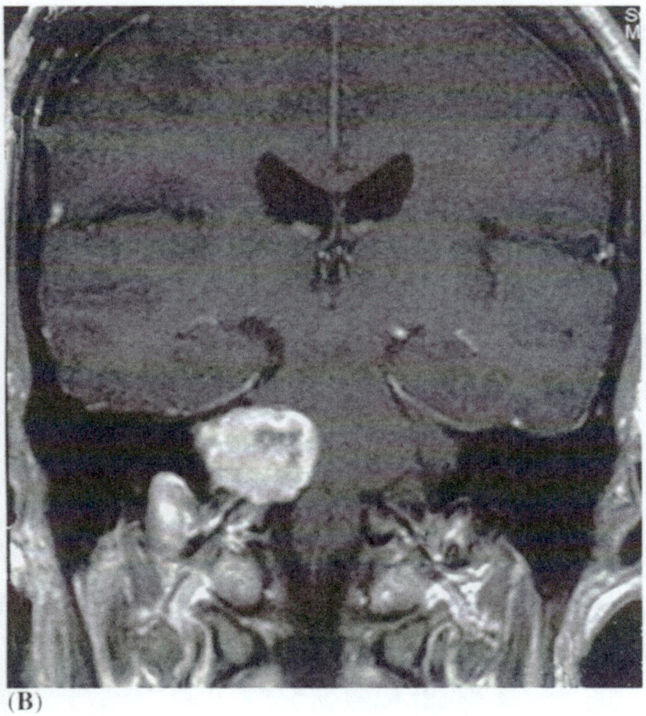

(B)

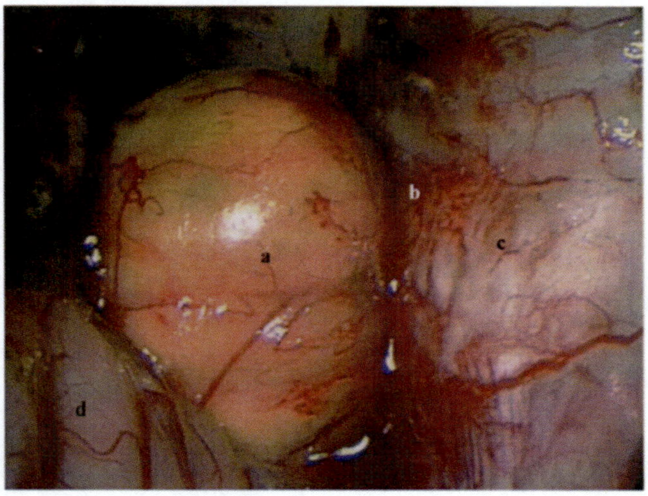

(C)

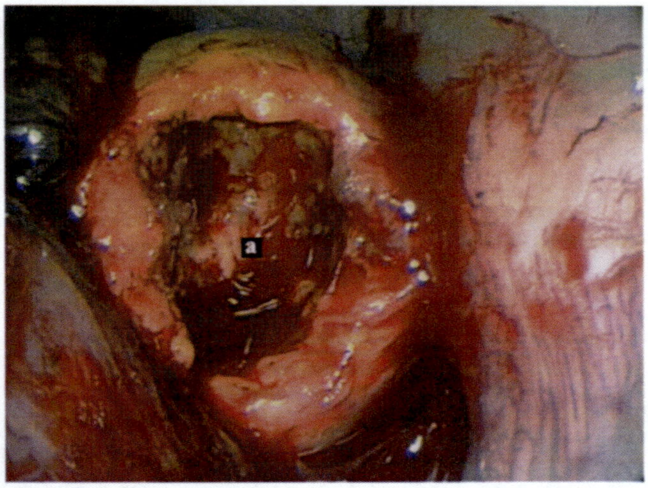

(D)

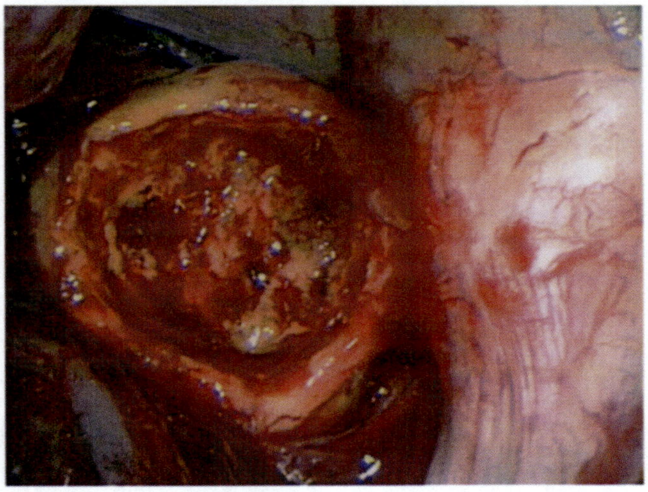

(E)

Fig. 25 (**A**) T_1-weighted, contrast-enhanced axial MRI showing a large acoustic neuroma. (**B**) T_1-weighted, contrast-enhanced coronal MRI showing a large acoustic neuroma. (**C**) Intraoperative endoscopic view showing the initial exposure of a large acoustic neuroma. (**C**)–(**H**) Intraoperative endoscopic view showing gradual resection of large acoustic neuroma. (**C**) *a* Acoustic neuroma. *b* Expanded internal auditory canal (IAC). *c* Petrous temporal bone. *d* Lateral aspect of cerebellum. (**D**) *a* Acoustic neuroma partly decompressed. (**F**) *a* Acoustic neuroma capsule. *b* Abducent nerve (VI). *c* Trigeminal nerve (V). (**G**) *a* Final remnants of acoustic neuroma capsule overlying the acousticofacial nerve bundle (VII, VIII). *b* Trigeminal nerve (V). (**H**) *a* Acousticofacial bundle (VII, VIII) after complete tumor removal. *b* Brainstem. *c* Trigeminal nerve (V). *d* Drilled posterior wall of internal auditory canal (IAC). *e* Trochlear nerve (IV). (**I**) Postoperative T_1-weighted, contrast-enhanced axial MRI. (**J**) Postoperative T_1-weighted, contrast-enhanced coronal MRI.

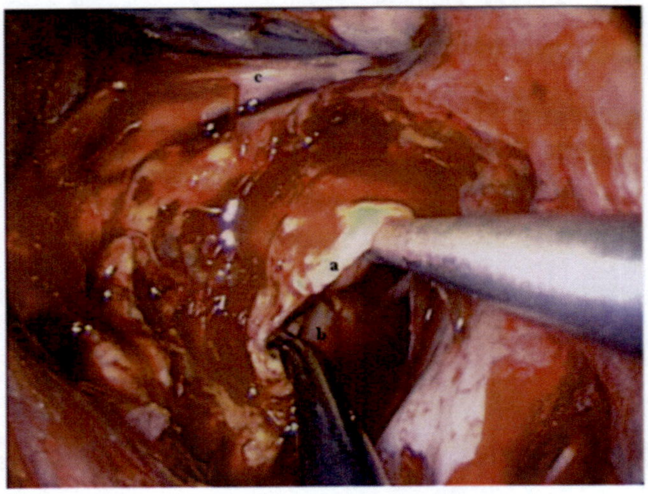

(F)

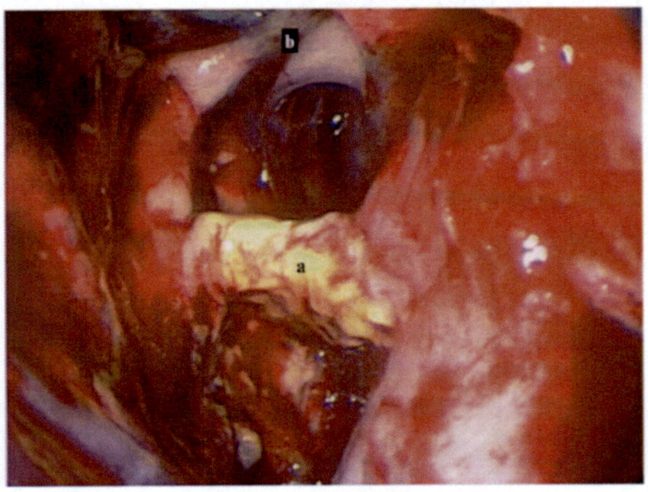

(G)

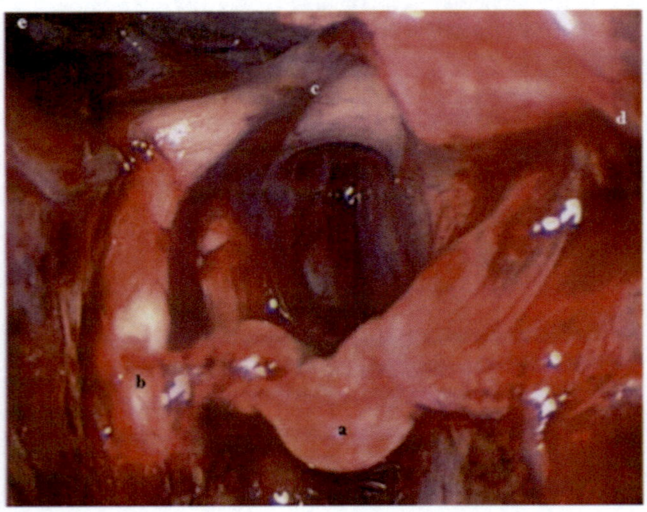

(H)

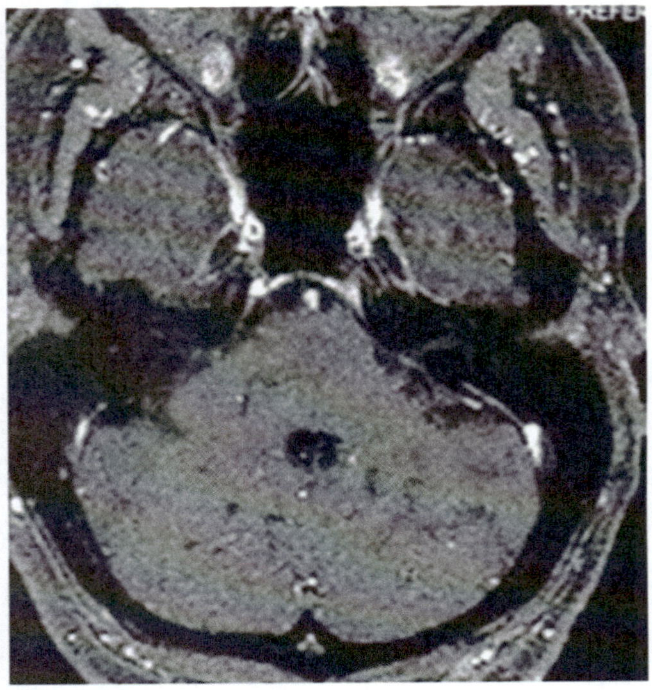
(I)

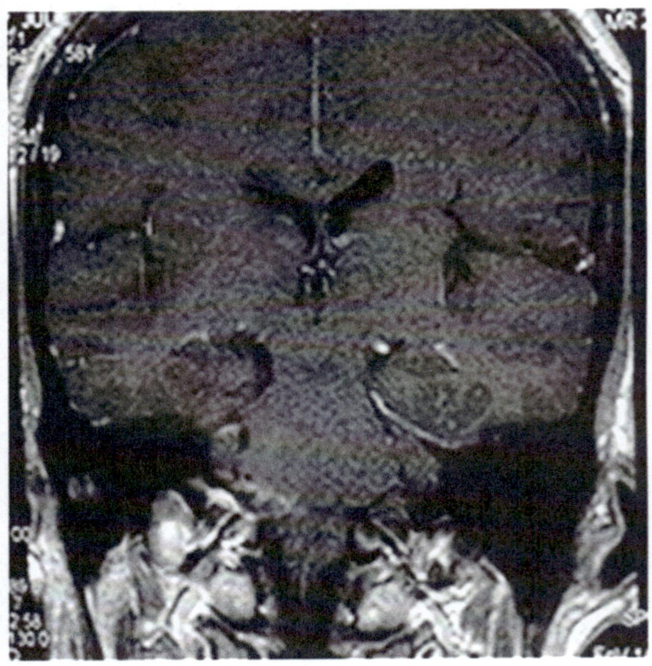
(J)

Fig. 25 (continued)

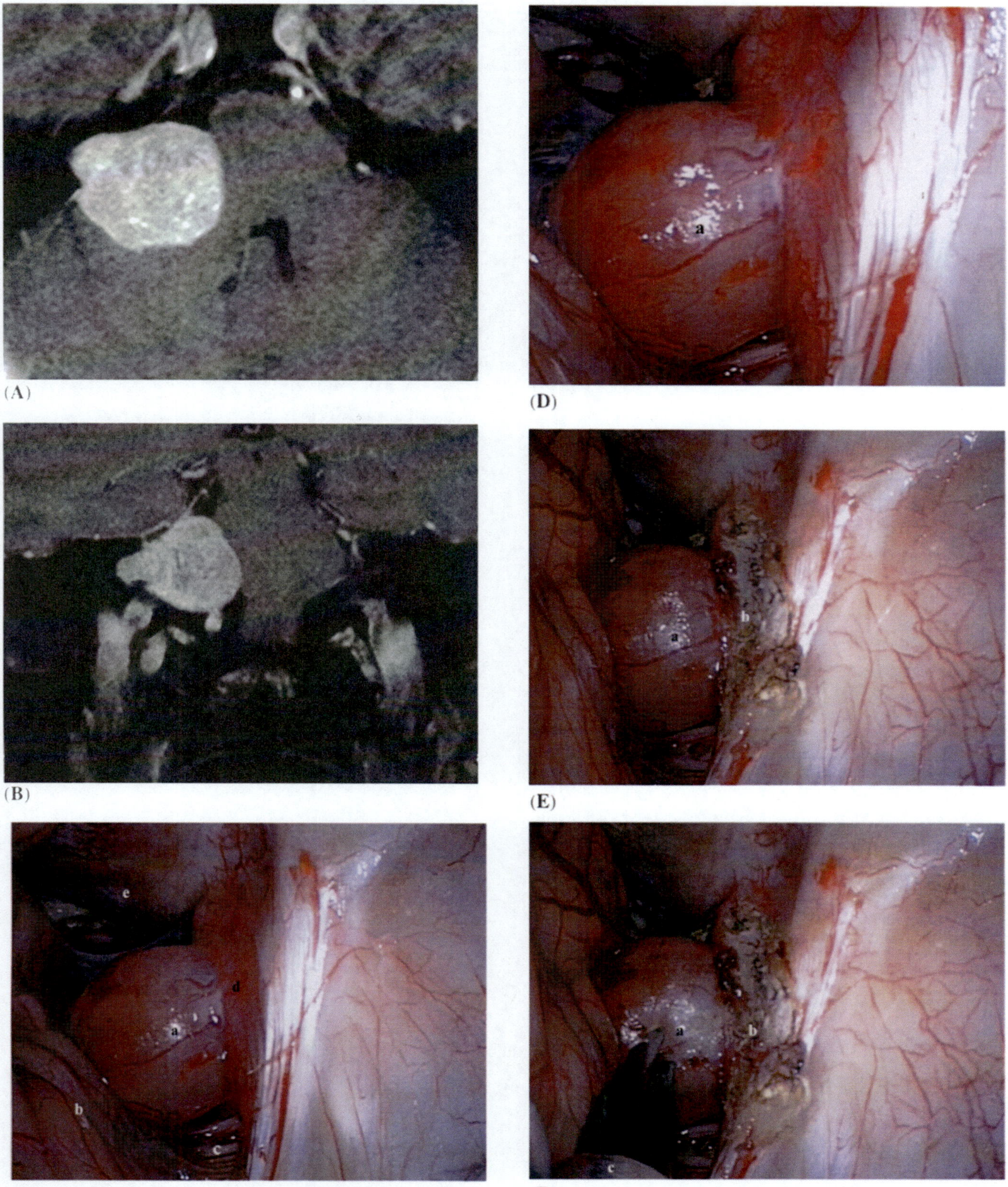

Fig. 26 (**A**) T_1-weighted, contrast-enhanced axial MRI showing large acoustic neuroma. (**B**) T_1-weighted, contrast-enhanced coronal MRI showing large acoustic neuroma. (**C**) and (**D**) Intraoperative endoscopic view showing the initial exposure of large acoustic neuroma. (**C**) *a* Acoustic neuroma. *b* Lateral aspect of cerebellum. *c* Lower cranial nerves (IX–XI). *d* Expanded internal auditory meatus (IAM). *e* Tentorium. (**D**) *a*. Close-up view of acoustic neuroma and regional anatomy. (**E**)–(**N**) Intraoperative endoscopic view showing gradual resection of large acoustic neuroma. (**E**) *a* Acoustic neuroma. *b* Cauterized dura. (**F**) *a* Acoustic neuroma. *b* Cauterized dura. *c* Bipolar diathermy tip. (**G**) *a* Acoustic neuroma. *b* Straight microscissors. (**I**) *a* Acoustic neuroma partly debulked. *b* MicroCUSA tip. (**L**) *a* Final remnants of acoustic neuroma capsule. *b* Drilled posterior wall of internal auditory canal (IAC). (**M**) *a* Final portion of acoustic neuroma capsule being dissected. *b* Upward-angled microhook. *c* Atraumatic suction. (**N**) *a* Vestibulocochlear nerve (VIII). *b* Facial nerve (VII). *c* Final portion of acoustic neuroma capsule being dissected. *d* Drilled posterior wall of internal auditory canal (IAC). *e* Upward-angled microhook. *f* Atraumatic suction. (**O**) and (**P**) Intraoperative endoscopic view following complete resection of large acoustic neuroma. (**O**) *a* Vestibulocochlear nerve following complete tumor resection (VIII). *b* Facial nerve (VII). *c* Trigeminal nerve (V). *d* Anterior wall of internal auditory canal (IAC). *e* Posterior wall.

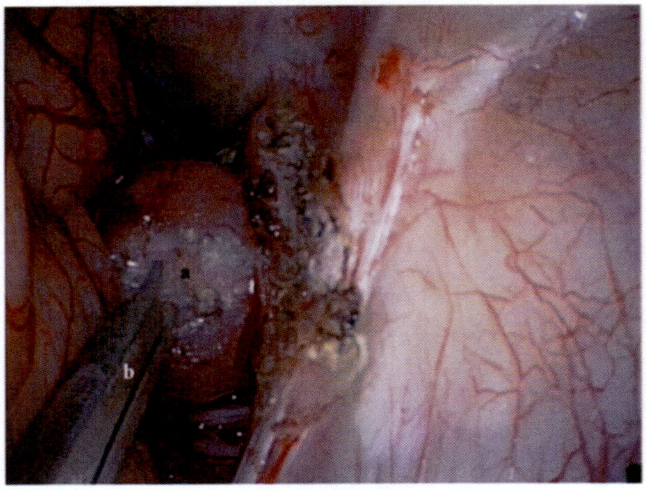

(G)

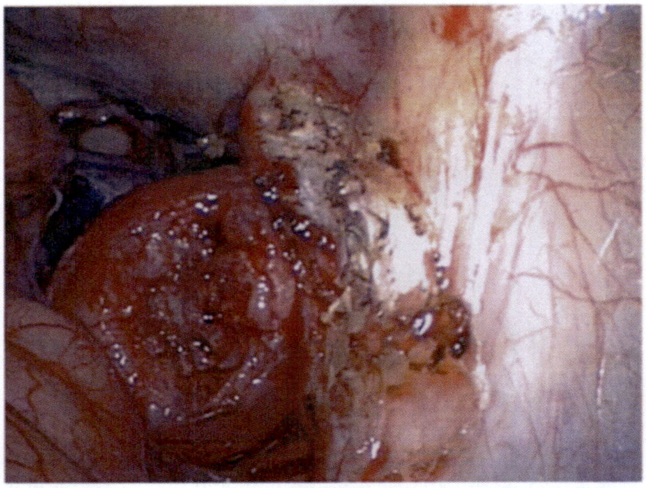

(H)

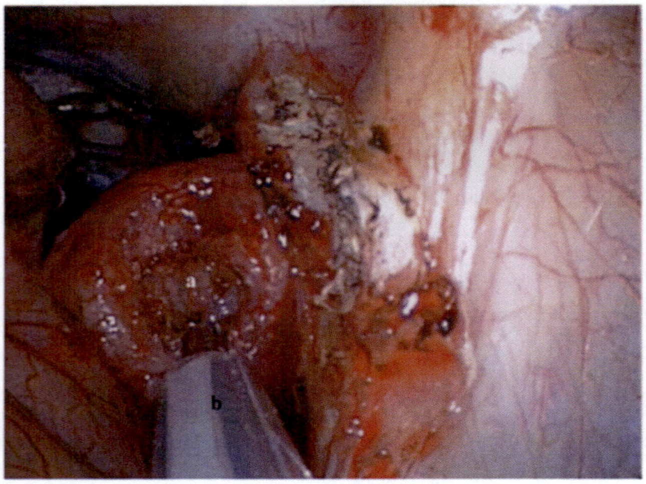

(I)

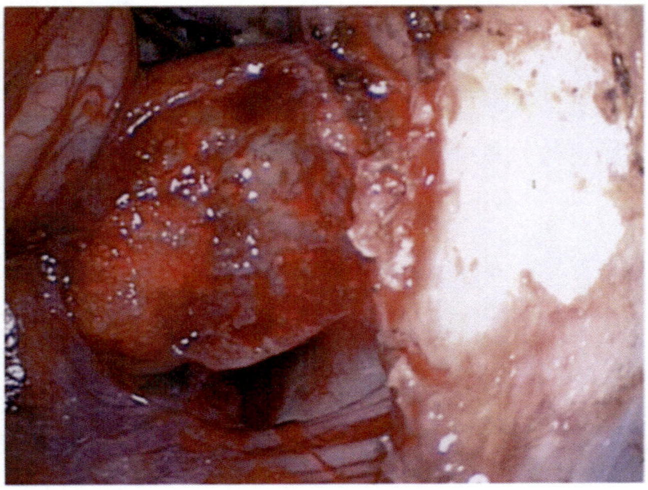

(J)

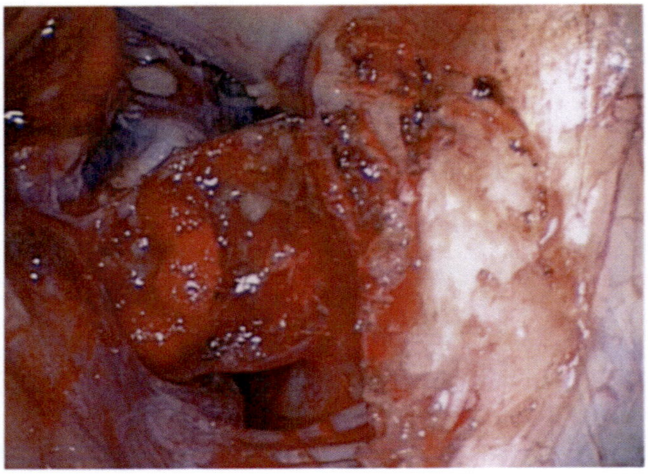

(K)

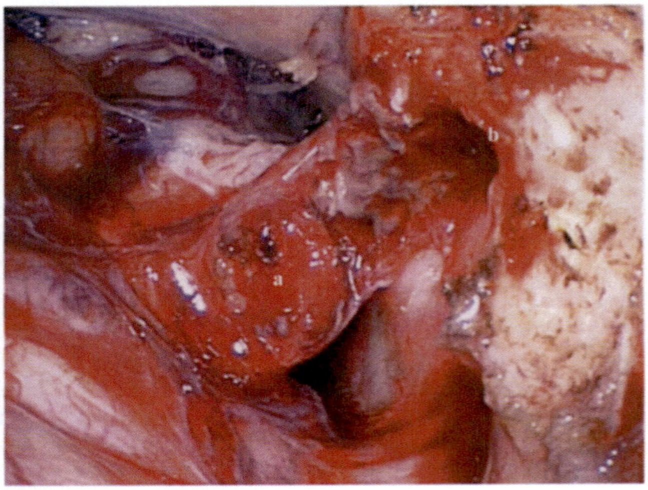

(L)

Fig. 26 (continued) of internal auditory canal (IAC). *f* Petrous temporal bone. *g* Lower cranial nerves (IX–XI). *h* Lateral aspect of cerebellum. *i* Brainstem. *j* Trochlear nerve (IV). *k* Tentorium. *l* Tentorial incisura. (**P**) *a* Close-up view of facial nerve (VII). *b* Close-up view of vestibulocochlear nerve (VIII). *c* Internal auditory canal (IAC). *d* Trigeminal nerve (V). *e* Meckel's cave. *f* Trochlear nerve (IV). *g* Tentorium. *h* Brainstem. (**Q**) Postoperative T_1-weighted, contrast-enhanced axial MRI. (**R**) Postoperative T1-weighted, contrast-enhanced coronal MRI.

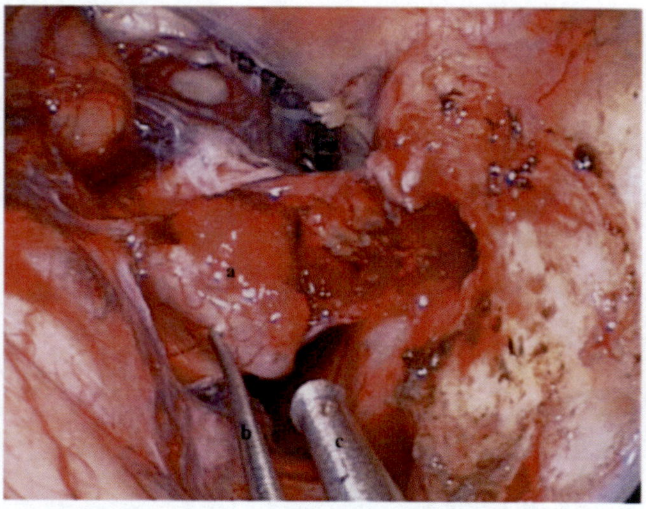

(M)

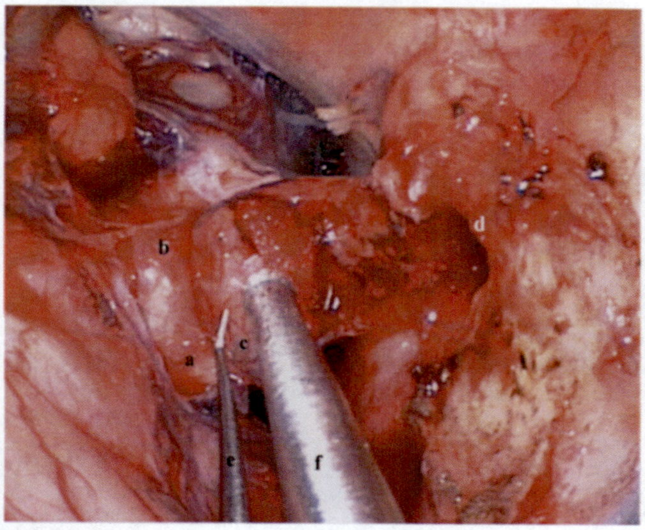

(N)

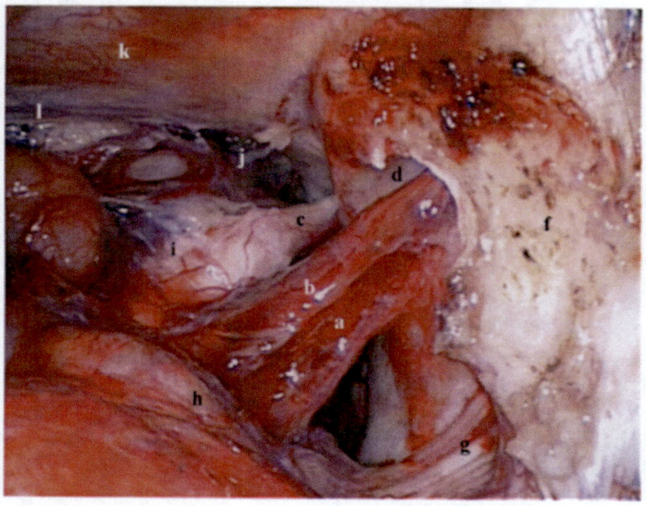

(O)

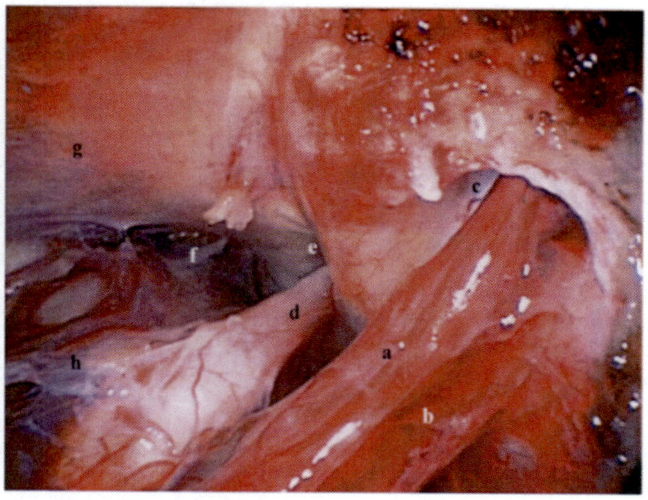

(P)

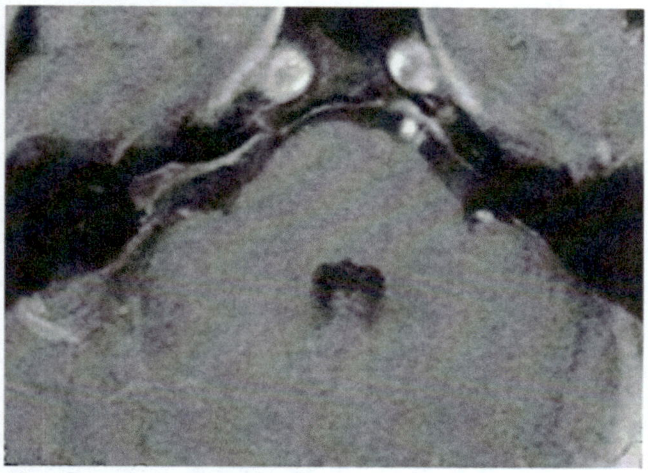
(Q)

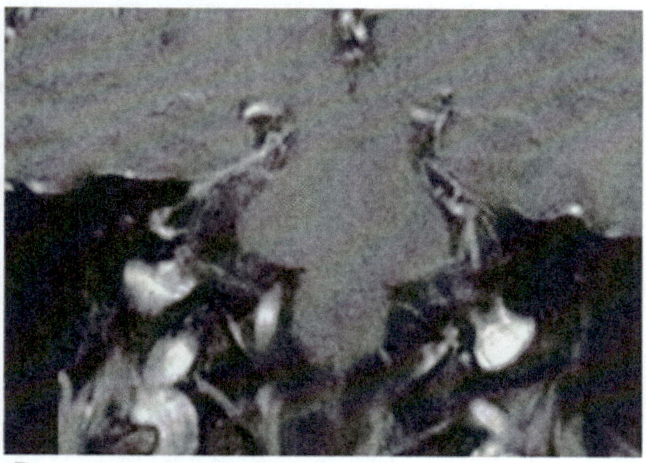
(R)

Fig. 26 (continued)

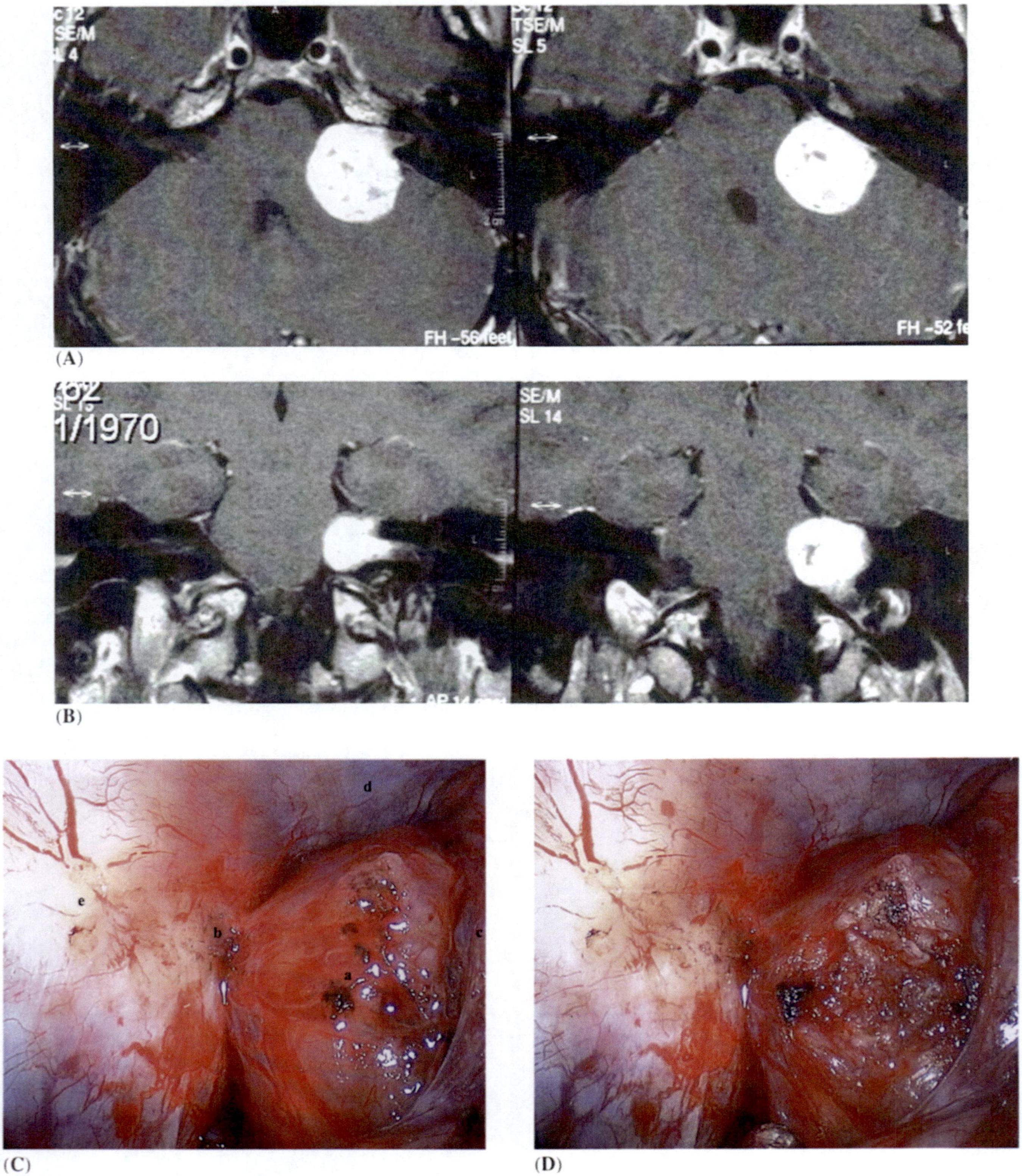

Fig. 27 (**A**) T_1-weighted, contrast-enhanced axial MRIs showing large acoustic neuroma. (**B**) T_1-weighted, contrast-enhanced coronal MRIs showing large acoustic neuroma. (**C**) Intraoperative endoscopic view showing the initial exposure of large acoustic neuroma. *a* Acoustic neuroma. *b* Expanded internal auditory meatus (IAM). *c* Lateral aspect of cerebellum. *d* Tentorium. *e* Petrous temporal bone. (**D**)–(**L**) Intraoperative endoscopic view showing gradual resection of large acoustic neuroma. (**F**) *a* Acoustic neuroma debulked. *b* Lower cranial nerves (IX–XI). (**G**) *a* Anterior capsule of acoustic neuroma. *b* Trigeminal nerve (V). *c* Drilled posterior wall of internal auditory canal (IAC). (**H**) *a* Anterior capsule of acoustic neuroma. *b* Abducent nerve (VI). (**I**) *a* Close-up view of intracanalicular portion of acoustic neuroma. (**J**) *a* Intracanalicular portion of acoustic neuroma being removed. *b* Angled extended ring curette. (**K**) *a* Close-up view showing the removal of intracanalicular portion of acoustic neuroma. (**L**) *a* Close-up view showing clean internal auditory canal after removal of intracanalicular portion of acoustic neuroma. *b* Trigeminal nerve (V). *c* Acousticofacial nerve bundle (VII, VIII). (**M**) and (**N**) Intraoperative endoscopic view after complete resection of large acoustic neuroma. (**M**) *a* Acousticofacial nerve bundle (VII, VIII) after complete tumor removal. (**N**) *a* Acousticofacial nerve bundle (VII, VIII). *b* Trigeminal nerve (V). *c* Brainstem. *d* Anterior wall of internal auditory canal (IAC). *e* Posterior wall of internal auditory canal (IAC). *f* Lower cranial nerves (IX–XI). *g* Lateral aspect of cerebellum. *h* Tentorium. (**O**) Postoperative T_1-weighted, contrast-enhanced axial MRIs. (**P**) Postoperative T_1-weighted, contrast-enhanced coronal MRIs.

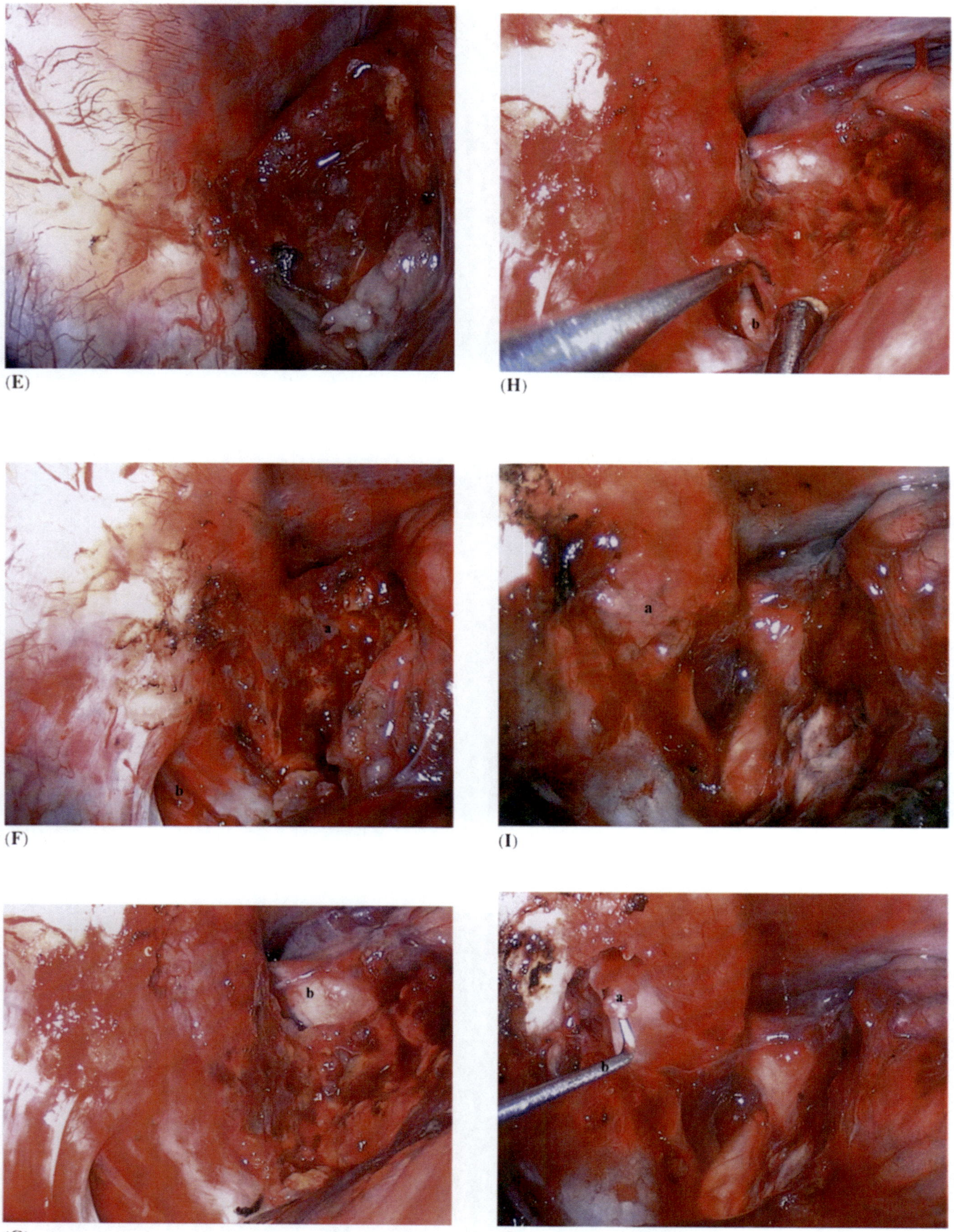

Fig. 27 (continued)

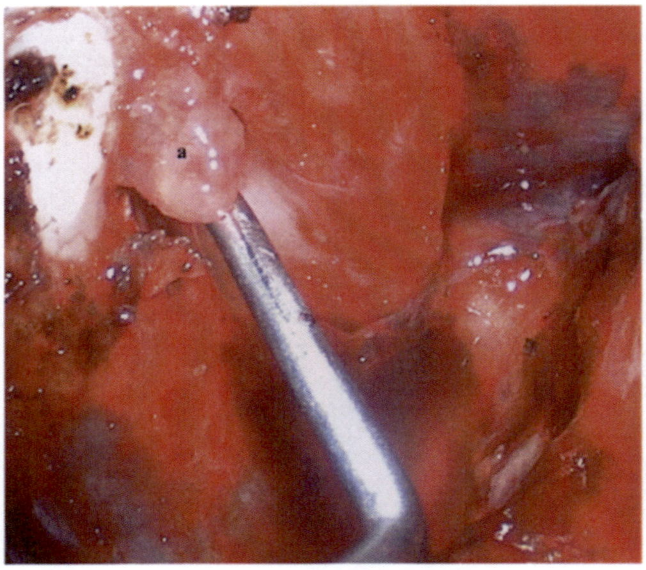

(K)

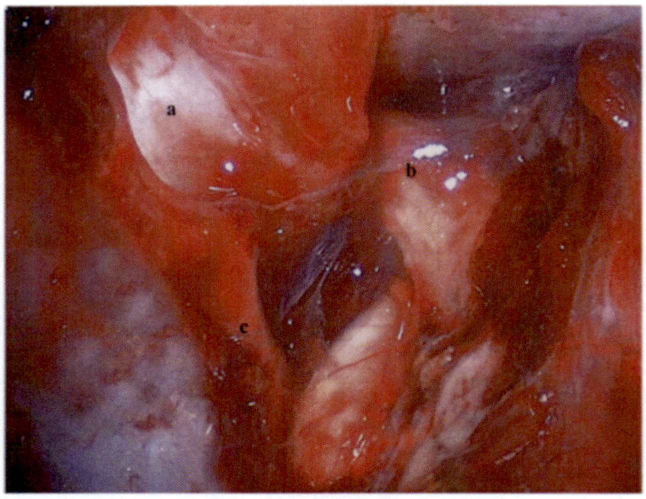

(L)

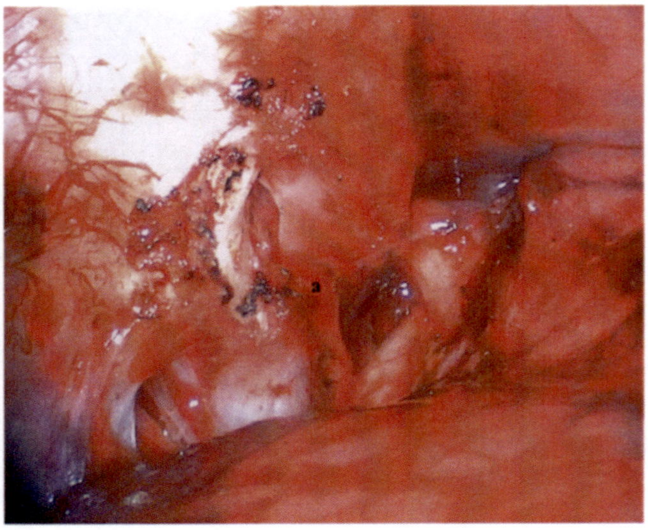

(M)

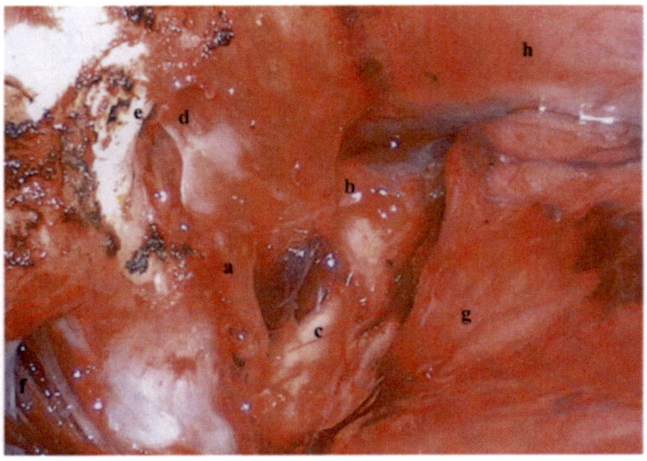

(N)

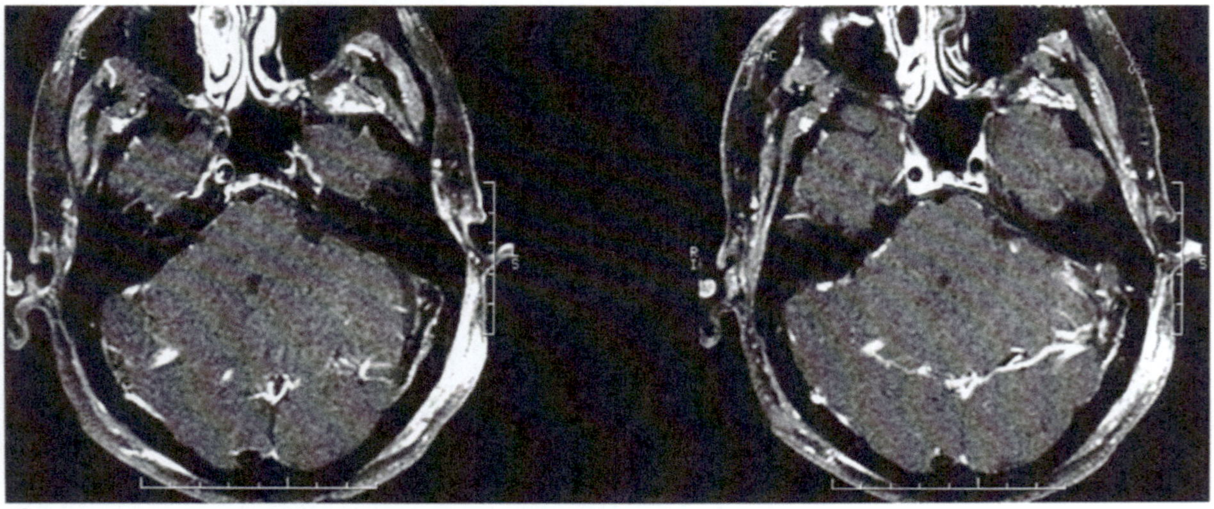

(O)

Fig. 27 (continued)

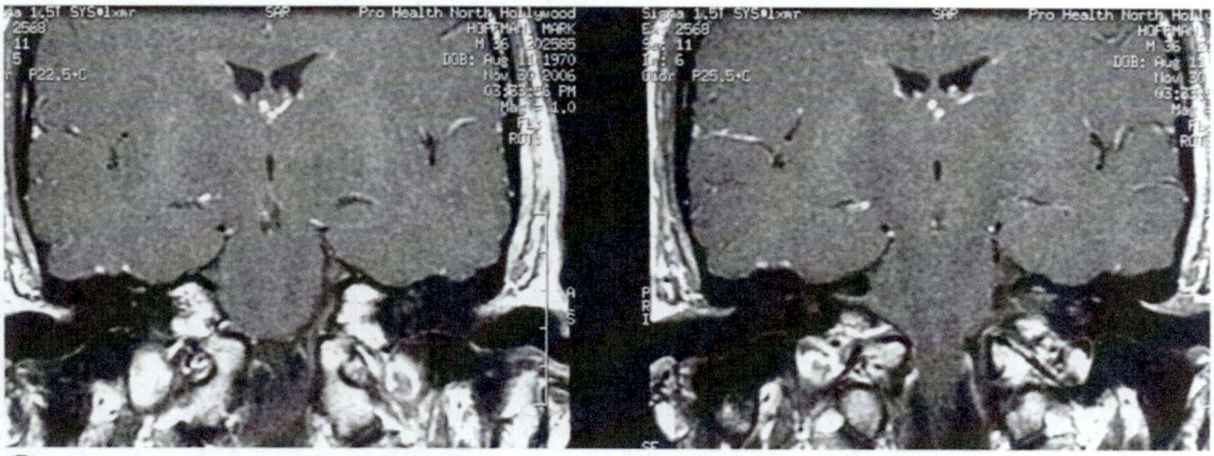

(P)

Fig. 27 (continued)

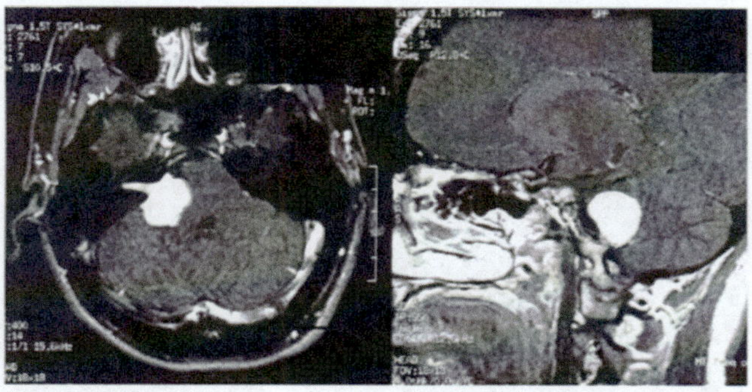

(A)

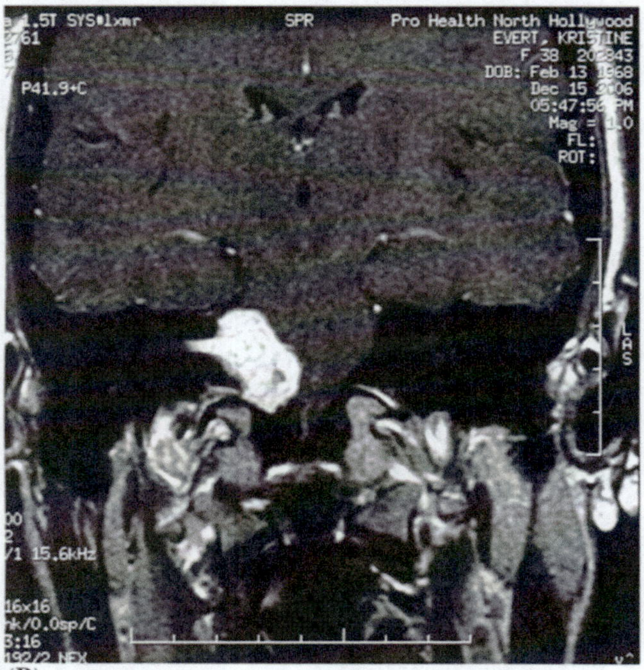

(B)

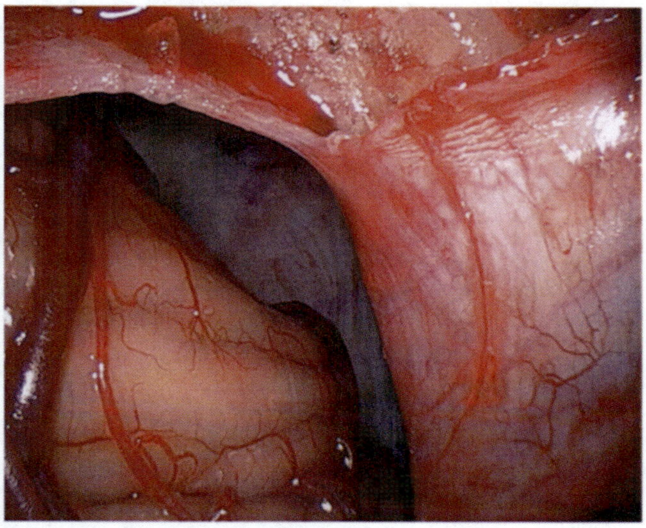

(C)

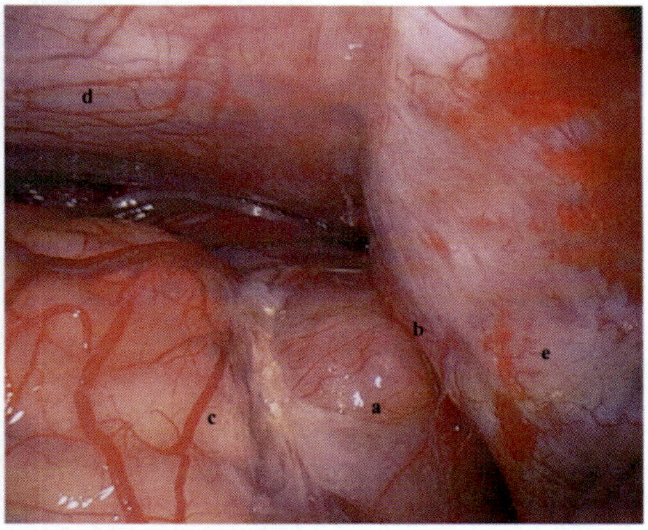

(D)

Fig. 28 (**A**) T_1-weighted, contrast-enhanced axial and sagittal MRIs showing large acoustic neuroma. (**B**) T_1-weighted, contrast-enhanced coronal MRI showing large acoustic neuroma. (**C**) and (**D**) Intraoperative endoscopic view showing the initial exposure of large acoustic neuroma. (**D**) *a* Acoustic neuroma. *b*. Expanded internal auditory meatus (IAM). *c*. Lateral aspect of cerebellum. *d*. Tentorium. *e*. Petrous temporal bone. (**E**)–(**T**) Intraoperative endoscopic view showing gradual resection of large acoustic neuroma. (**E**) *a* Acoustic neuroma. *b* Bipolar diathermy tip. *c* Atraumatic suction. (**I**) *a* Acoustic neuroma partly debulked. *b* MicroCUSA tip. (**L**) *a* Anterior capsule of acoustic neuroma. *b* Trigeminal nerve (V). (**M**) *a* Anterior capsule of acoustic neuroma. *b* Drilled posterior wall of internal auditory canal (IAC). (**N**) *a* Anterior capsule of acoustic neuroma. *b* Abducent nerve (VI). (**P**) *a* Anterior capsule of acoustic neuroma. *b* MicroCUSA tip. (**S**) *a* Final portion of anterior capsule of acoustic neuroma. *b* Acousticofacial nerve bundle (VII, VIII). *c* Brainstem. *d* Trigeminal nerve (V). *e* Abducent nerve (VI). (**T**) *a* Acousticofacial nerve bundle (VII, VIII) after complete tumor removal. *b* Brainstem. *c* Lateral aspect of cerebellum. *d* Trigeminal nerve (V). (**U**) Postoperative T_1-weighted, contrast-enhanced axial and sagittal MRIs. (**V**) Postoperative T_1-weighted, contrast-enhanced coronal MRI.

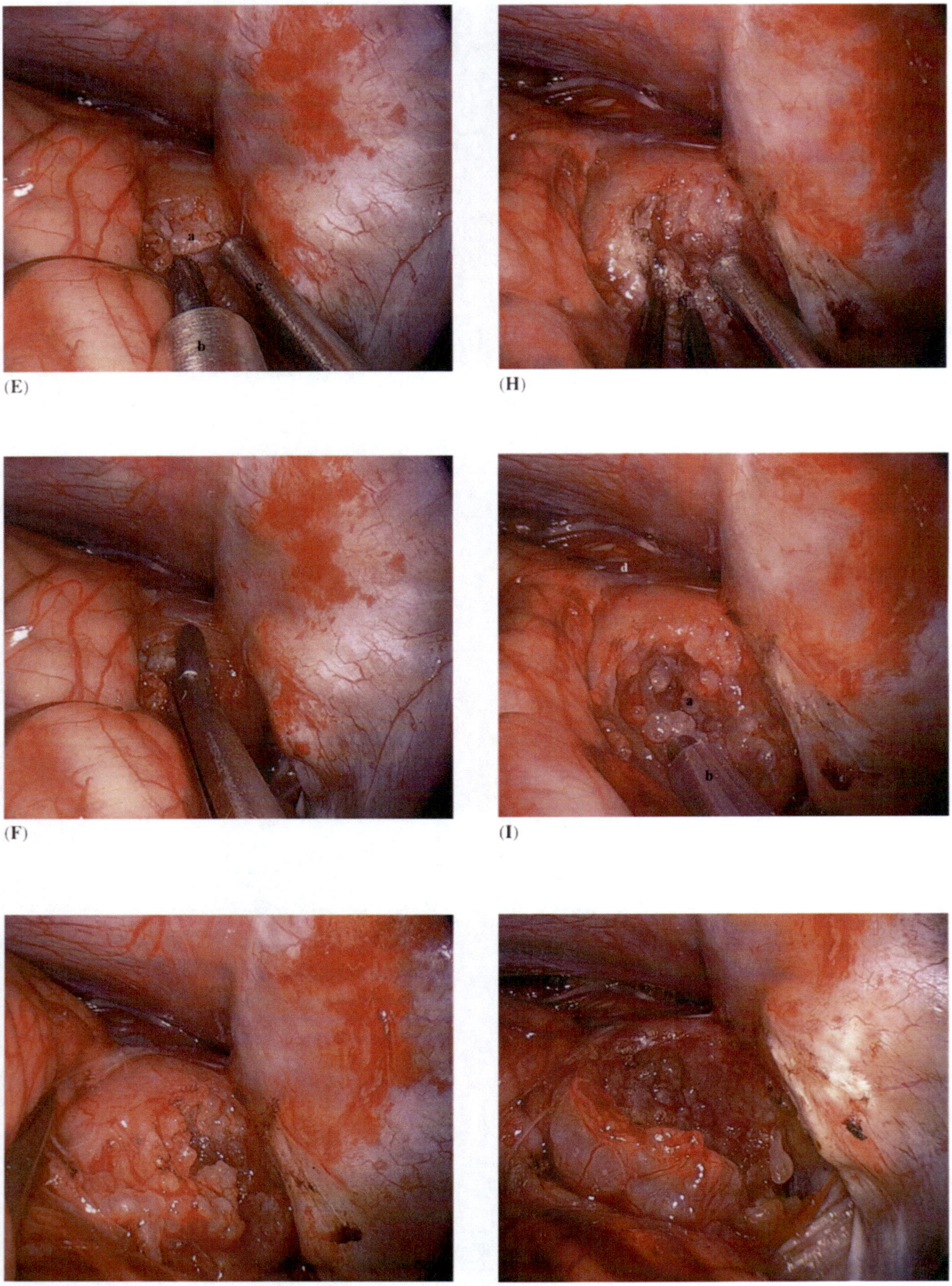

Fig. 28 (continued)

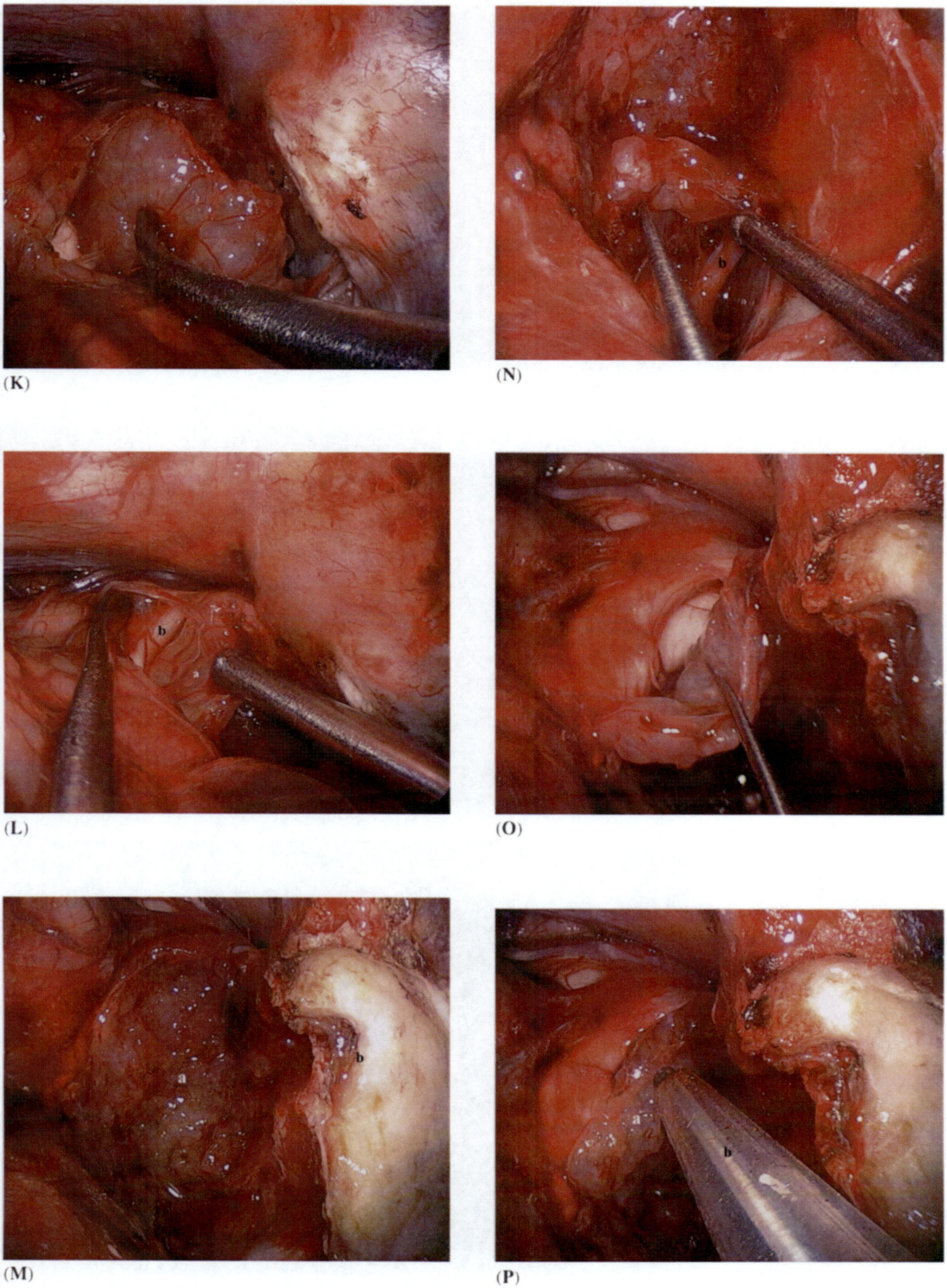

Fig. 28 (continued)

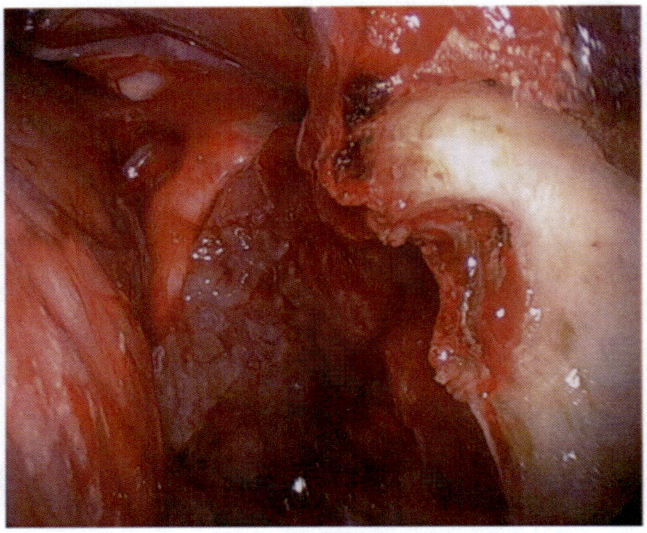

(Q)

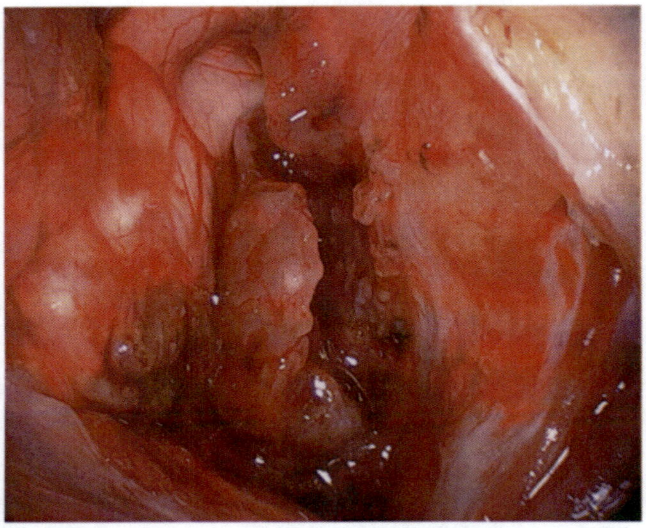

(R)

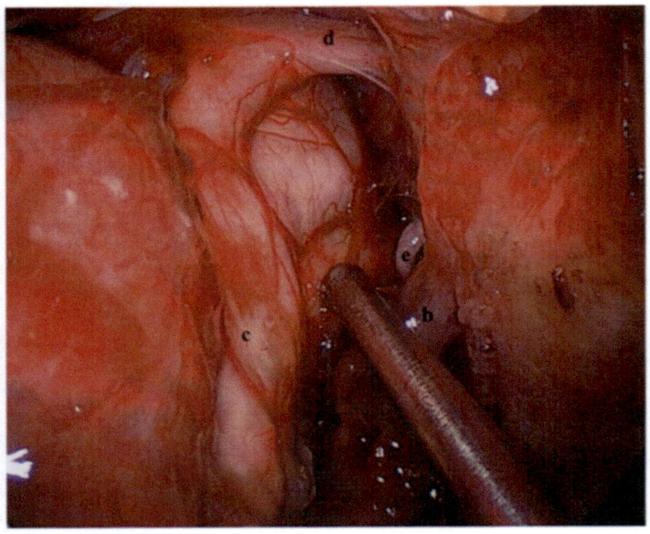

(S)

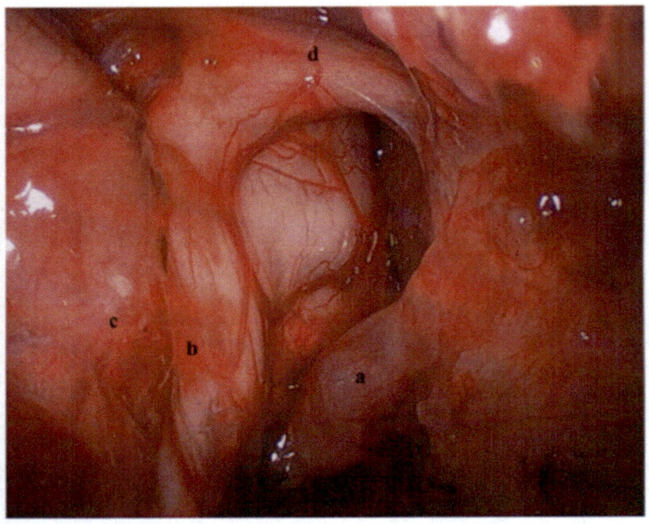

(T)

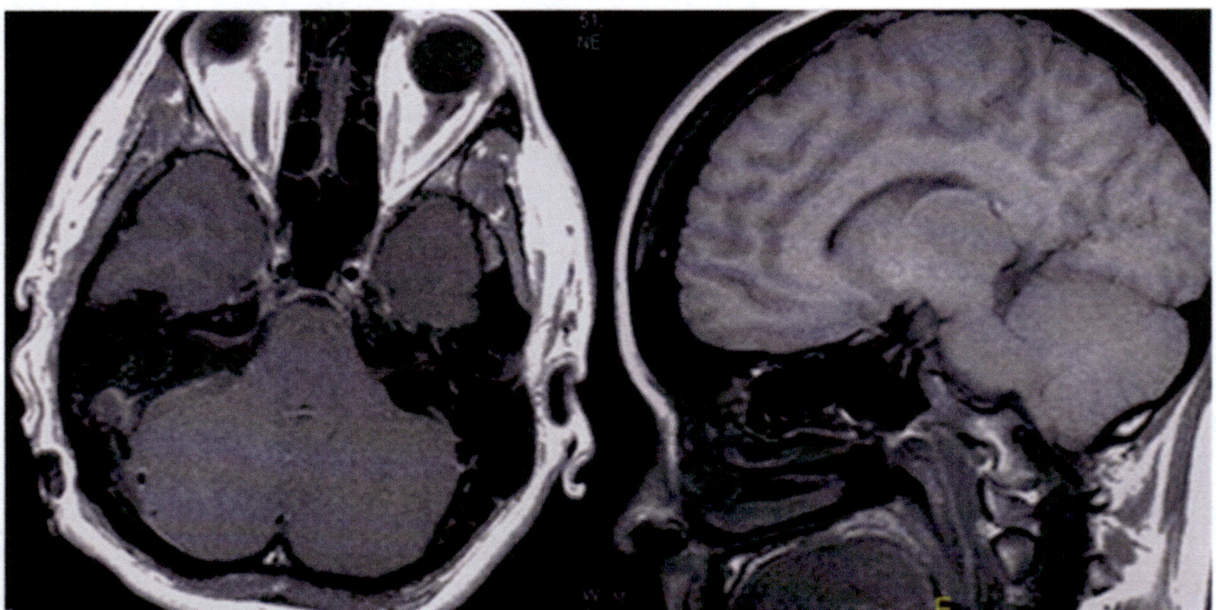

(U)

Fig. 28 (continued)

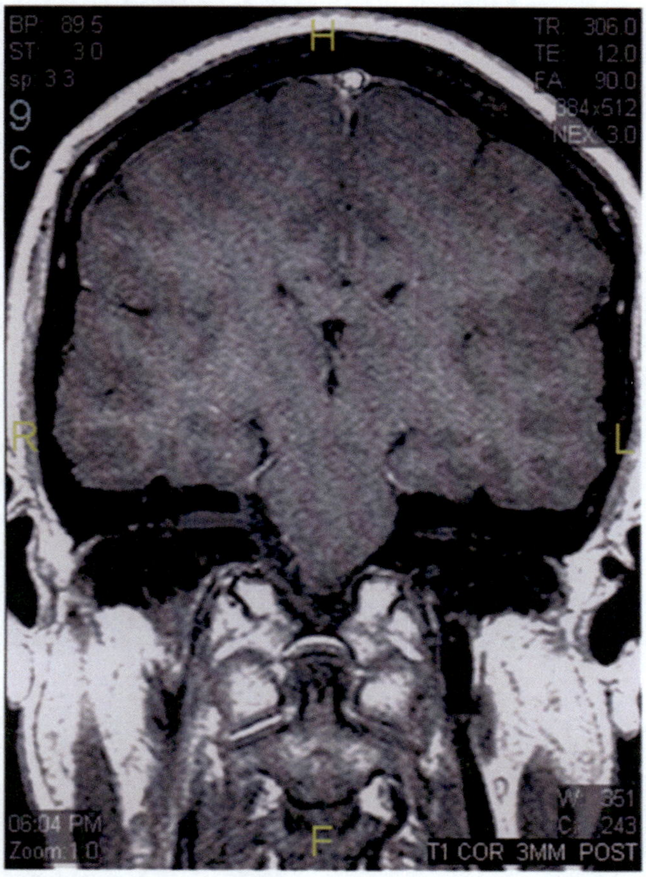

(V)

Fig. 28 (continued)

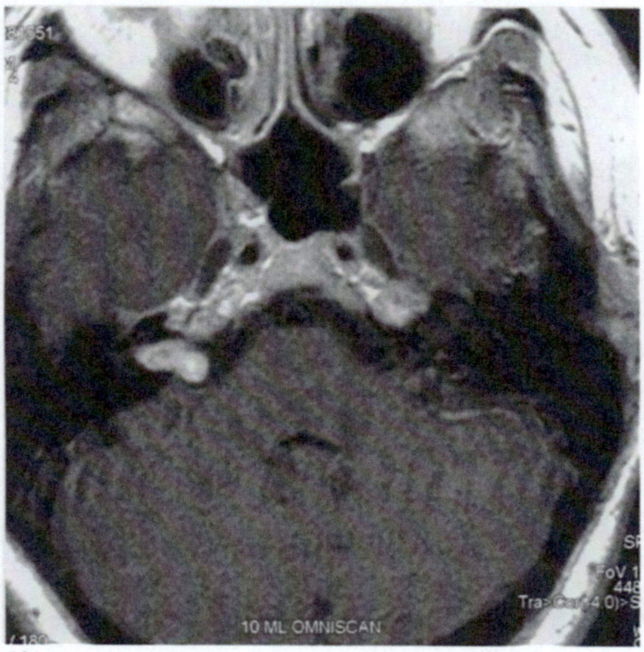

(A)

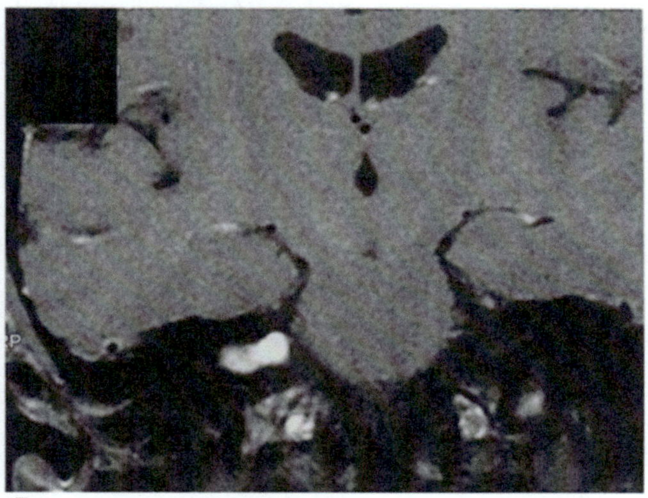
(B)

Fig. 29 (**A**) T_1-weighted, contrast-enhanced axial MRI showing medium-size acoustic neuroma. (**B**) T_1-weighted, contrast-enhanced coronal MRI showing medium-size acoustic neuroma. (**C**) Intraoperative endoscopic view showing initial exposure of medium-size acoustic neuroma. *a* Acoustic neuroma. *b* Acousticofacial nerve bundle (VII, VIII). *c* Expanded internal canal (IAC). *d* Petrous temporal bone. *e* Lateral aspect of cerebellum. *f* Tentorium. (**D**)–(**L**) Intraoperative endoscopic view showing gradual resection of medium-size acoustic neuroma. (**F**) *a* Acoustic neuroma. *b* Acousticofacial nerve bundle (VII, VIII). *c* Trigeminal nerve (V). (**H**) *a* Drilled posterior wall of internal auditory canal (IAC). *b* Acoustic neuroma. *c* Acousticofacial nerve bundle (VII, VIII). *d* Trigeminal Nerve (V). (**I**) *a* Intracanalicular Acoustic neuroma. (**J**) *a* Facial nerve (VII).

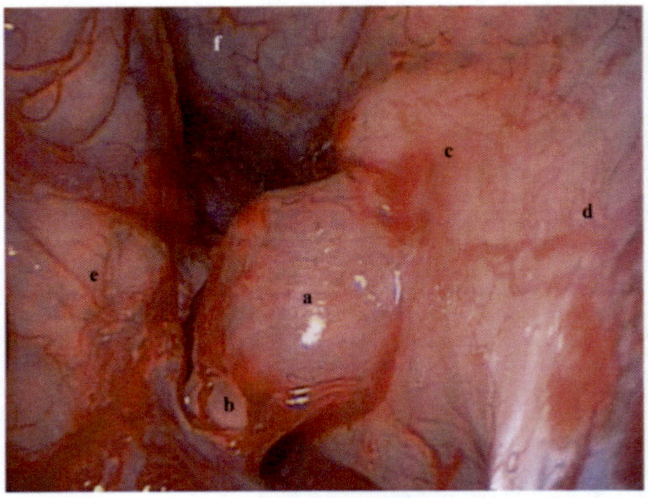

(C)

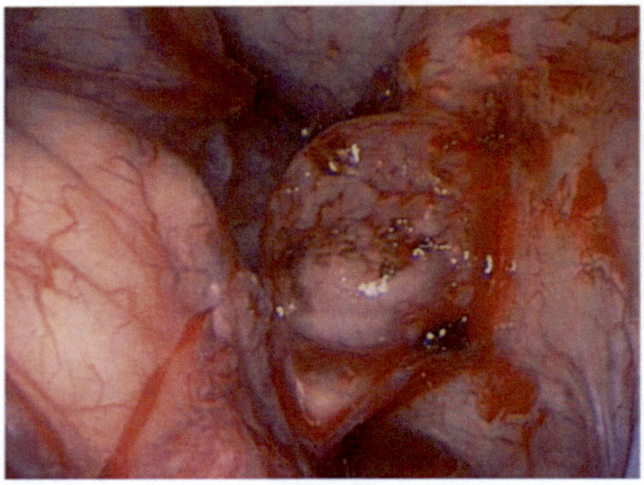

(D)

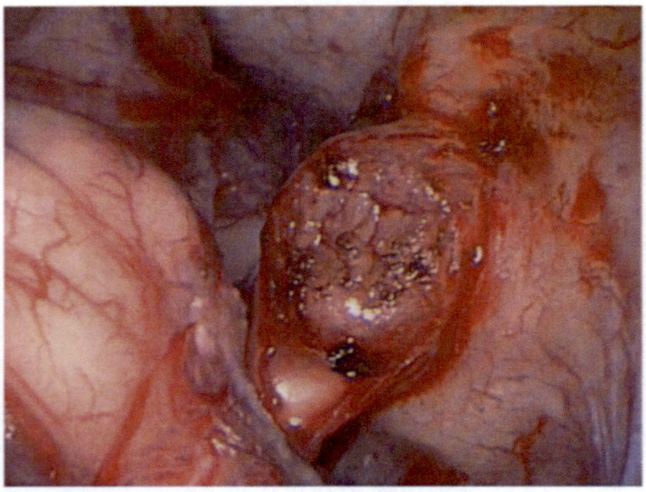

(E)

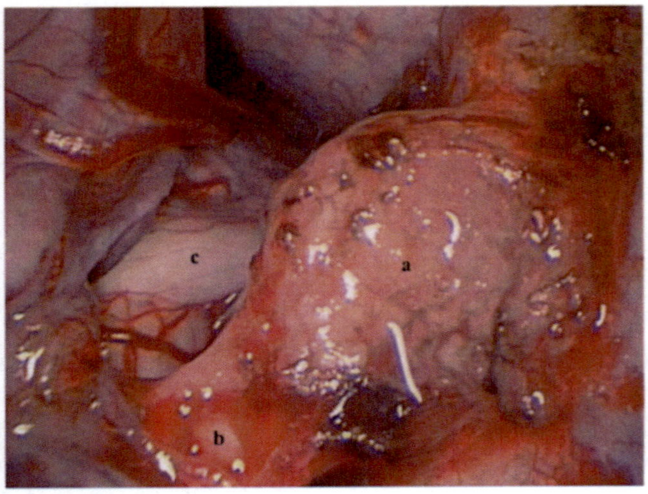

(F)

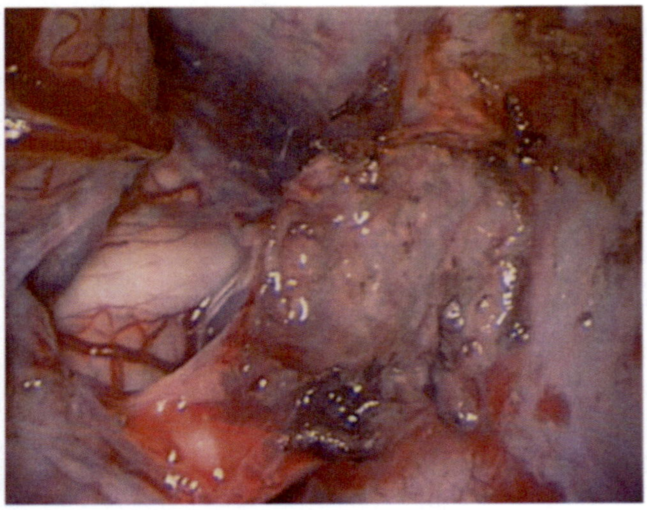

(G)

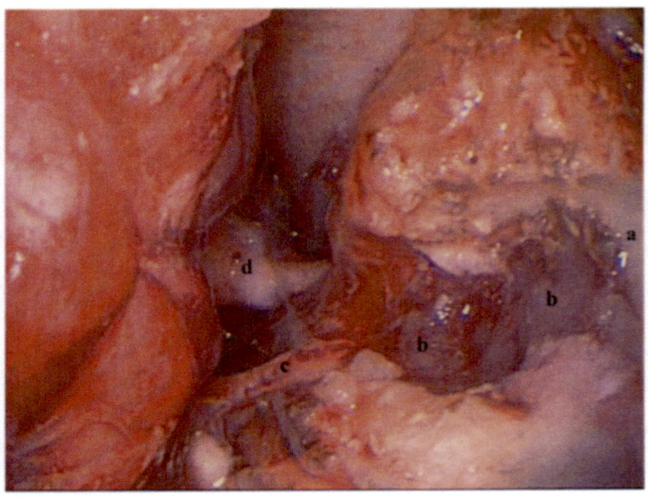

(H)

Fig. 29 (continued) (VIII). *b* Vestibulocochlear nerve (VIII). *c* Anterior wall of internal auditory canal. (**L**) *a* Facial nerve (VII). *b* Vestibulocochlear nerve (VIII). *c* Anterior wall of internal auditory canal (IAC). *d* Drilled posterior wall of internal auditory canal (IAC). *e* Trigeminal nerve (V). (**M**) Postoperative T_1-weighted, contrast-enhanced axial MRI. (**N**) Postoperative T_1-weighted, contrast-enhanced coronal MRI.

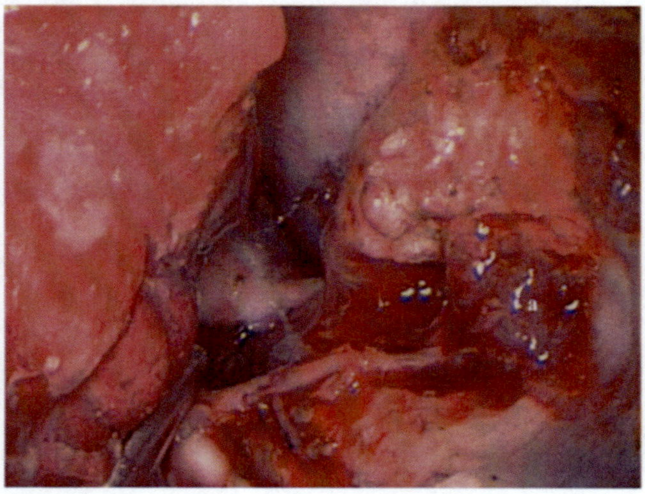

(I)

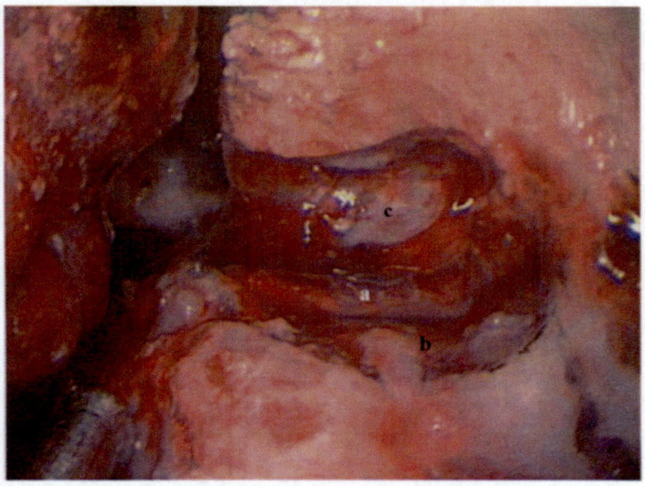

(J)

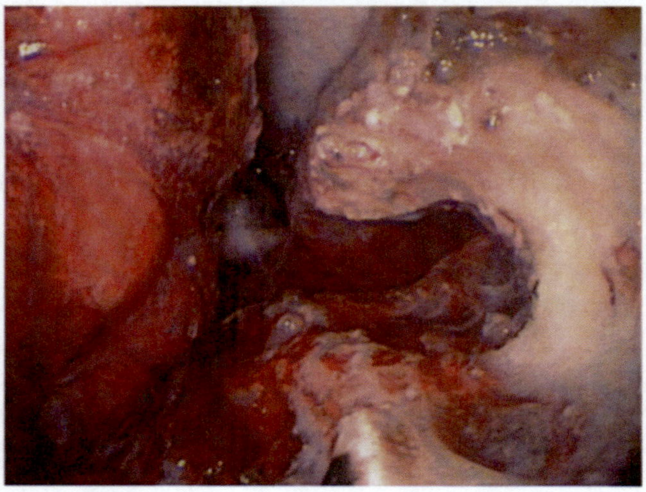

(K)

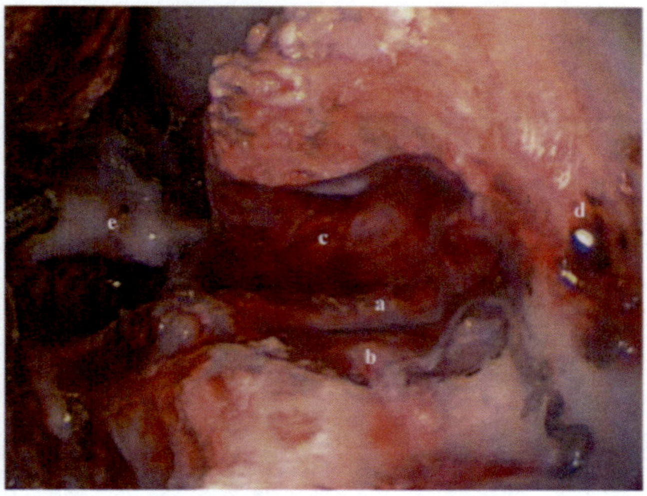

(L)

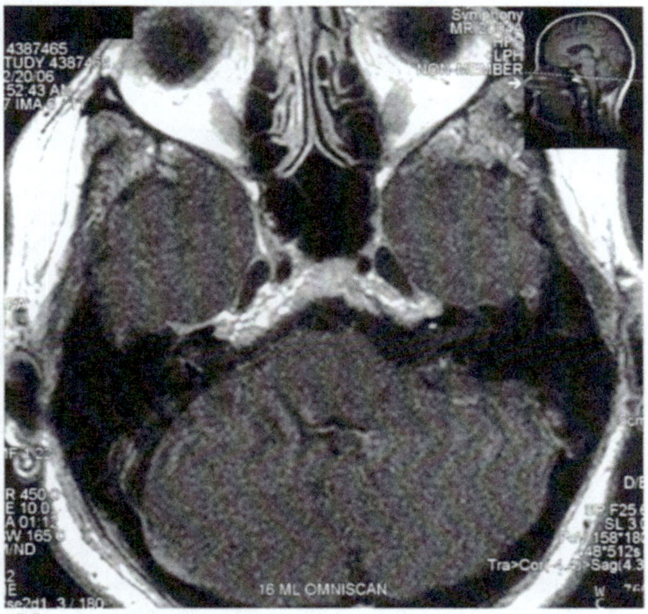

(M)

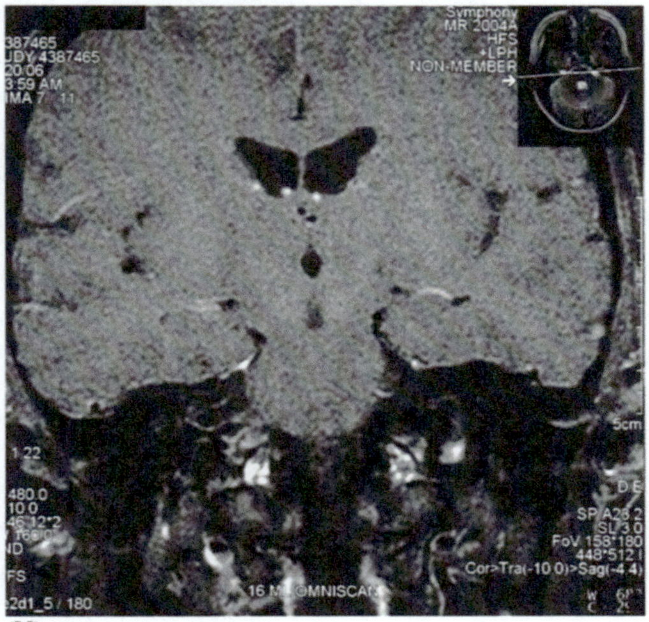

(N)

Fig. 29 (continued)

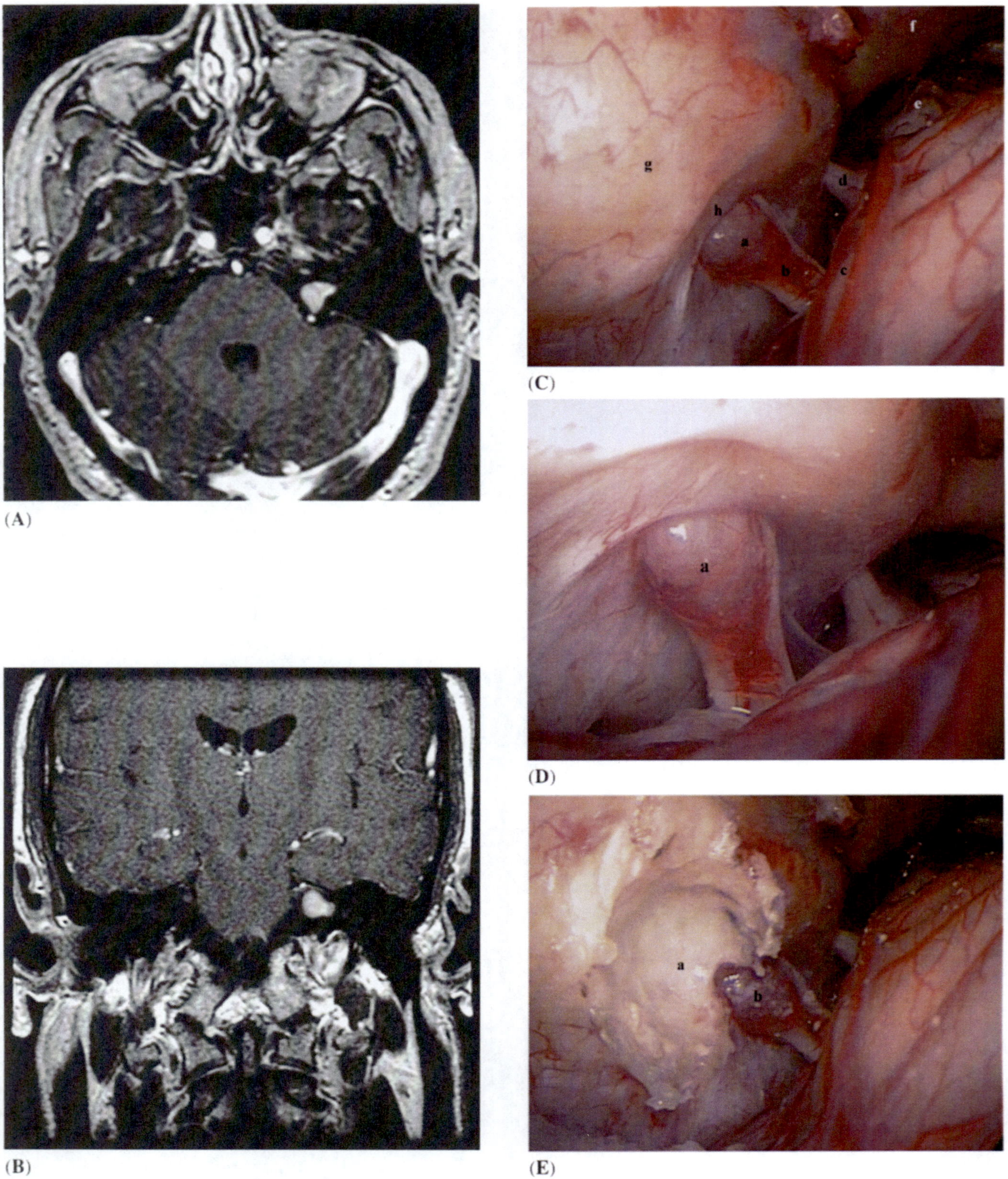

Fig. 30 (**A**) T_1-weighted, contrast-enhanced axial MRI showing medium-size acoustic neuroma. (**B**) T_1-weighted, contrast-enhanced coronal MRI showing medium-size acoustic neuroma. (**C**) and (**D**) Intraoperative endoscopic view showing initial exposure of medium-size acoustic neuroma. (**C**) *a* Acoustic neuroma. *b* Acousticofacial nerve bundle (VII, VIII). *c* Lateral aspect of cerebellum. *d* Trigeminal nerve (V). *e* Brainstem. *f* Tentorium. *g* Petrous temporal bone. *h* Expanded internal meatus (IAM). (**D**) *a* Close-up view of acoustic neuroma and regional anatomy. (**E**)–(**N**) Intraoperative endoscopic view showing gradual resection of medium-size acoustic neuroma. (**E**) *a* Drilled posterior wall of internal auditory canal (IAC). *b* Acoustic neuroma. (**F**) *a* Intracanalicular portion of acoustic neuroma. (**G**) *a* Acoustic neuroma. *b* Ring curette. (**L**) *a* Acoustic neuroma. *b* MicroCUSA tip. (**M**) *a* Final intracanalicular portion of acoustic neuroma. *b* Vestibulocochlear nerve (VIII). *c* Facial nerve (VII). (**N**) *a* Acoustic neuroma. *b* Angled extended ring curette. (**O**)–(**R**) Intraoperative endoscopic view after complete resection of medium-size acoustic neuroma. (**O**) *a* Vestibulocochlear nerve (VIII). *b* Facial nerve (VII). *c* Lateral limit of drilled posterior wall of internal auditory canal (IAC). (**P**) *a* Measurement (1-mm intervals). (**Q**) *a* Vestibulocochlear nerve (VIII) (view using 30° endoscope). *b* Facial nerve (VII) (view using 30° endoscope). *c* Trigeminal (V) nerve. (**R**) *a* Vestibulocochlear nerve (VIII) (close-up view using 30° endoscope). *b* Facial nerve (VII) (close-up view using 30° endoscope). (**S**) Postoperative T_1-weighted, contrast-enhanced axial MRI. (**T**) Postoperative T_1-weighted, contrast-enhanced coronal MRI.

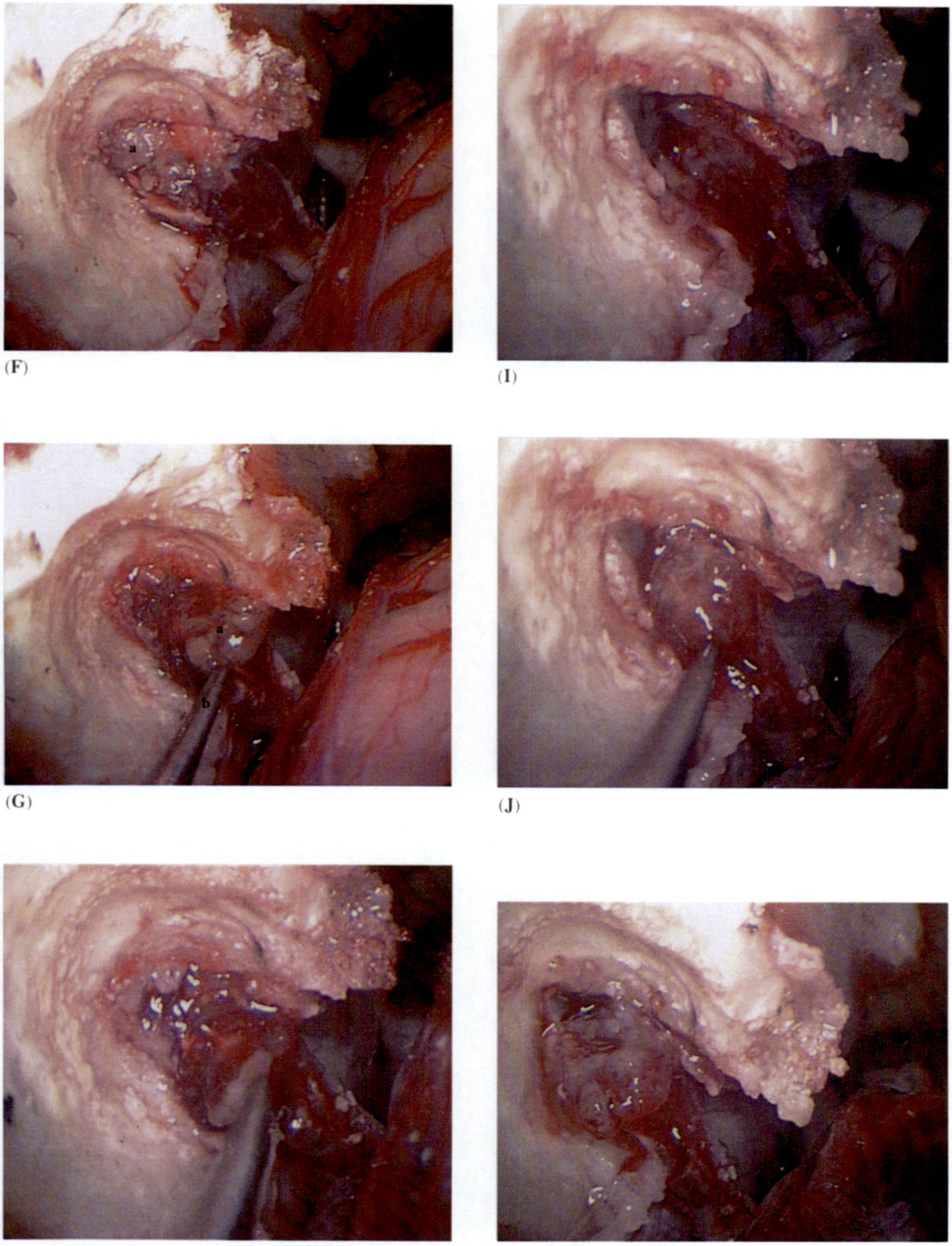

Fig. 30 (continued)

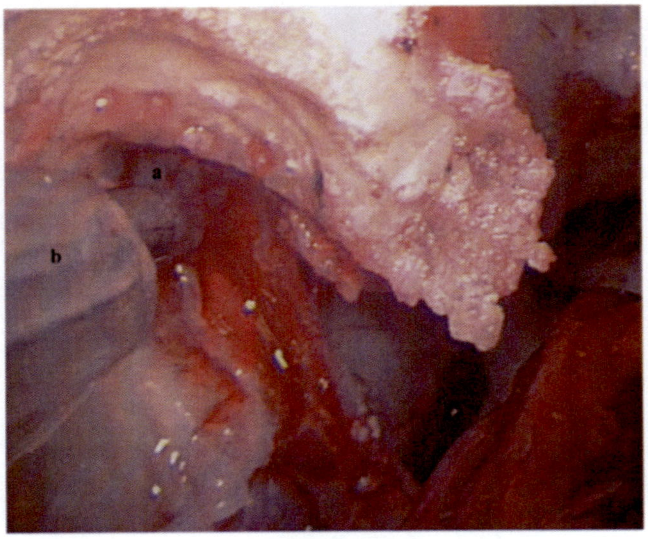

(L)

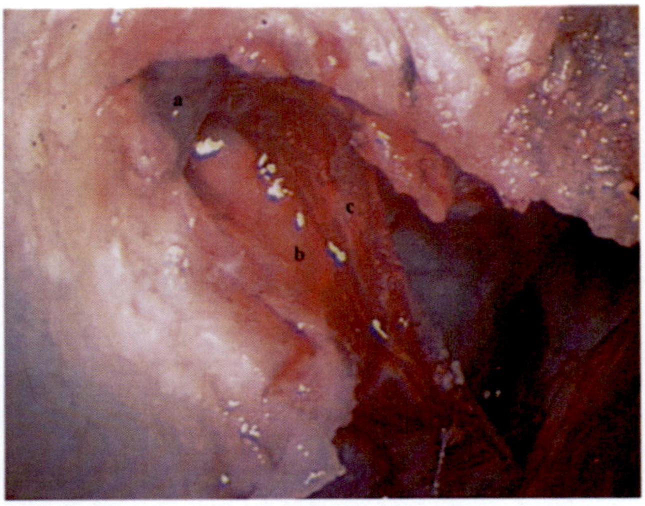

(M)

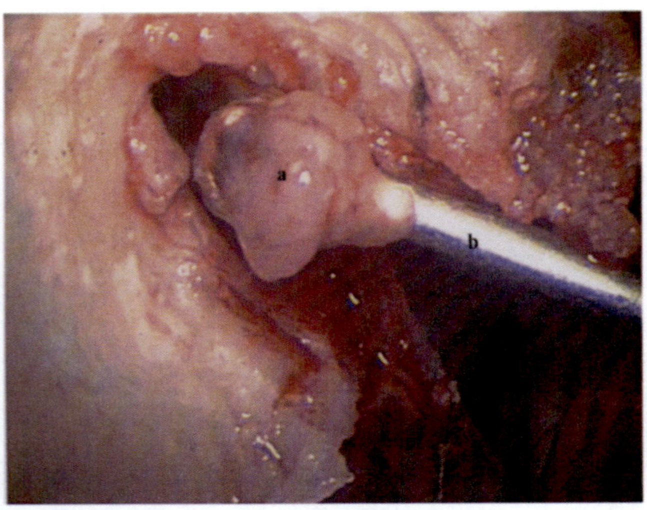

(N)

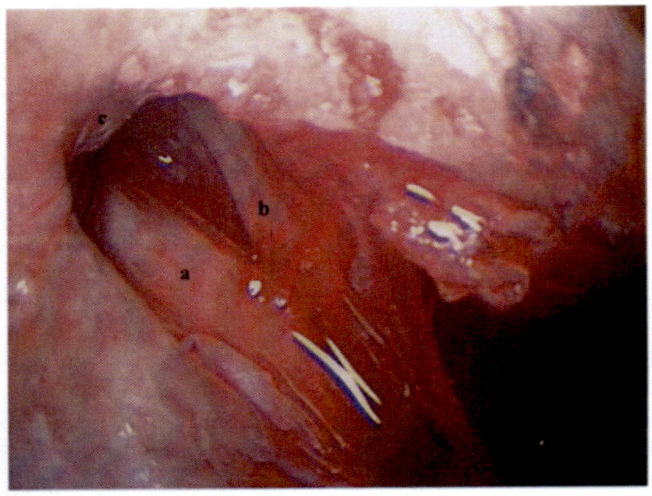

(O)

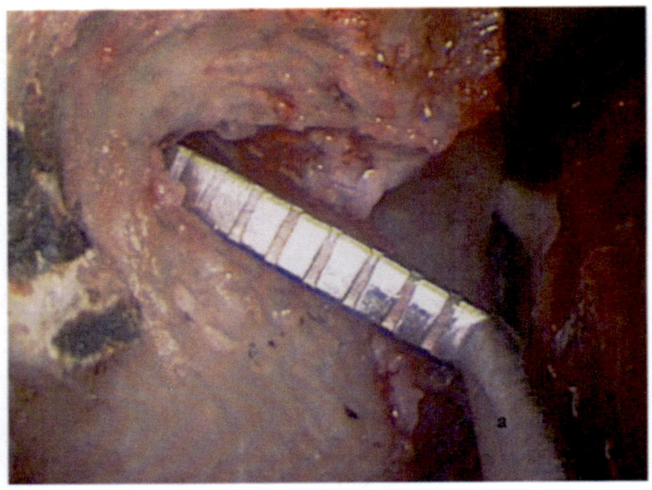

(P)

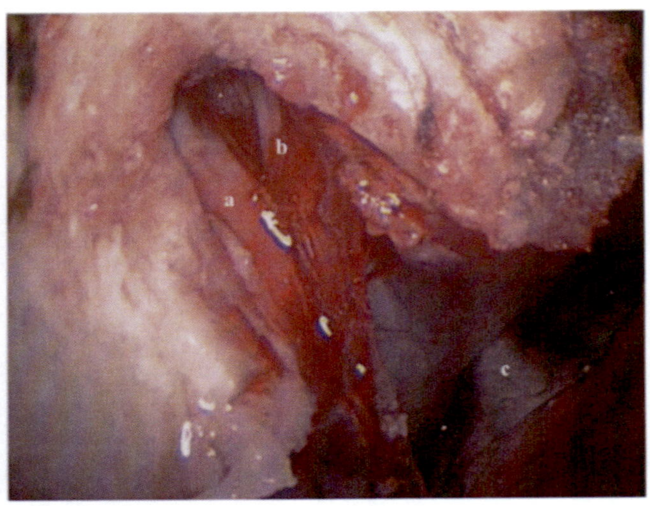

(Q)

Fig. 30 (continued)

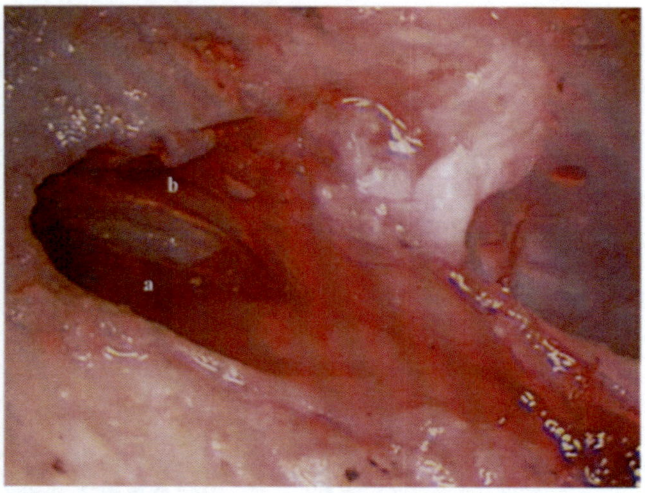

(R)

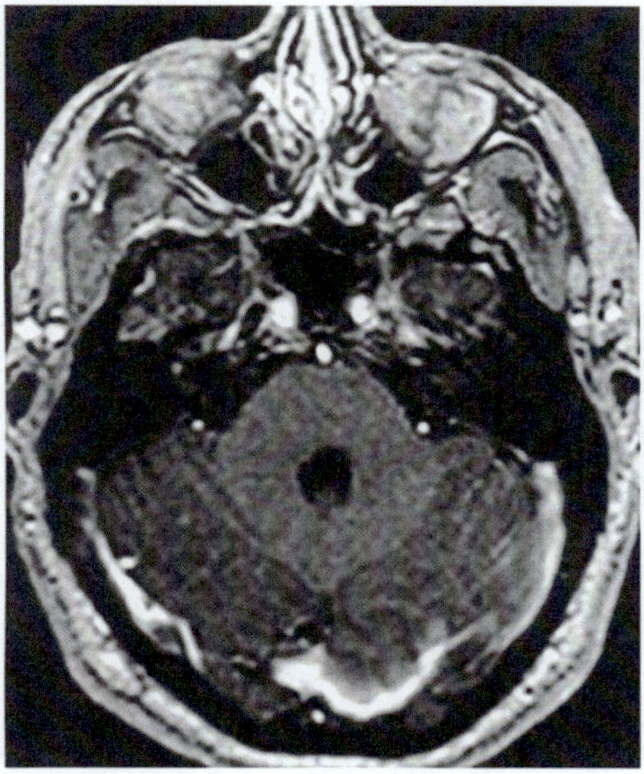

(S)

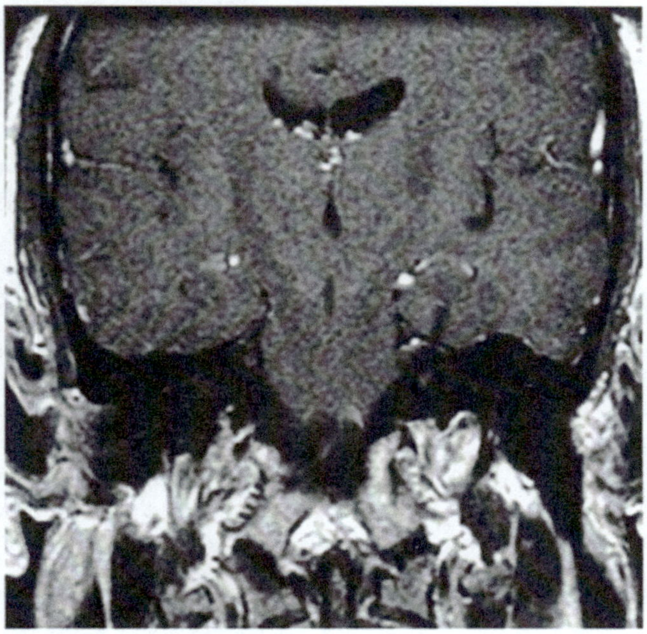

(T)

Fig. 30 (continued)

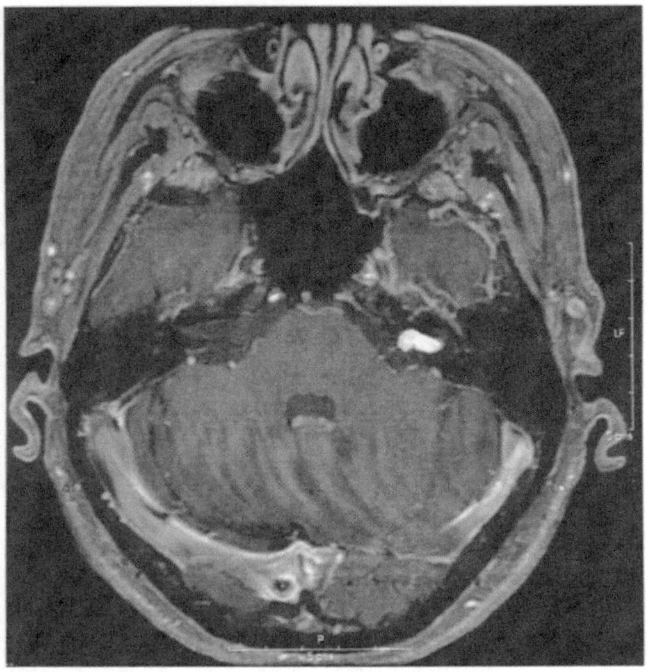

(A)

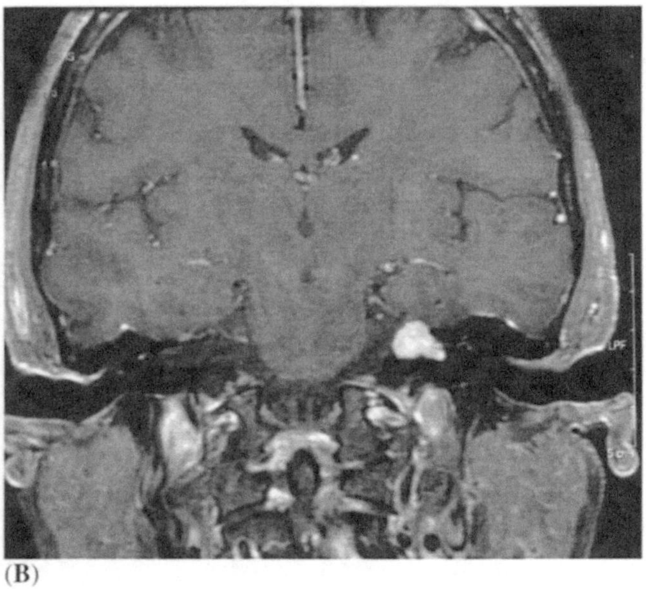

(B)

Fig. 31 (**A**) T_1-weighted, contrast-enhanced axial MRI showing medium-size acoustic neuroma. (**B**) T_1-weighted, contrast-enhanced coronal MRI showing medium-size acoustic neuroma. (**C**) and (**D**) Intraoperative endoscopic view showing initial exposure of medium-size acoustic neuroma. (**C**) *a* Acoustic neuroma. *b* Superior aspect of cerebellum. *c* Expanded internal meatus (IAM). *d* Tentorium. *e* Trigeminal nerve (V). *f* Brainstem. (**D**) *a* Acoustic neuroma. *b* Acousticofacial nerve bundle (VII, VIII). (**E**)–(**K**) Intraoperative endoscopic view showing gradual resection of medium-size acoustic neuroma. (**E**) *a*. Acoustic neuroma. *b*. Left curved microscissors. (**H**) *a* Drilled posterior wall of internal auditory canal (IAC). *b* Acoustic neuroma. *c* Acousticofacial nerve bundle (VII, VIII). *d* Trigeminal nerve (V). (**I**) *a* Close-up view of final portions of acoustic neuroma. (**L**) and (**M**) Intraoperative endoscopic view after complete resection of medium-size acoustic neuroma. (**L**) *a* Close-up view of vestibulocochlear nerve (VII, VIII). *b* Close-up view of facial nerve (VII). *c* Lateral limit of drilled posterior wall of internal auditory canal (IAC). (**M**) *a* Vestibulocochlear nerve (VIII) (close-up view using 30° endoscope). *b* Facial nerve (VII) (close-up view using 30° endoscope). (**N**) Postoperative T_1-weighted, contrast-enhanced axial MRI. (**O**) Postoperative T_1-weighted, contrast-enhanced coronal MRI.

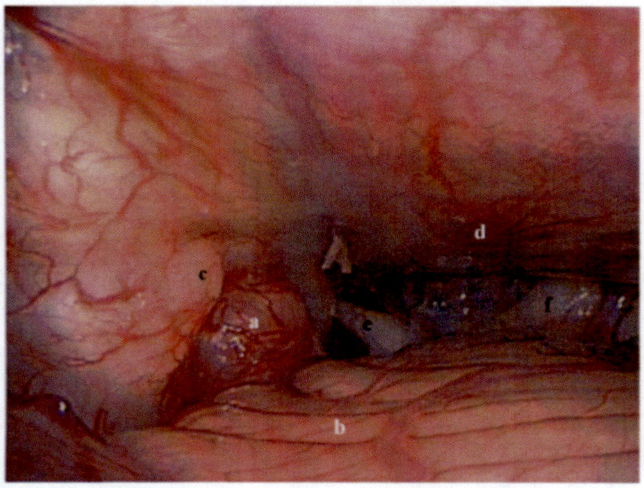

(C)

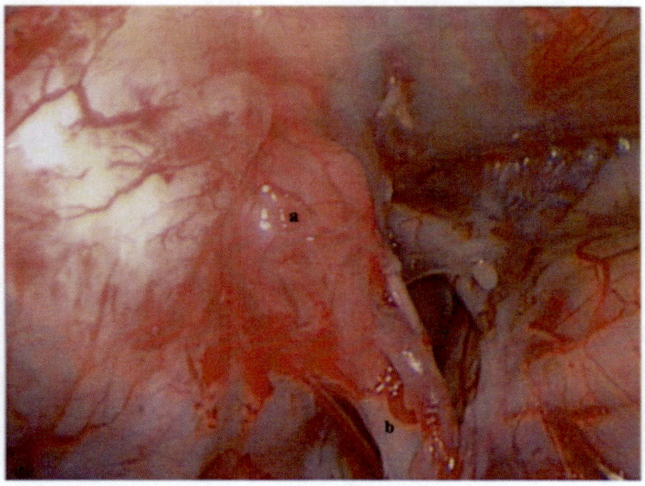

(D)

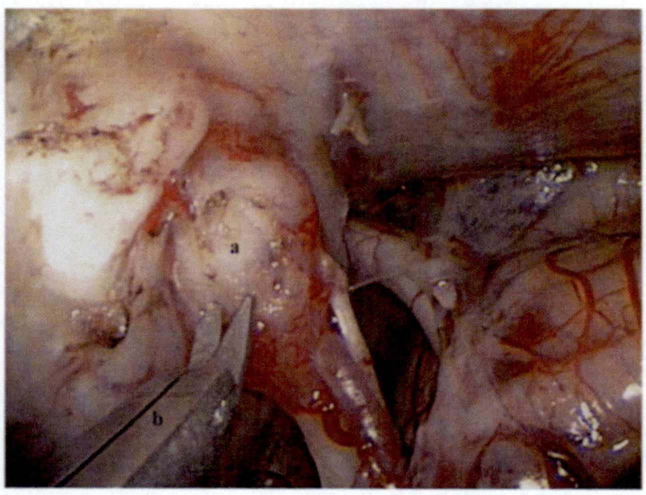

(E)

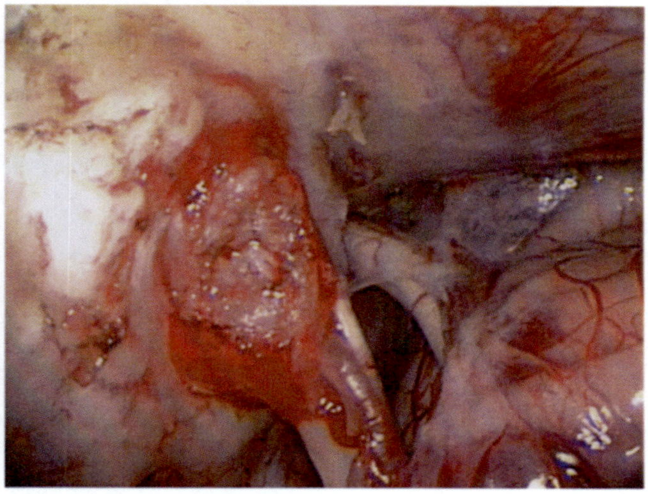
(F)

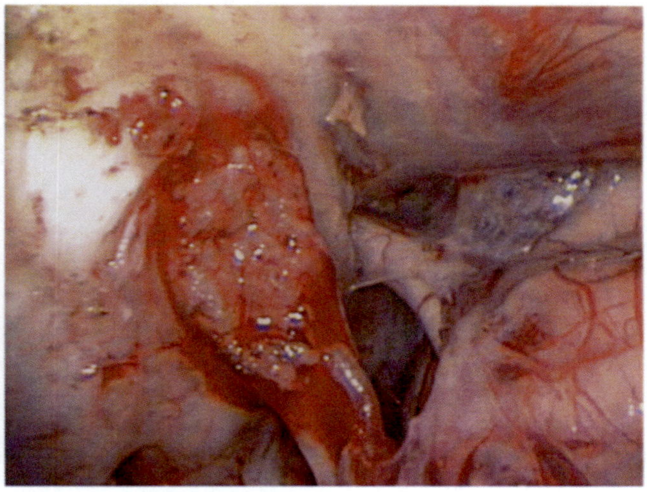
(G)

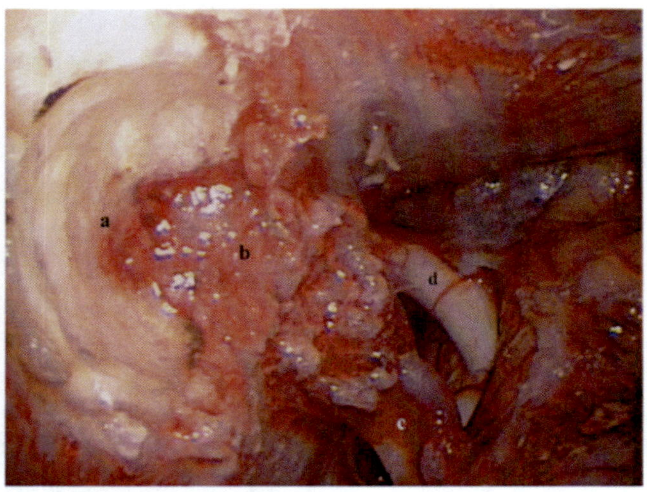

(H)

Fig. 31 (continued)

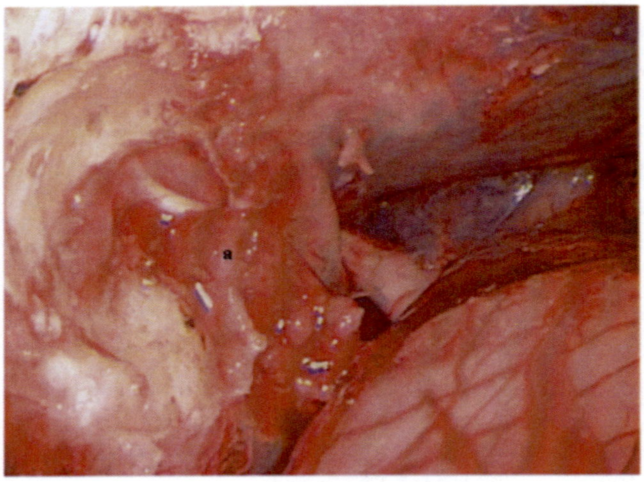

(I)

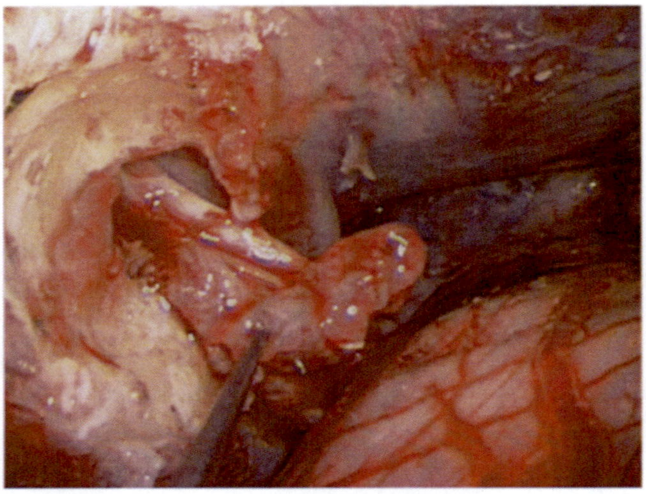

(J)

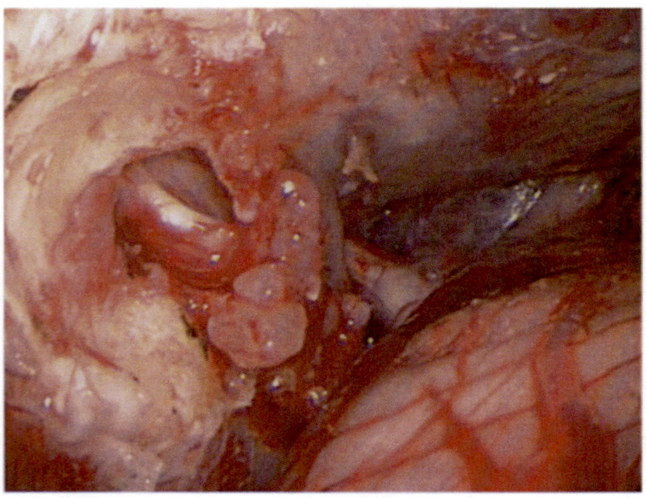

(K)

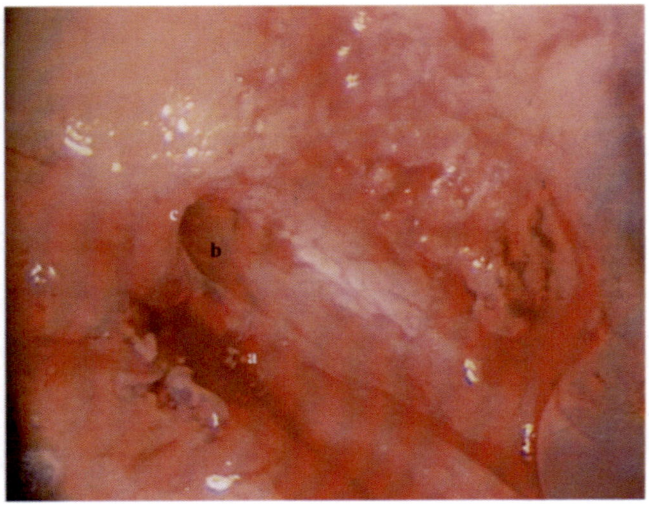

(L)

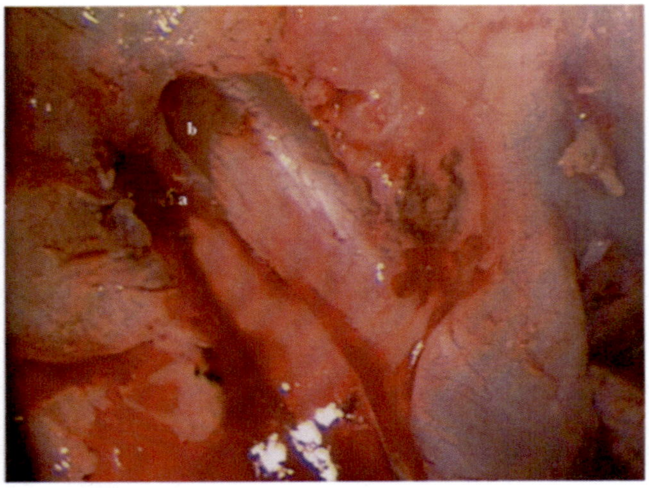

(M)

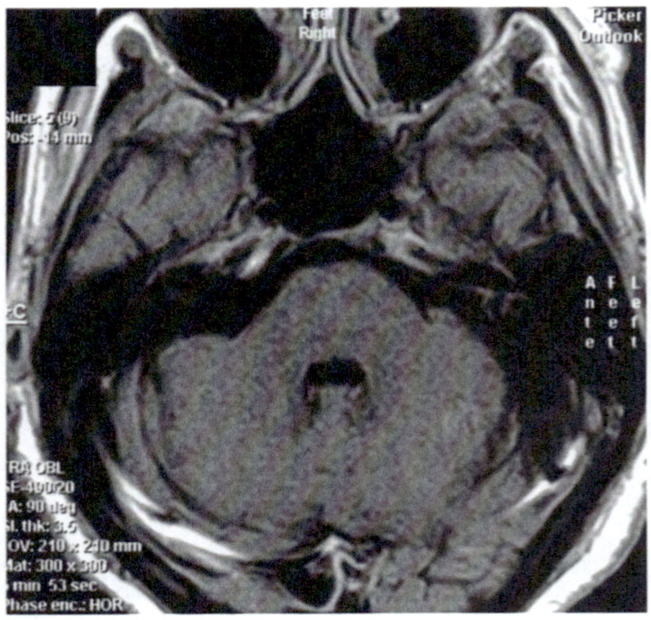

(N)

Fig. 31 (continued)

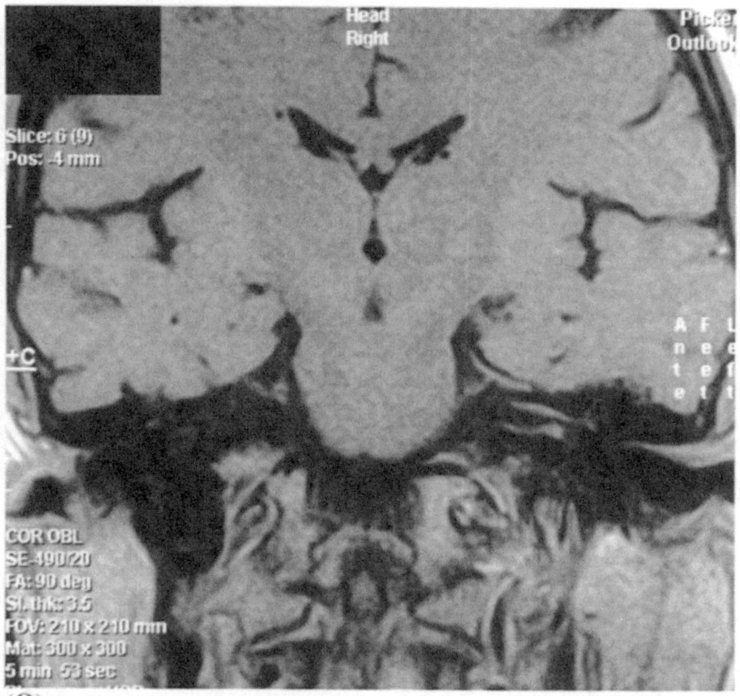

(O)

Fig. 31 (continued)

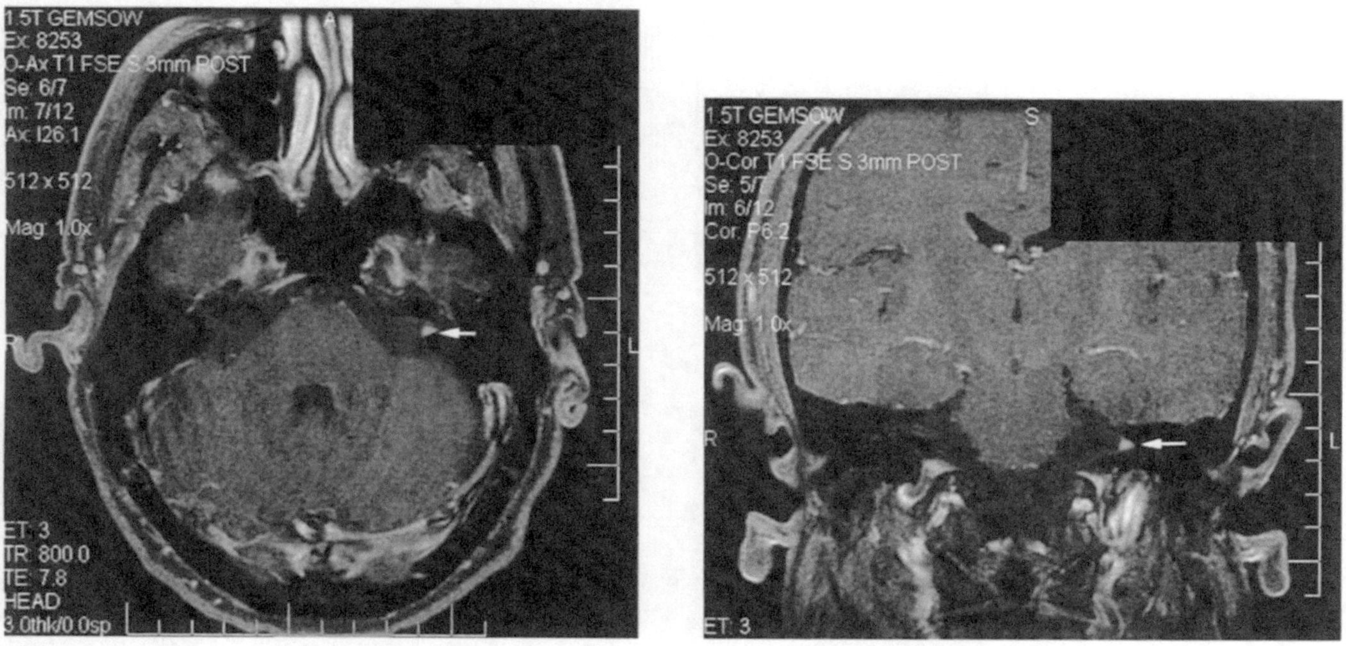

(A) (B)

Fig. 32 (**A**) T_1-weighted, contrast-enhanced axial MRI showing a purely intracanalicular acoustic neuroma. (**B**) T_1-weighted, contrast-enhanced coronal MRI showing a purely intracanalicular acoustic neuroma. (**C**)–(**J**) Intraoperative endoscopic view showing exposure and resection of a purely intracanalicular acoustic neuroma. (**C**) *a* Vestibulocochlear nerve (VIII). *b* Facial nerve (VII). *c* Lateral aspect of cerebellum. *d* Expanded internal meatus (IAM). *e* Petrous temporal bone. (**D**) *a* Close-up view of vestibulocochlear nerve (VIII). *b* Facial nerve (VII). (**E**) *a* Drilling of posterior wall of internal auditory canal (IAC). (**H**) *a* Acoustic neuroma. (**J**) *a* Intracanlicular vestibulocochlear nerve (VIII) after complete tumor resection. *b* Facial nerve (VII). *c*. Lateral limit of drilled internal auditory canal (IAC). *d*. Brainstem. (**K**) Postoperative T_1-weighted, contrast-enhanced axial MRI. (**L**) Postoperative T_1-weighted, contrast-enhanced coronal MRI.

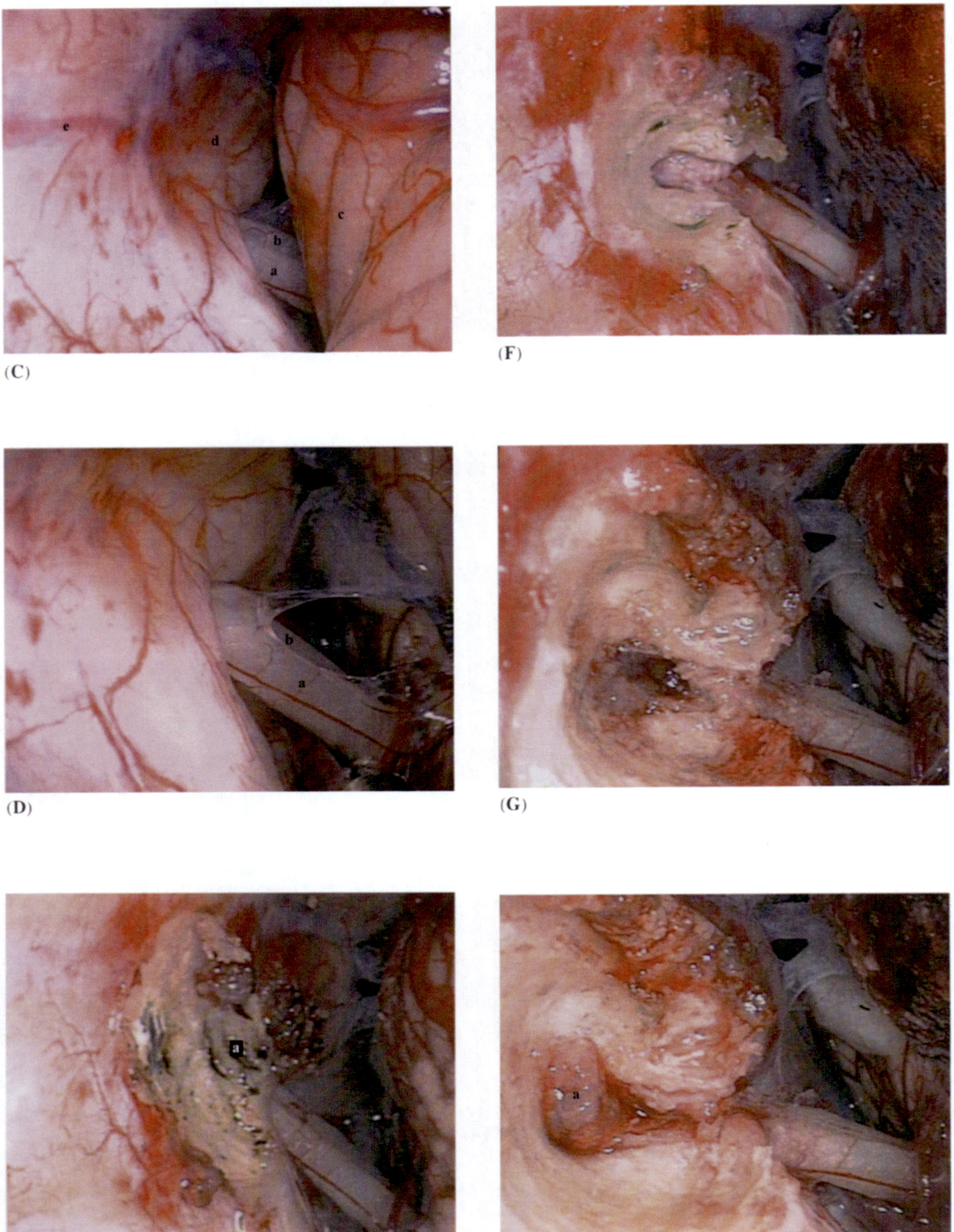

(C) (F) (D) (G) (E) (H)

Fig. 32 (continued)

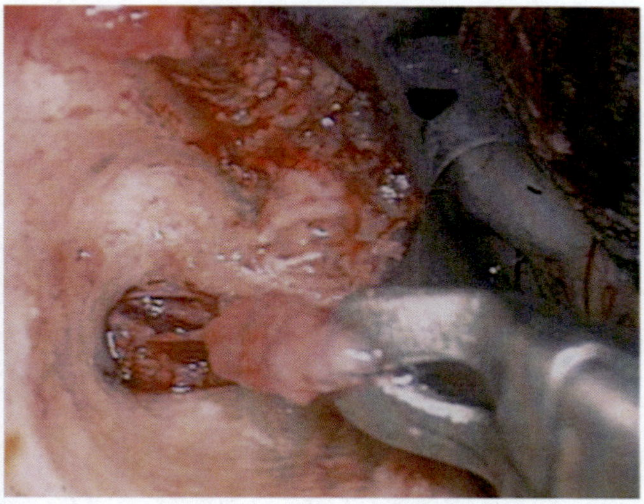

(I)

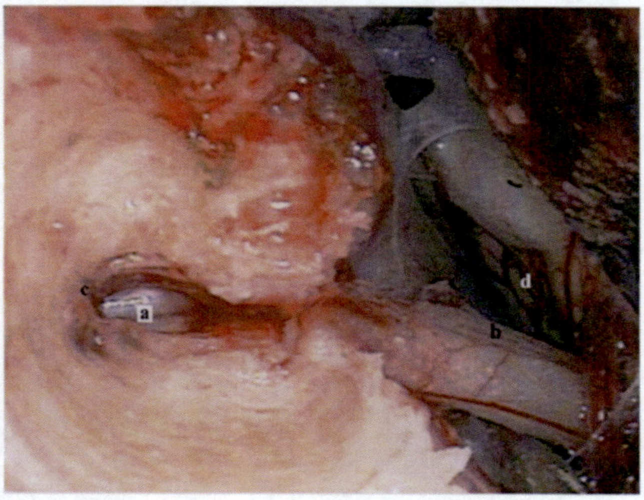

(J)

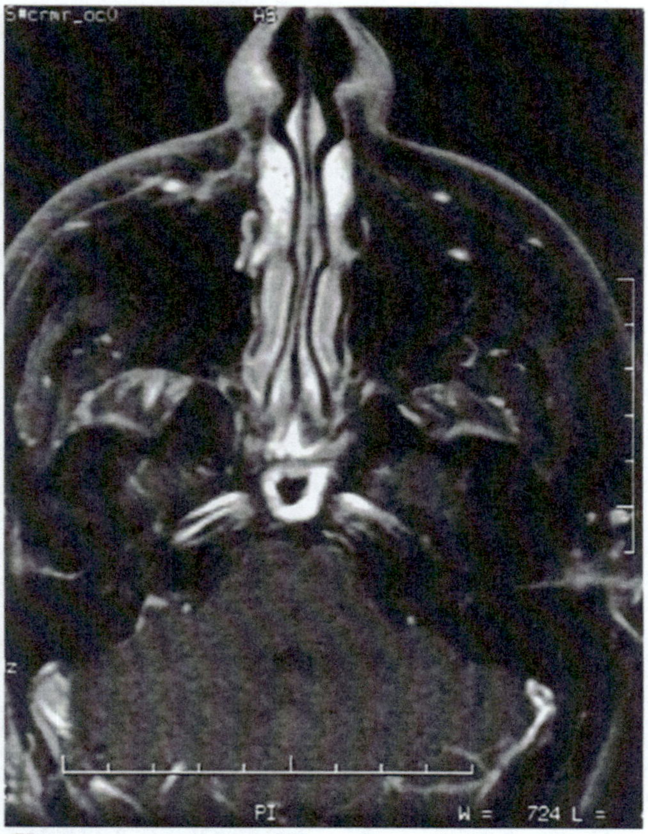

(K)

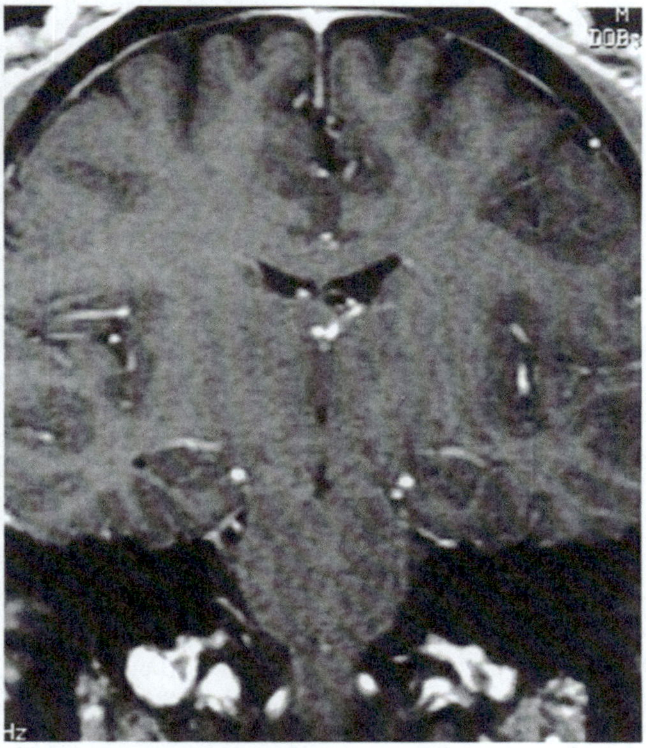

(L)

Fig. 32 (continued)

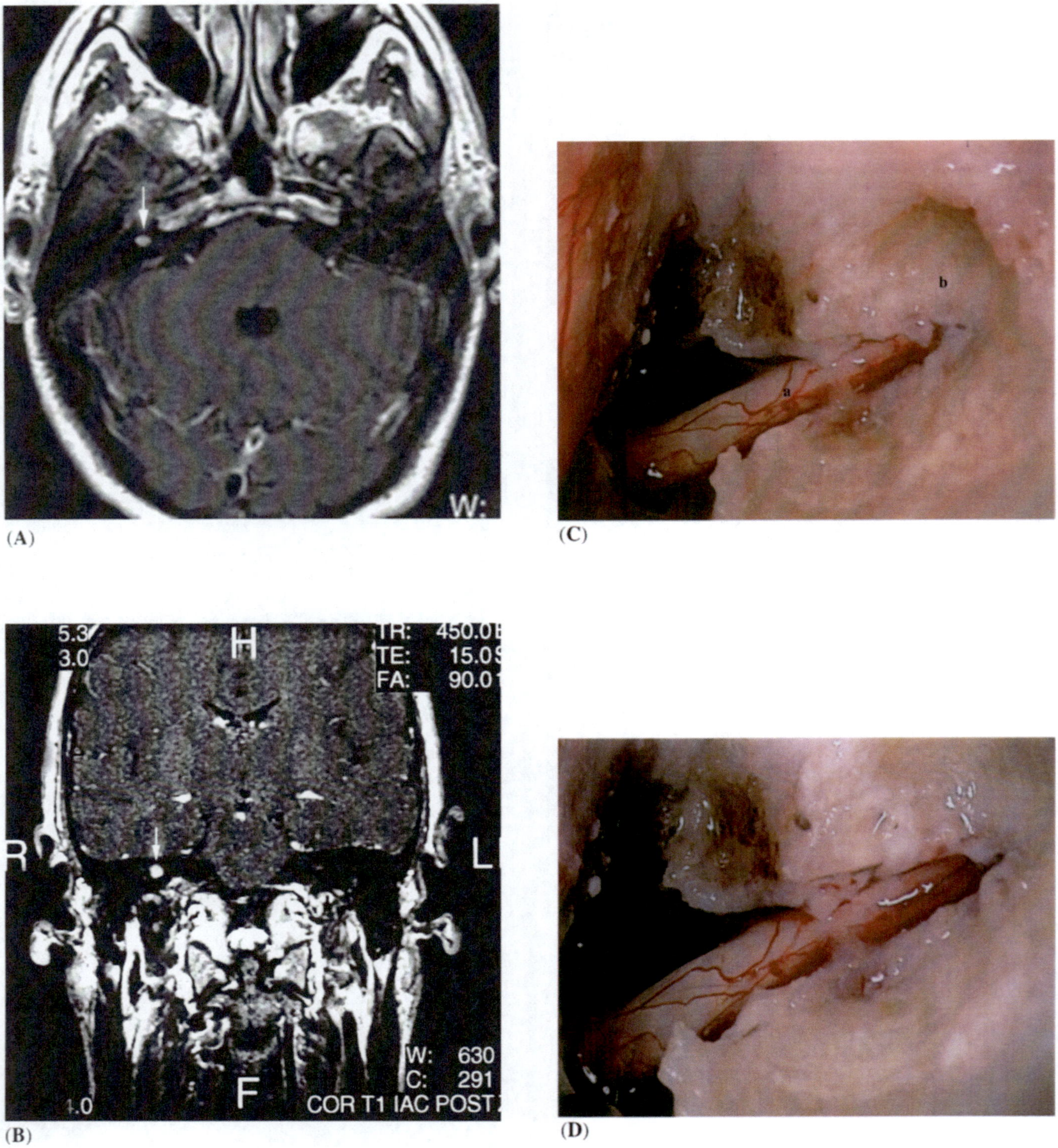

Fig. 33 (**A**) T_1-weighted, contrast-enhanced axial MRI showing a purely intracanalicular acoustic neuroma. (**B**) T_1-weighted, contrast-enhanced coronal MRI showing a purely intracanalicular acoustic neuroma. (**C**)–(**G**) Intraoperative endoscopic view showing exposure and resection of a purely intracanalicular acoustic neuroma. (**C**) *a* Vestibulocochlear nerve (VIII). *b* Drilling of posterior wall of internal auditory canal (IAC). (**E**) *a* Acoustic neuroma. *b* Vestibulocochlear nerve (VIII). (**F**) *a* Acoustic neuroma. *b* Right-curved microcupped forceps tip. *c* Atraumatic suction. (**G**) *a* Acoustic neuroma cavity after complete tumor resection. (**H**) Postoperative T_1-weighted, contrast-enhanced axial MRI. (**I**) Postoperative T_1-weighted, contrast-enhanced coronal MRI.

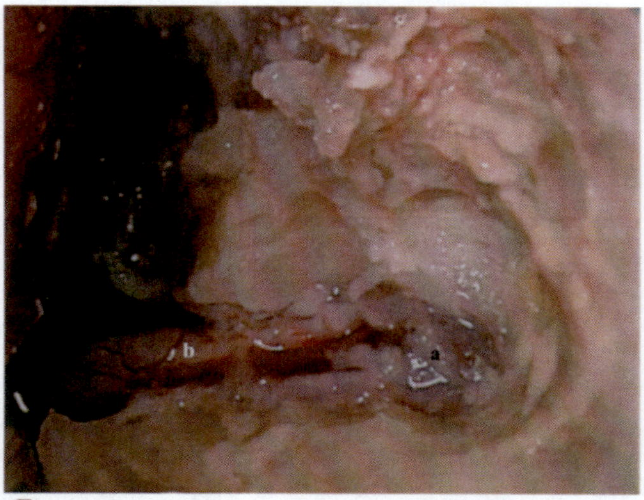

(E)

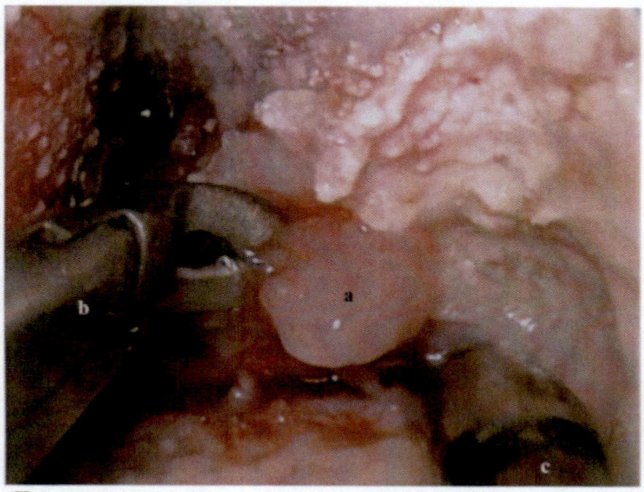

(F)

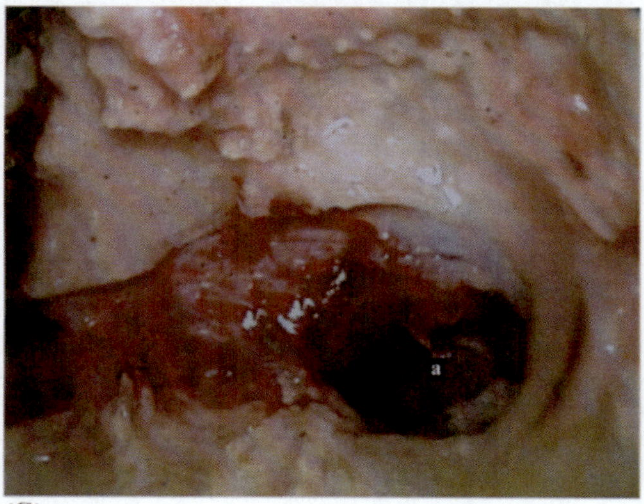

(G)

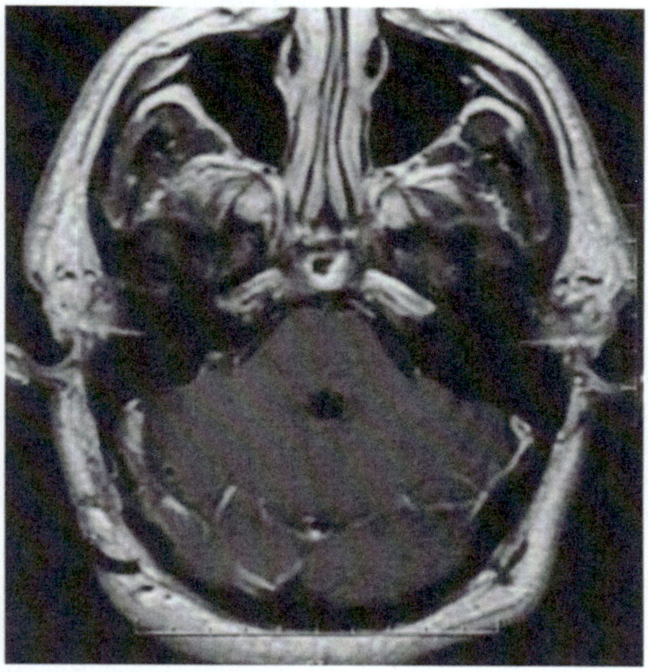

(H)

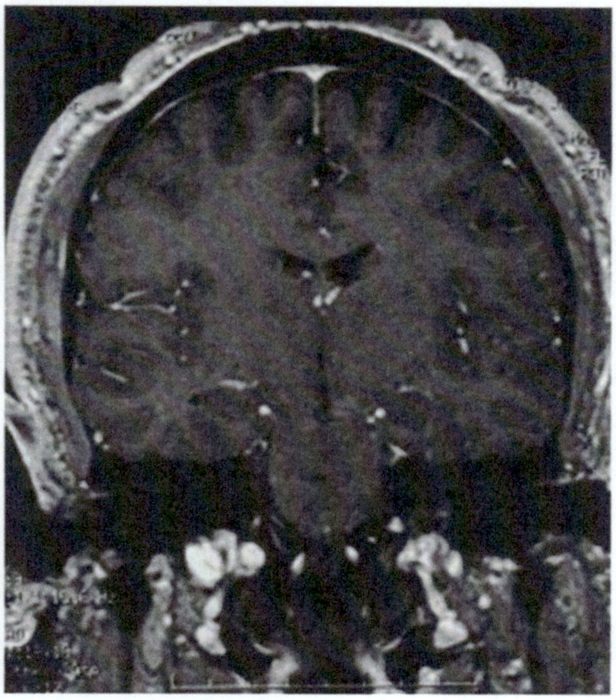

(I)

Fig. 33 (continued)

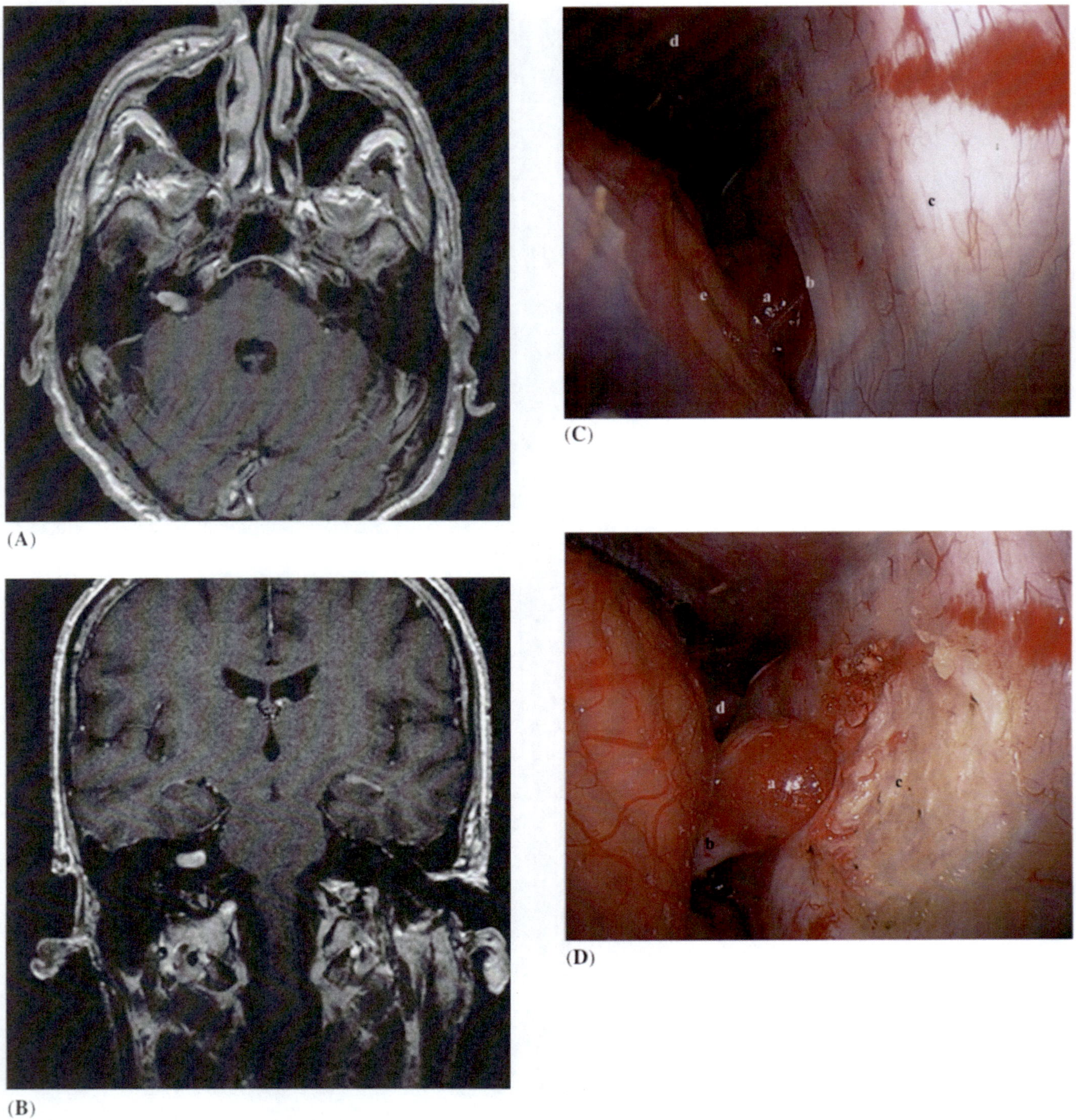

Fig. 34 (**A**) T_1-weighted, contrast-enhanced axial MRI showing intracanalicular acoustic neuroma. (**B**) T_1-weighted, contrast-enhanced coronal MRI showing intracanalicular acoustic neuroma. (**C**)–(**N**) Intraoperative endoscopic view showing exposure and resection of intracanalicular acoustic neuroma. (**C**) *a* Acoustic neuroma. *b* Expanded internal meatus (IAM). *c* Petrous temporal bone. *d* Tentorium. *e* Lateral aspect of cerebellum. (**D**) *a* Acoustic neuroma. *b* Vestibulocochlear nerve (VIII). *c* Drilling of posterior wall of internal auditory canal (IAC). *d* Trigeminal nerve (V). (**F**) *a* Acoustic neuroma. *b* Straight microscissors. (**I**) *a* Acoustic neuroma. *b* Upward-angled microhook. *c* Atraumatic suction. (**L**) *a* Final portions of acoustic neuroma. *b* Vestibulocochlear nerve (VIII). (**M**) *a* Final portions of acoustic neuroma being removed. *b* Extended angled ring curette. (**O**)–(**Q**) Intraoperative endoscopic view after complete resection of intracanalicular acoustic neuroma. (**O**) *a* Vestibulocochlear nerve (VIII). *b* Facial nerve (VII). *c* Lateral Limit of drilled posterior wall of internal auditory canal (IAC). *d* Lateral aspect of cerebellum. (**P**) *a* Close-up view of vestibulocochlear nerve (VIII) and regional anatomy. *b* facial nerve (**Q**) *a* Close-up view of vestibulocochlear nerve (VIII) and regional anatomy using 30° endoscope. (**R**) Postoperative T_1-weighted, contrast-enhanced axial MRI. (**S**) Postoperative T_1-weighted, contrast-enhanced coronal MRI.

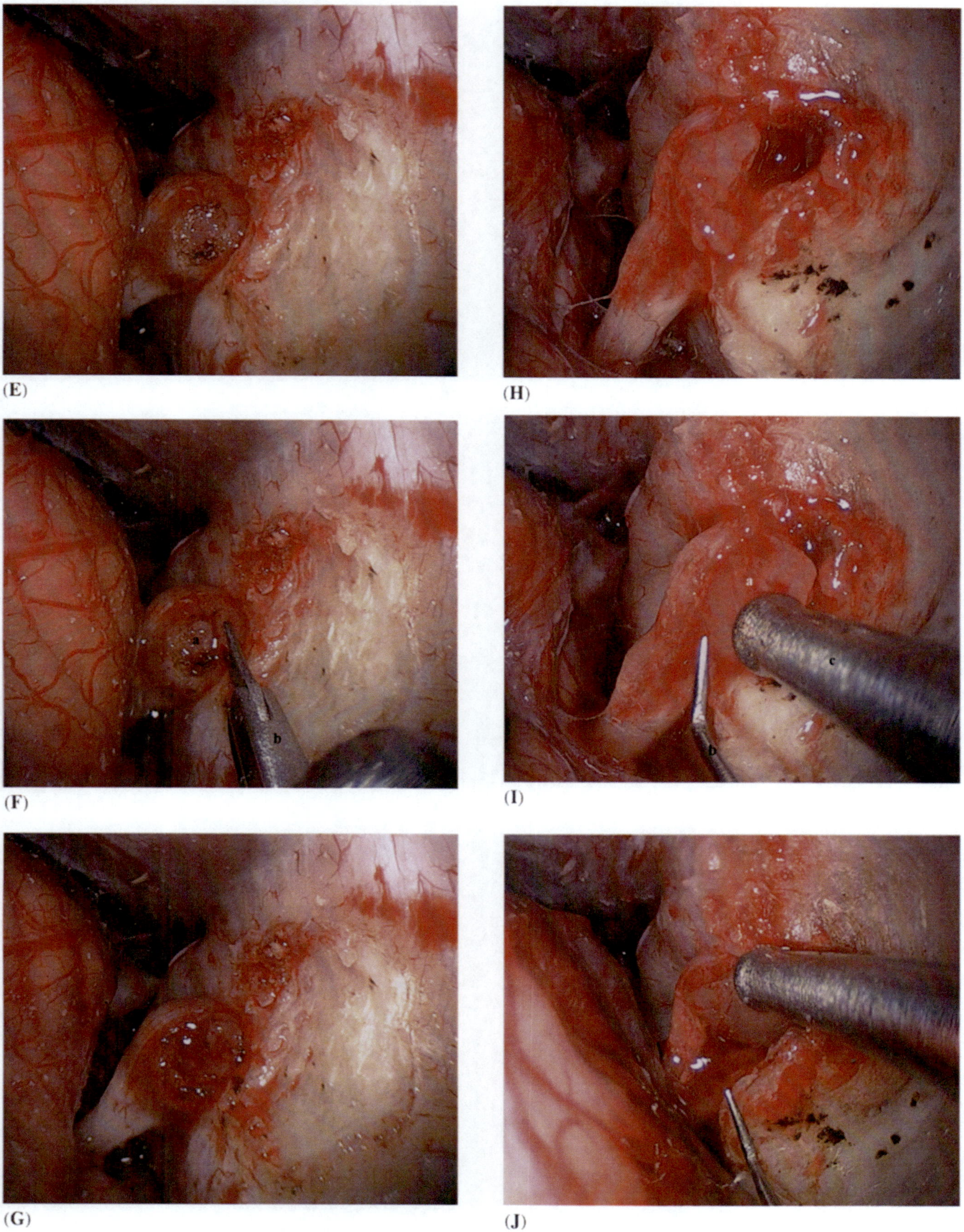

Fig. 34 (continued)

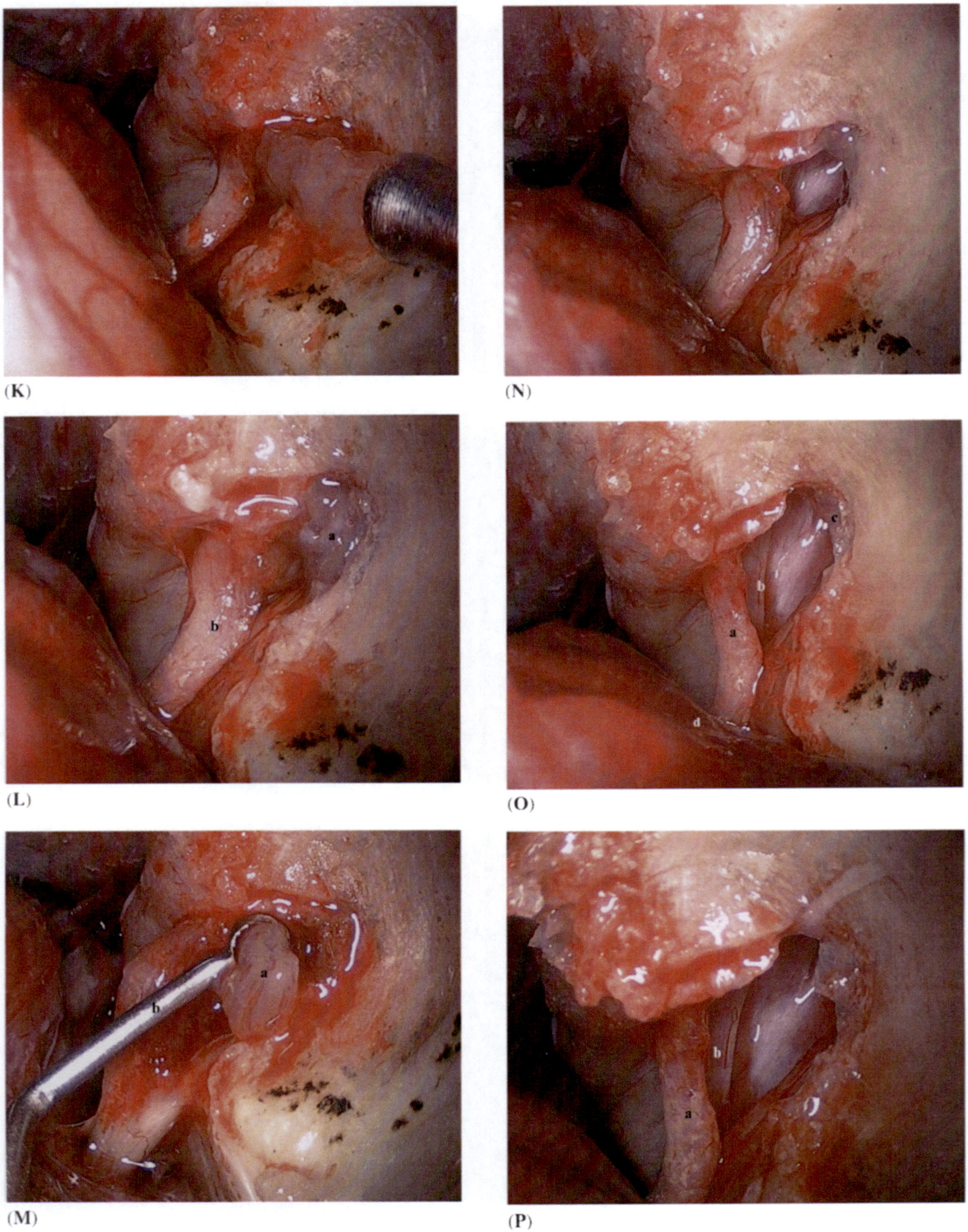

Fig. 34 (continued)

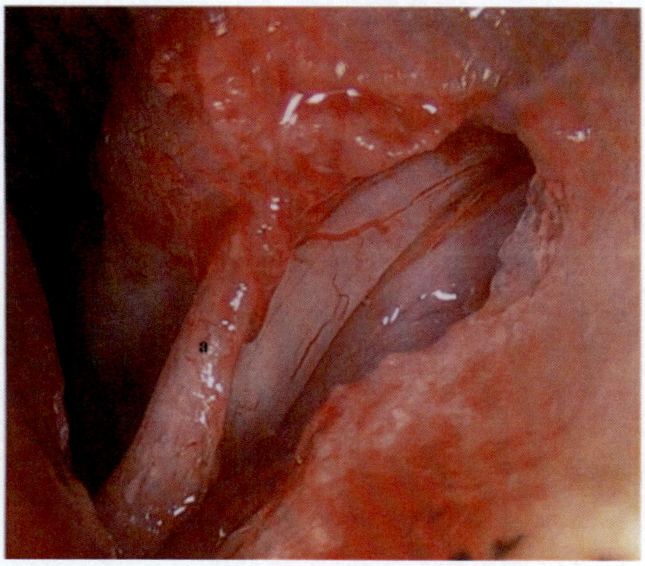

(**Q**)

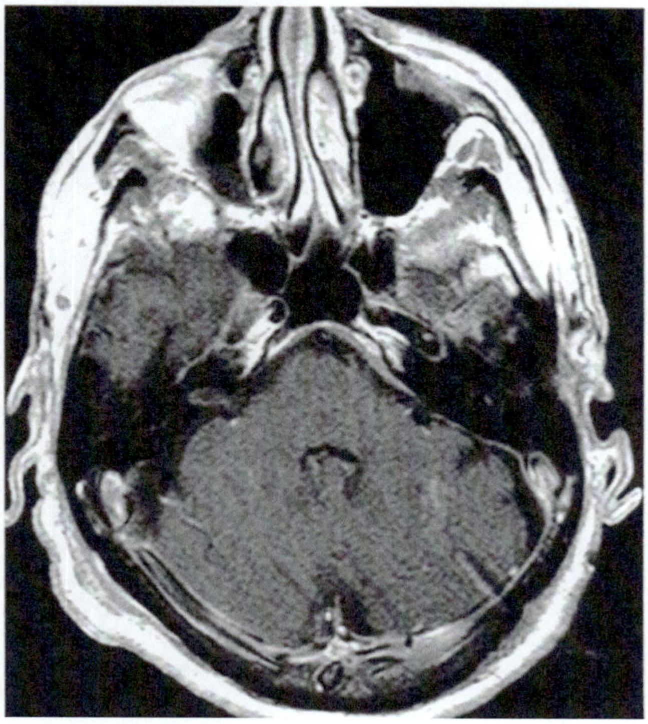

(**R**)

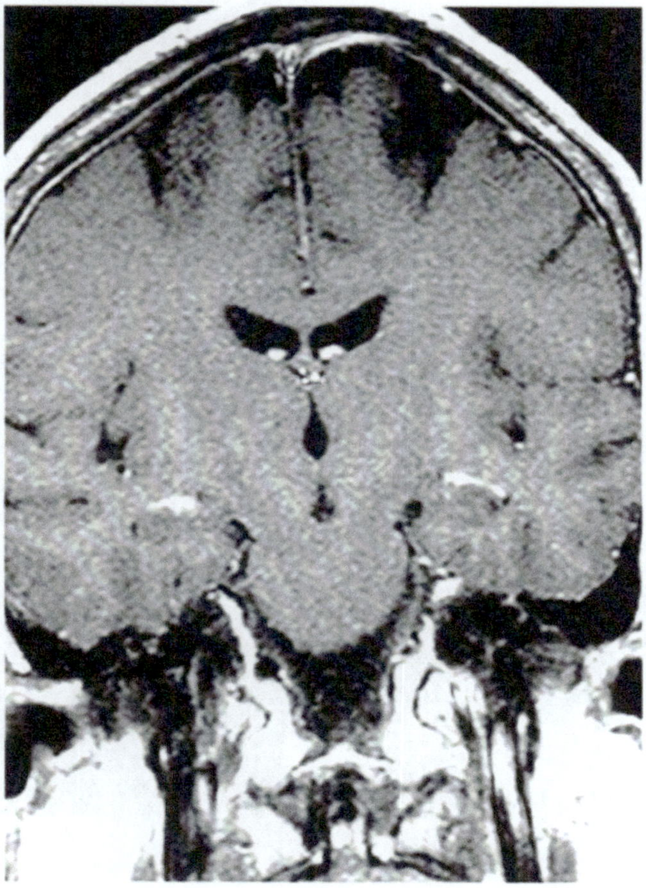

(**S**)

Fig. 34 (continued)

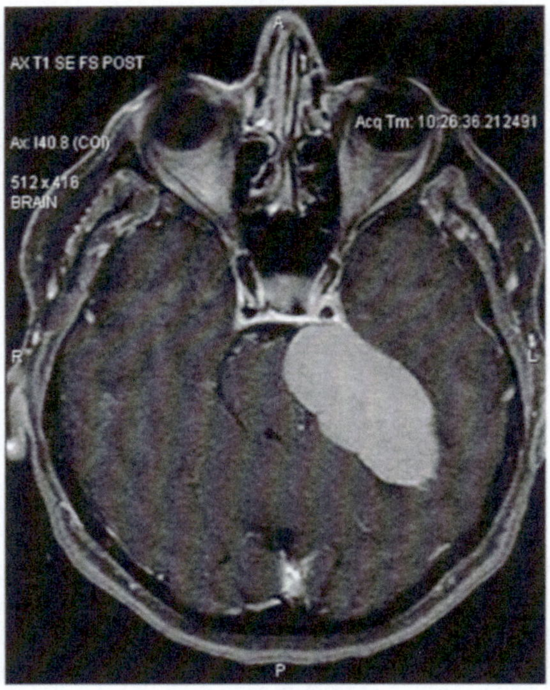

(A)

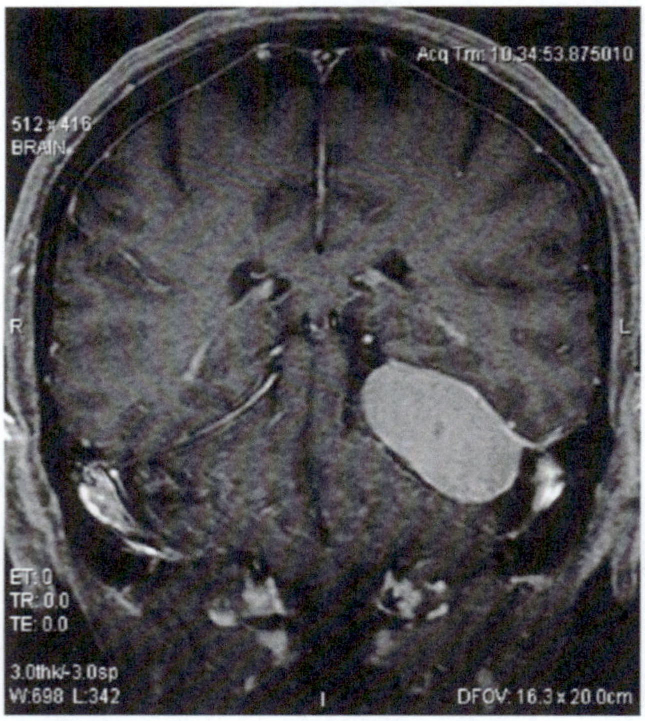

(B)

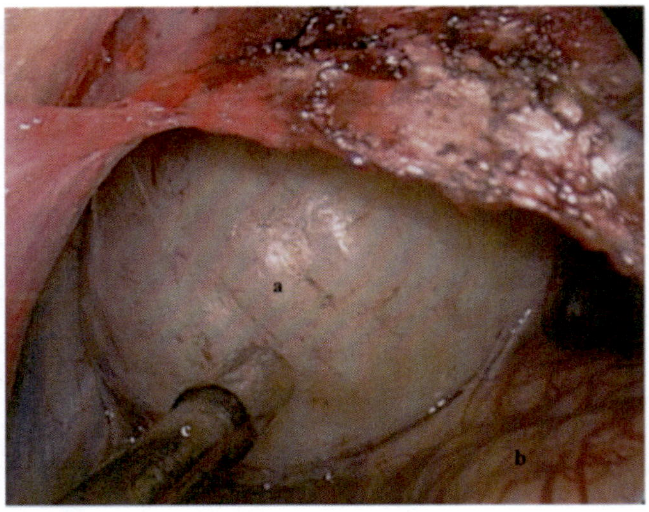

(C)

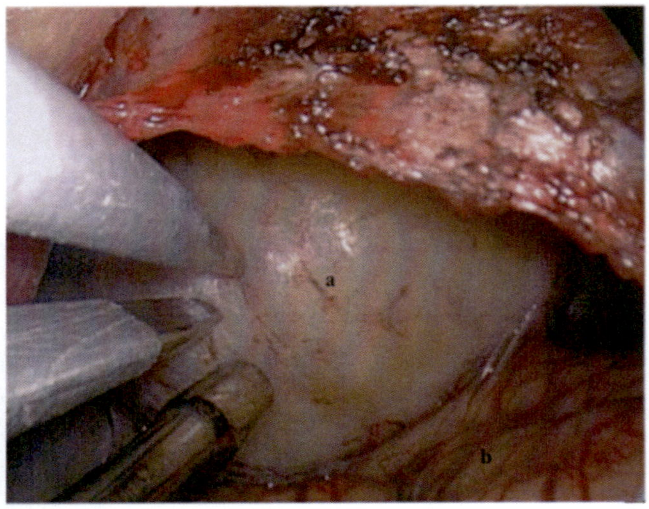

(D)

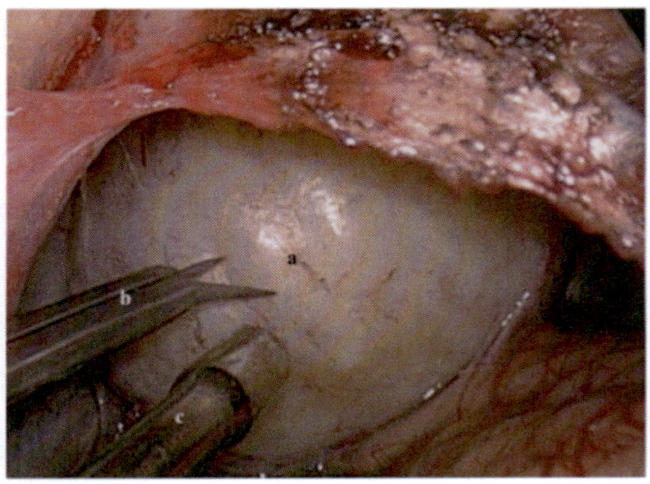

(E)

Fig. 35 (**A**) T_1-weighted, contrast-enhanced axial MRI showing a superior cerebellar convexity meningioma extending to cerebellopontine angle (CPA). (**B**) T_1-weighted, contrast-enhanced coronal MRI showing a superior cerebellar convexity meningioma extending to CPA. (**C**) Intraoperative endoscopic view showing initial exposure of a superior cerebellar convexity meningioma extending to CPA. *a* Meningioma. *b* Superolateral aspect of cerebellum. *c* Atraumatic suction. (**D**)–(**J**) Intraoperative endoscopic view showing gradual resection of a superior cerebellar convexity meningioma extending to CPA. (**D**). *a* Meningioma. *b* Superolateral aspect of cerebellum. (**E**) *a* Meningioma. *b* Straight microscissors. *c* Atraumatic suction. (**F**) *a* Meningioma biopsied. (**G**) *a* Meningioma partly debulked. *b* MicroCUSA tip. (**I**) *a* Meningioma attachment being cauterized and resected. *b* Facial nerve (VII). *c* Superior aspect of cerebellum. (**J**) *a* Meningioma attachment after complete tumor resection. *b* Tentorium. *c* Trochlear nerve (IV). *d* Trigeminal nerve (V). *e* Acousticofacial nerve bundle (VII, VIII). *f* Superior aspect of cerebellum. (**K**) Postoperative T_1-weighted, contrast-enhanced axial MRI. (**L**) Postoperative T_1-weighted, contrast-enhanced coronal MRI.

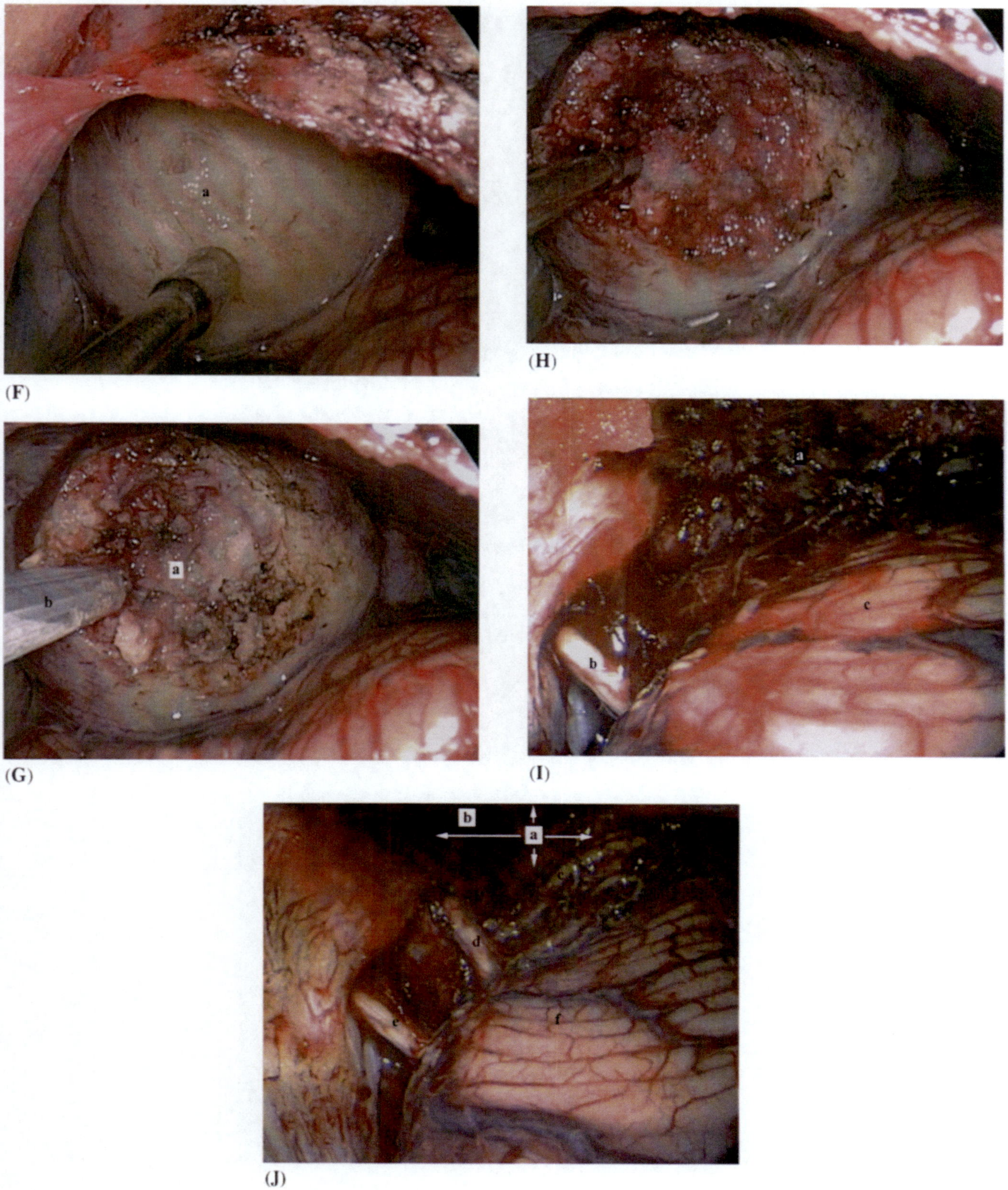

Fig. 35 (continued)

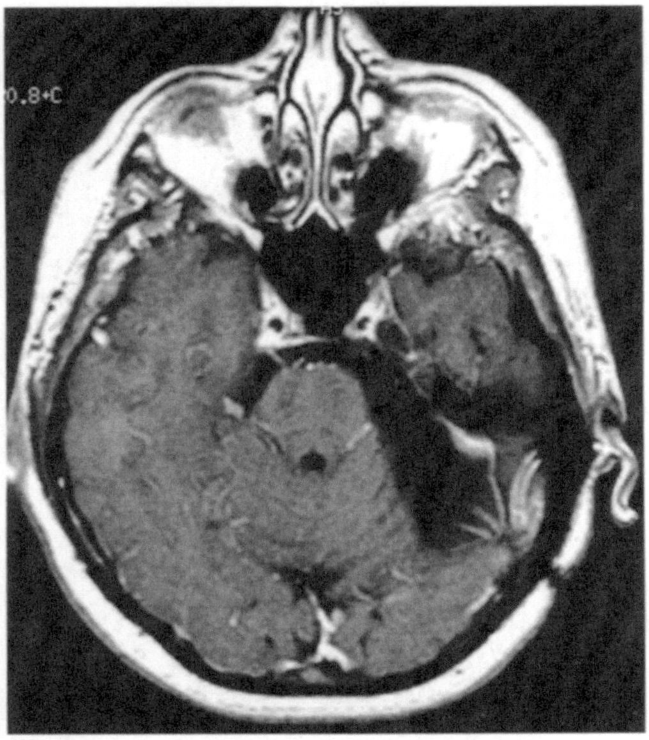

(K)

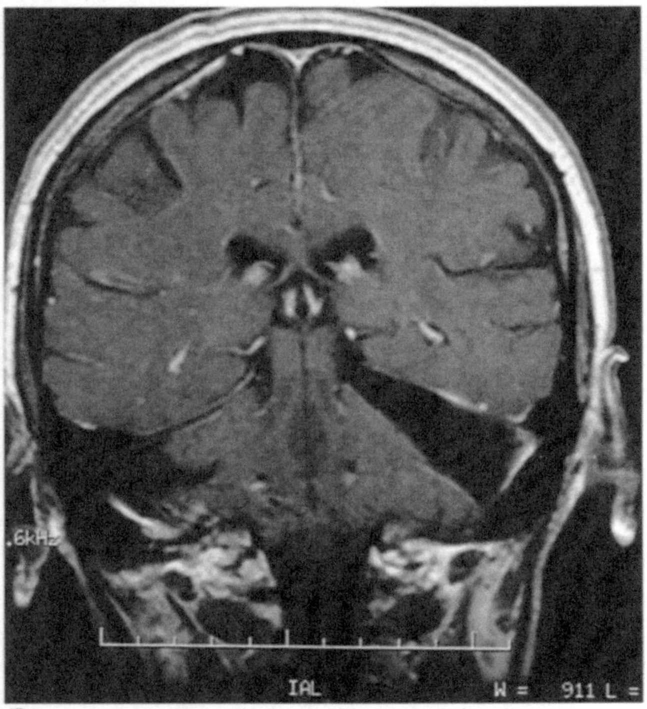

(L)

Fig. 35 (continued)

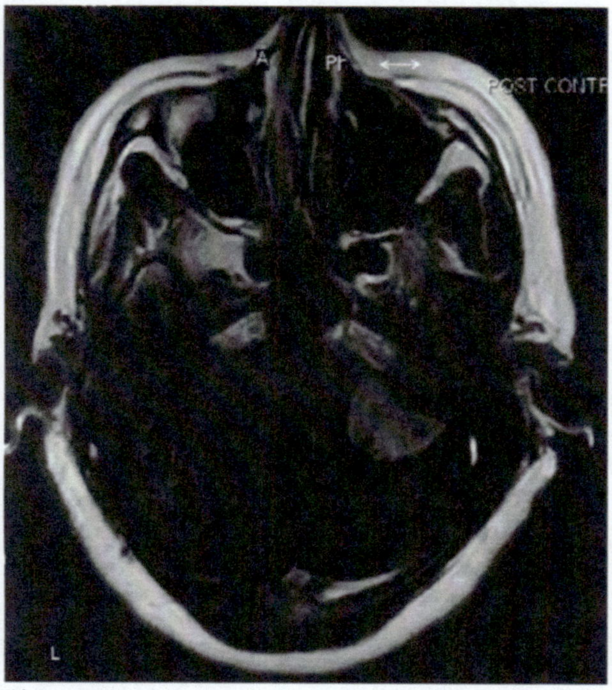

(A)

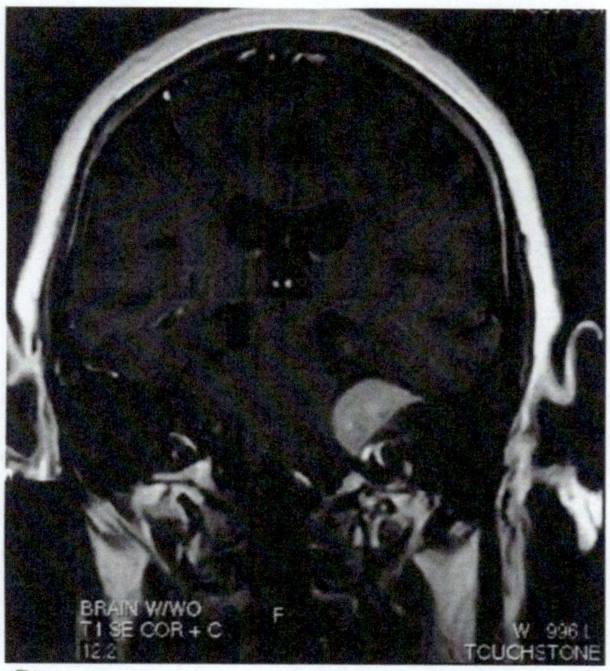

(B)

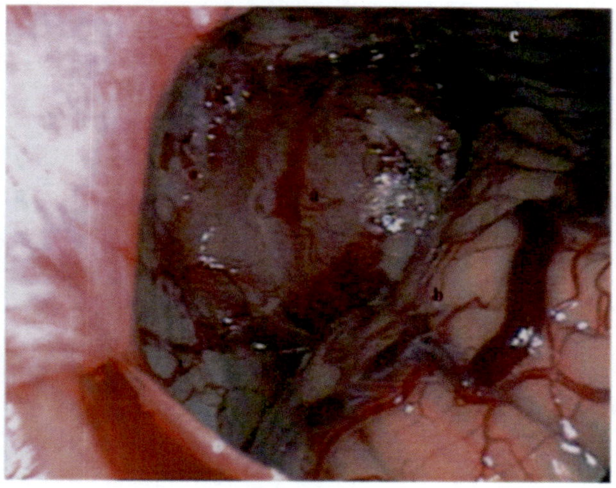

(C)

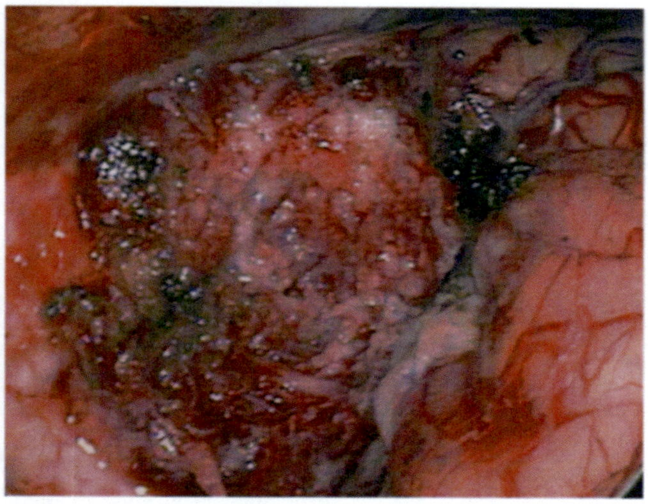

(D)

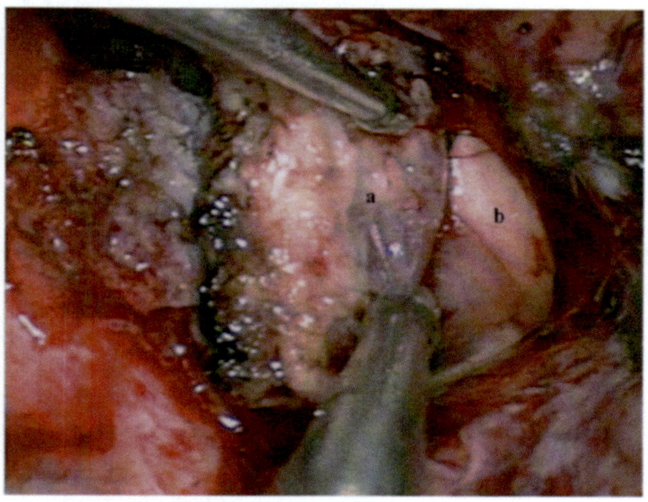

(E)

Fig. 36 (**A**) T_1-weighted, contrast-enhanced axial MRI showing a lateral cerebellopontine angle (CPA) meningioma. (**B**) T_1-weighted, contrast-enhanced coronal MRI showing a lateral CPA meningioma. (**C**) Intraoperative endoscopic view showing initial exposure of a lateral CPA meningioma. *a* Meningioma. *b* Lateral aspect of cerebellum. *c* Tentorium. (**D**)–(**N**) Intraoperative endoscopic view showing gradual resectionof a lateral CPA meningioma. (**E**) *a* Meningioma. *b* Acousticofacial nerve bundle (VII, VIII) stretched by tumor. (**F**) *a* Meningioma capsule. *b* Acousticofacial nerve bundle (VII, VIII). *c* Trigeminal nerve (V). *d* Brainstem. (**G**) *a* Meningioma. (**H**) *a* Close-up view of final portion of meningioma attached to petrous temporal bone. (**I**) *a* Final portion of meningioma attached to petrous temporal bone. *b* Acousticofacial nerve bundle (VII, VIII). *c* Trigeminal nerve (V). *d* abducent nerve (VI). *e* Brainstem. *f* Lateral aspect of cerebellum. *g* Clivus. (**J**) *a* Clean petrous bone after complete meningioma resection. *b* Acousticofacial nerve bundle (VII, VIII). *c* Trigeminal nerve (V). *d* Tentorium. *e* Brainstem. *f* Lateral aspect of cerebellum. (**K**) Postoperative T_1-weighted, contrast-enhanced axial MRI. (**L**) Postoperative T_1-weighted, contrast-enhanced coronal MRI.

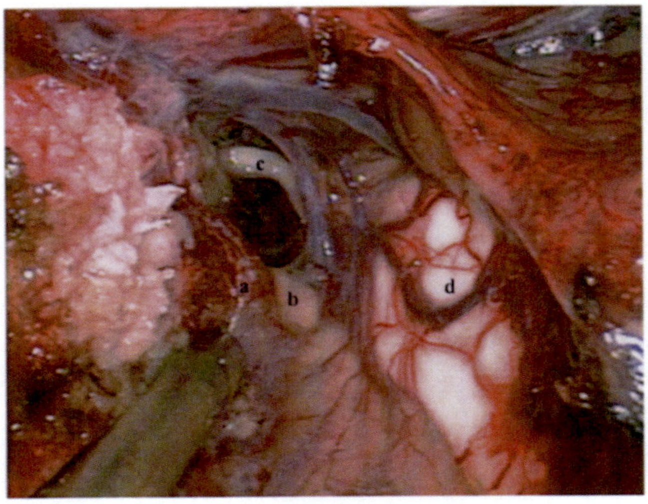

(F)

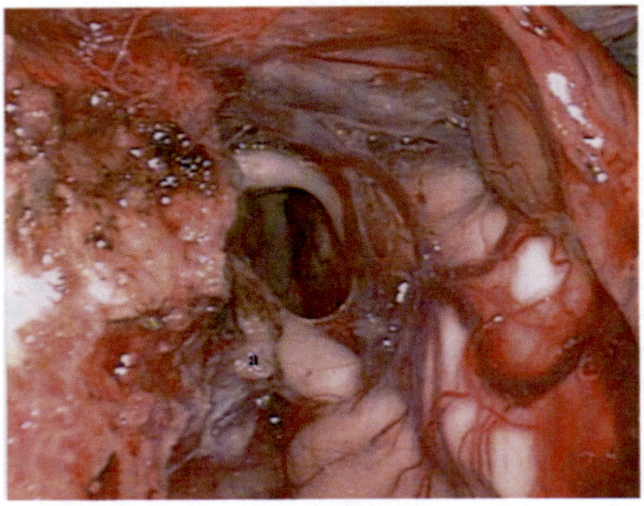

(G)

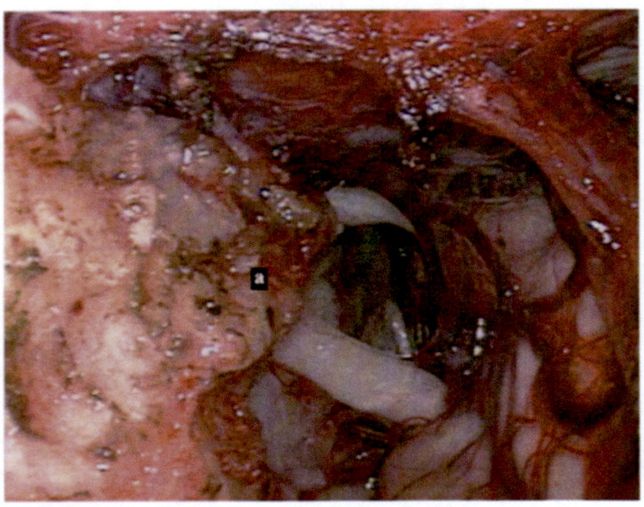

(H)

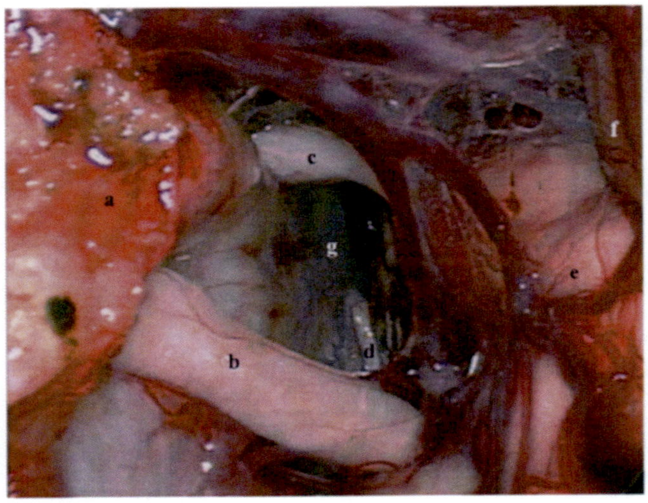

(I)

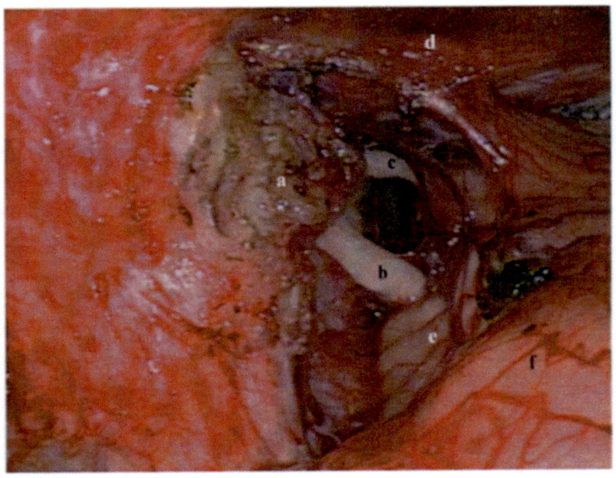

(J)

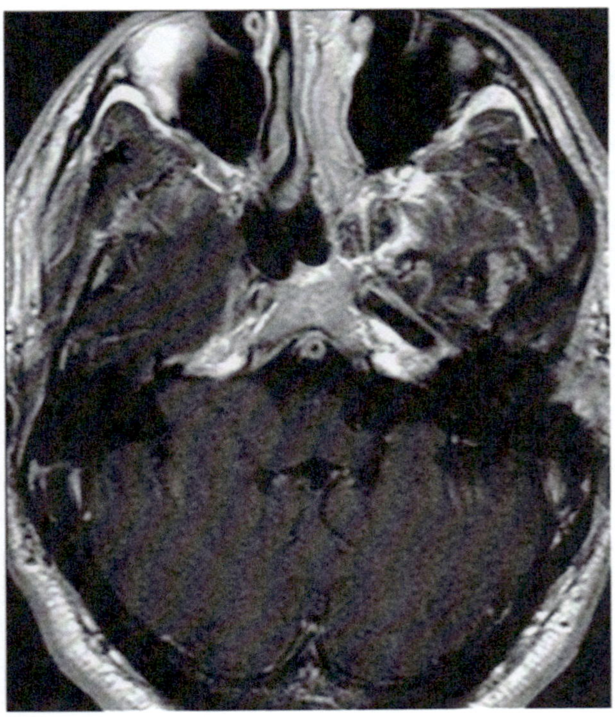

(K)

Fig. 36 (continued)

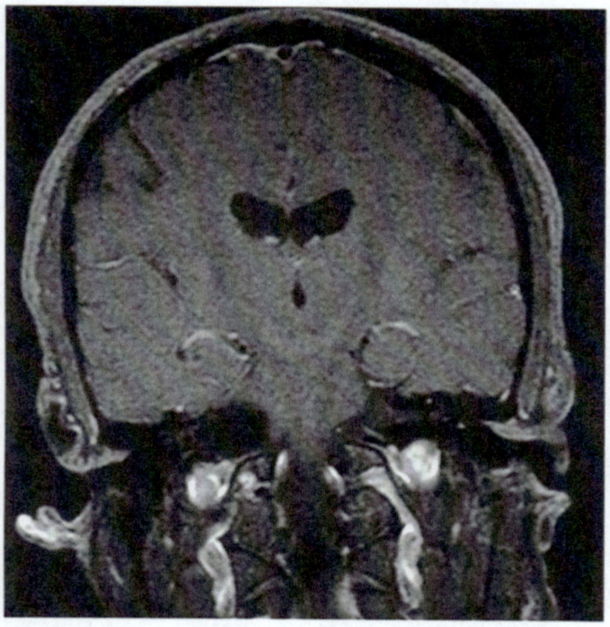

(L)

Fig. 36 (continued)

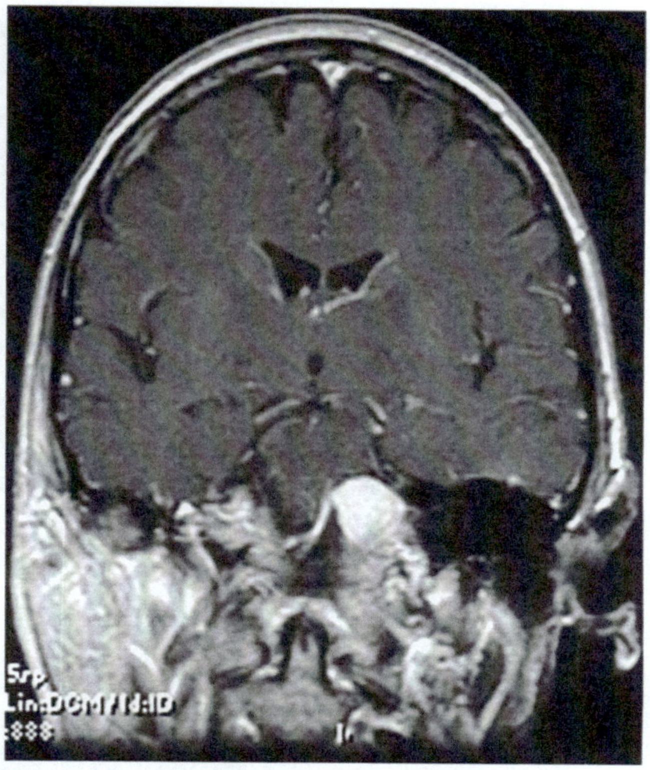

(B)

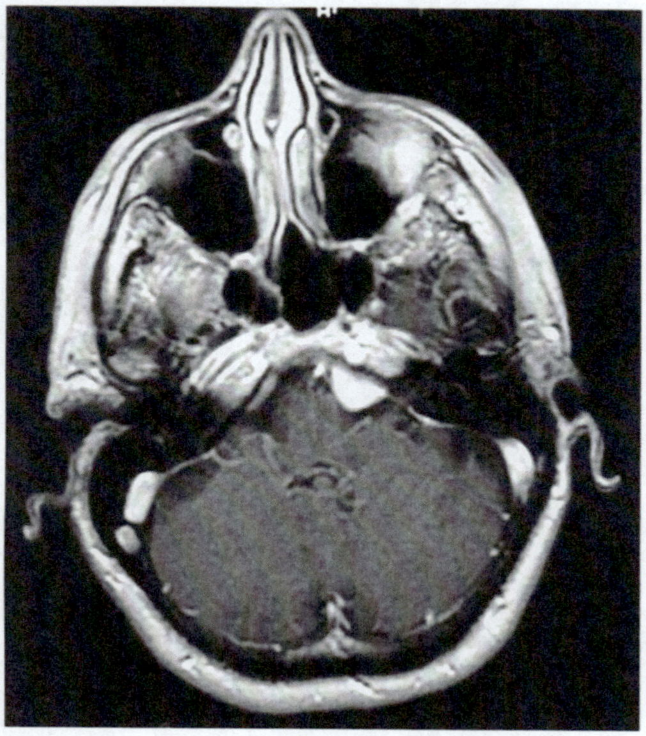

(A)

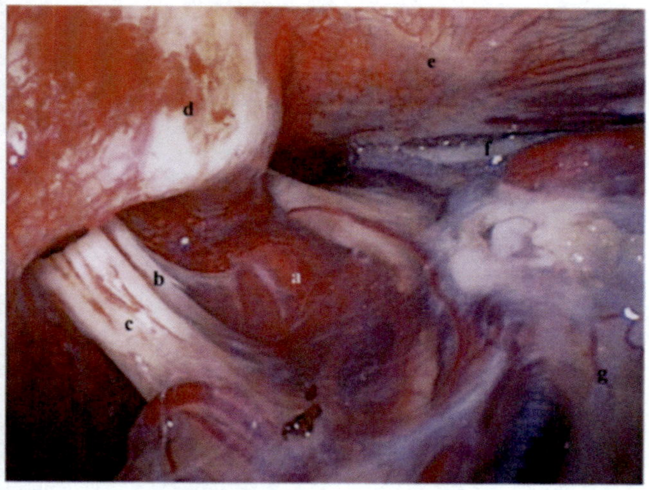

(C)

Fig. 37 (**A**) T_1-weighted, contrast-enhanced axial MRI showing a medial cerebellopontine angle (CPA) meningioma. (**B**) T_1-weighted, contrast-enhanced coronal MRI showing a medial CPA meningioma. (**C**) Intraoperative endoscopic view showing initial exposure of a medial CPA meningioma. *a* Meningioma. *b* Facial nerve (VII). *c* Vestibulocochlear nerve (VIII). *d* Petrous apex. *e* Tentorium. *f* Trochlear nerve (IV). *g* Lateral aspect of cerebellum. (**D**)–(**R**) Intraoperative endoscopic view showing gradual resection of a medial CPA meningioma. (**F**) *a* Meningioma capsule. *b* Acousticofacial nerve bundle (VII, VIII). *c* Bipolar diathermy tip. *d* Atraumatic suction. *e* Trigeminal nerve (V). *f* Trochlear nerve (IV). (**I**) *a* Meningioma. *b* Vestibulocochlear nerve (VIII). *c* Facial nerve (VII). *d* Internal auditory meatus (IAM). *e* MicroCUSA tip. *f* Atraumatic suction. *g* Trochlear nerve (IV). (**J**) *a* Meningioma capsule. (**N**) *a* Final portion of meningioma attached to petrous temporal bone. *b* Acousticofacial nerve bundle (VII, VIII). *c* Trigeminal nerve (V). *d* Trochlear nerve (IV). *e* Brainstem. *f* Lateral aspect of cerebellum. (**R**) *a* Clean petrous bone after complete meningioma resection. *b* Trigeminal nerve (V). *c* Meckel's cave. *d* Tentorium. *e* Trochlear nerve (IV). *f* Brainstem. (**S**) Postoperative T_1-weighted, contrast-enhanced axial MRI. (**T**) Postoperative T_1-weighted, contrast-enhanced coronal MRI.

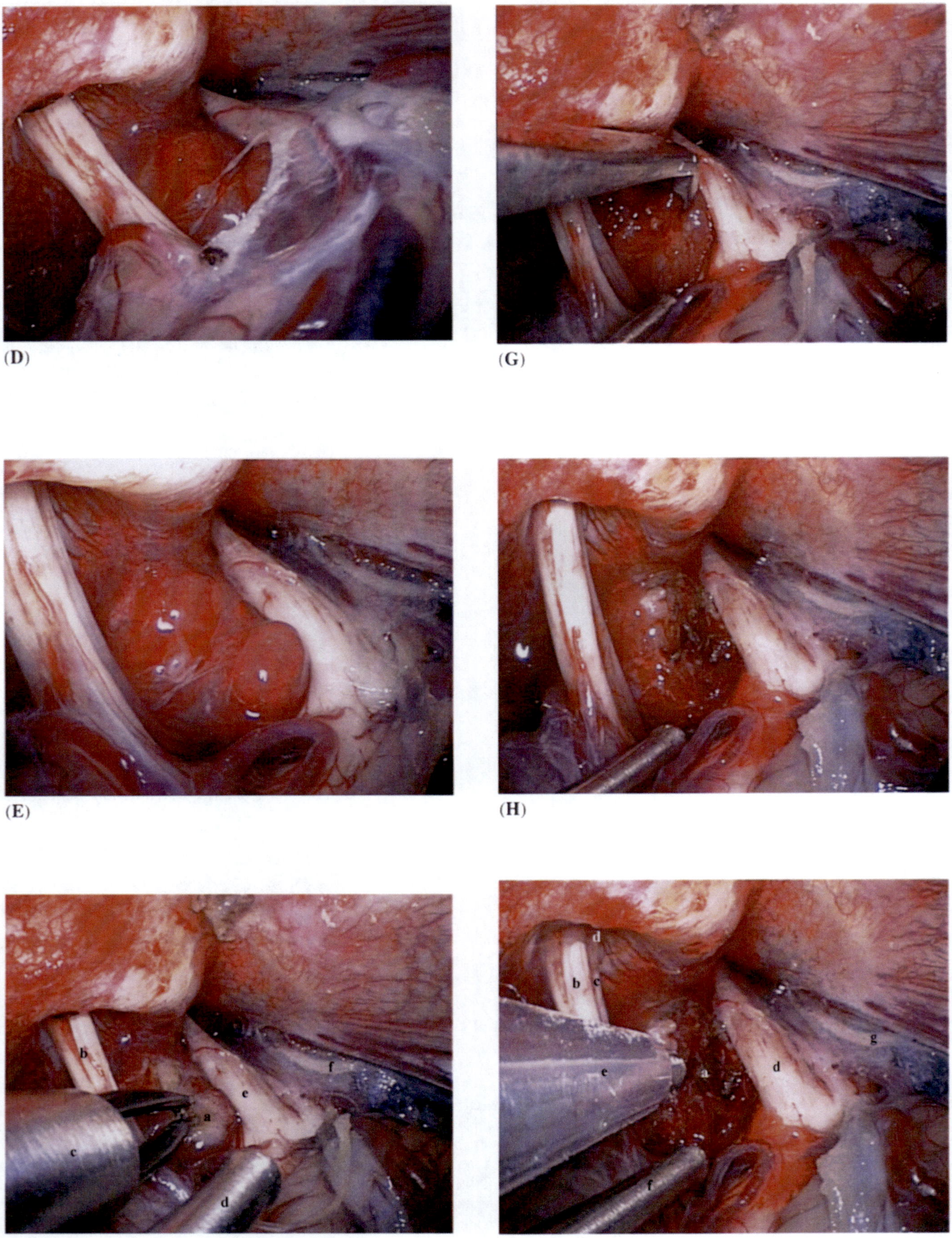

(D) (G)

(E) (H)

(F) (I)

Fig. 37 (continued)

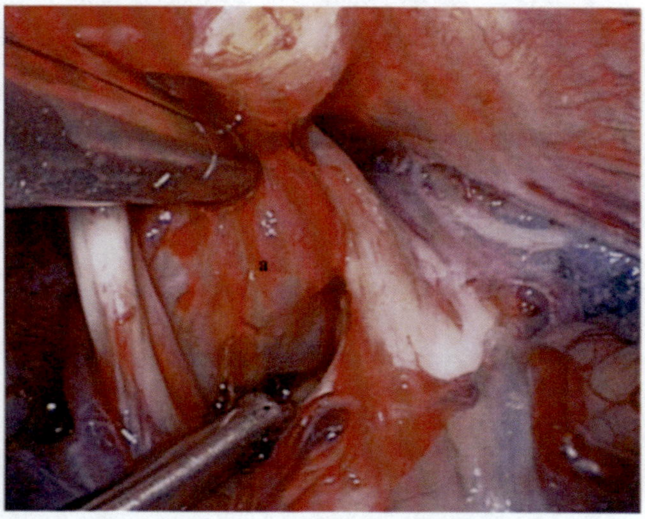

(J)

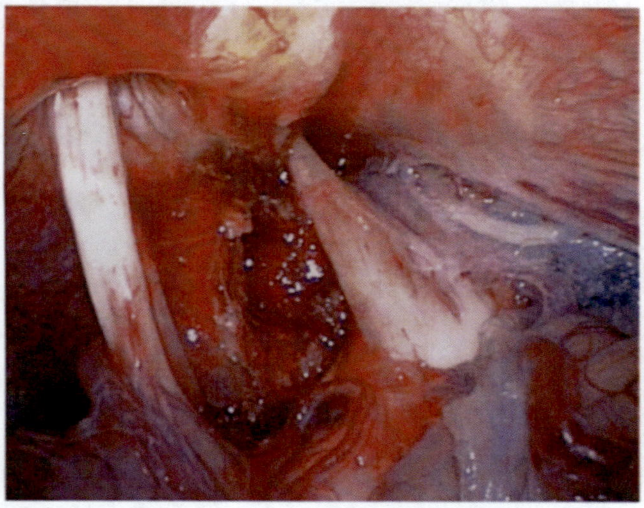

(K)

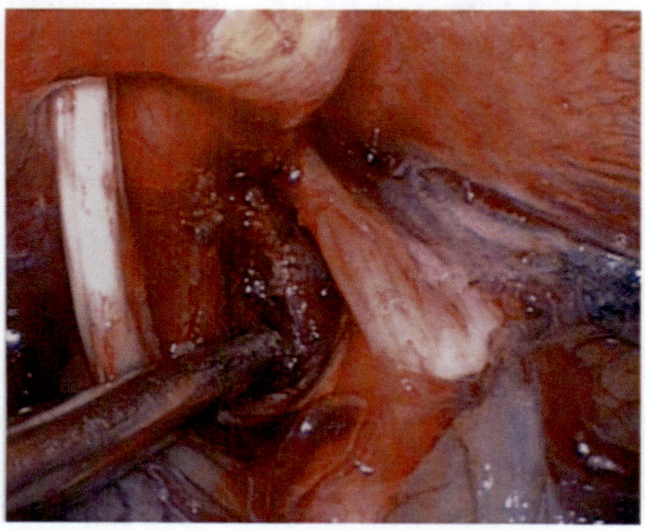

(L)

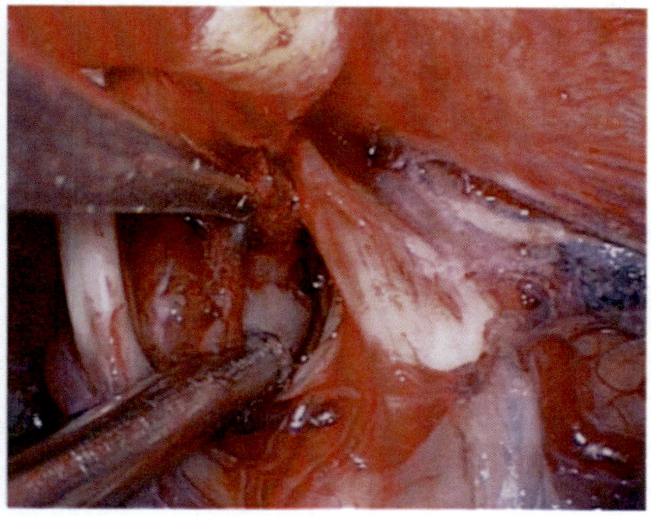

(M)

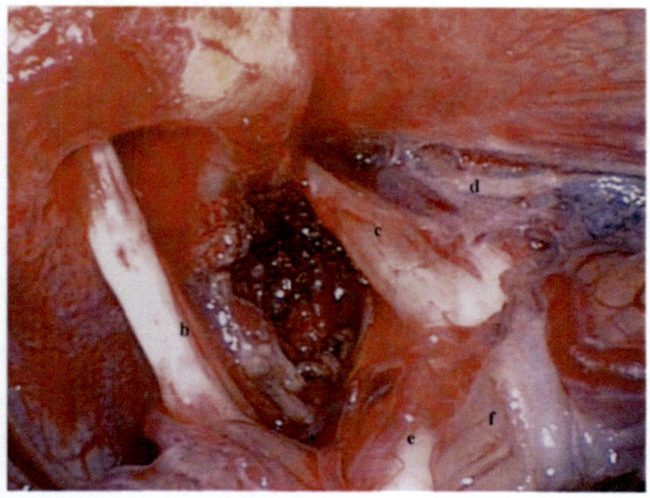

(N)

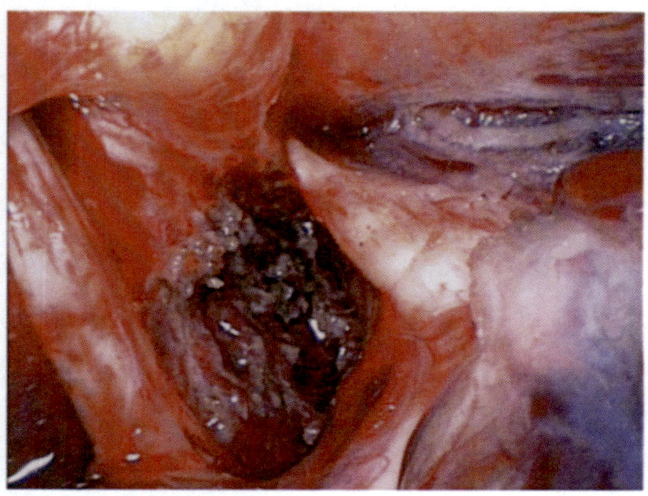

(O)

Fig. 37 (continued)

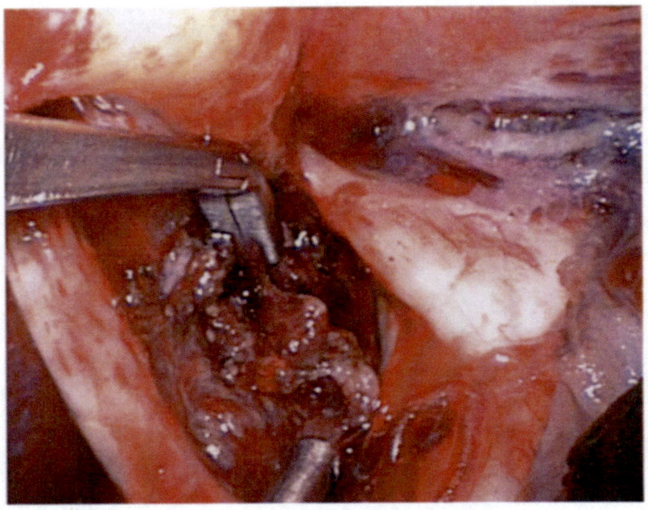

(P)

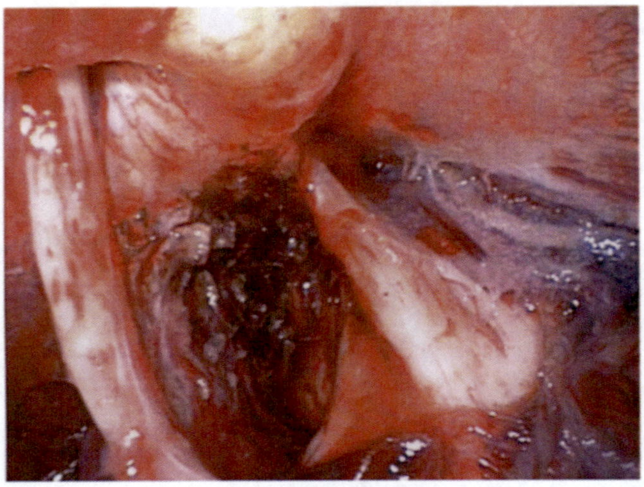

(Q)

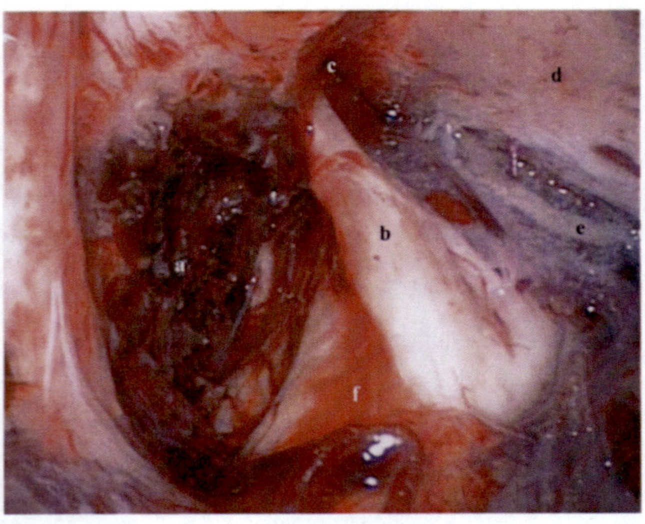

(R)

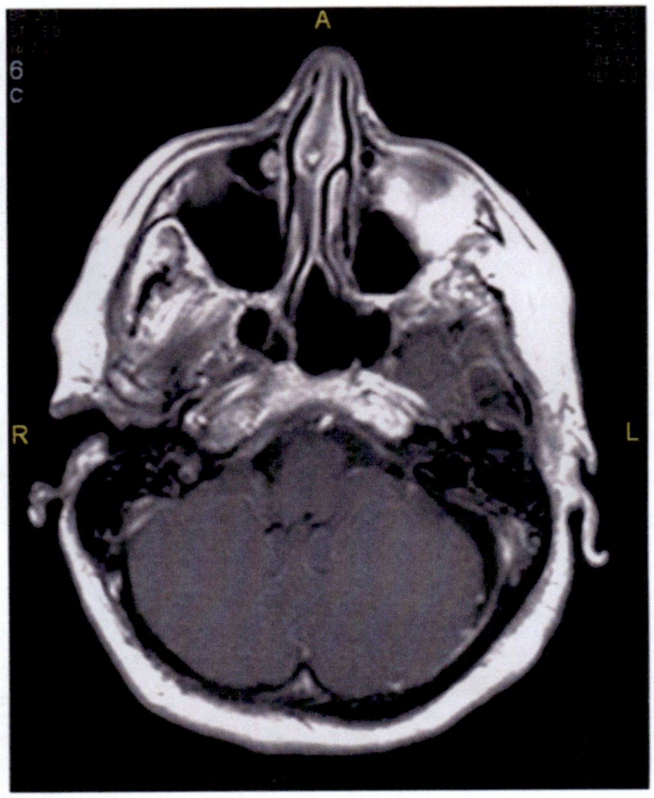

(S)

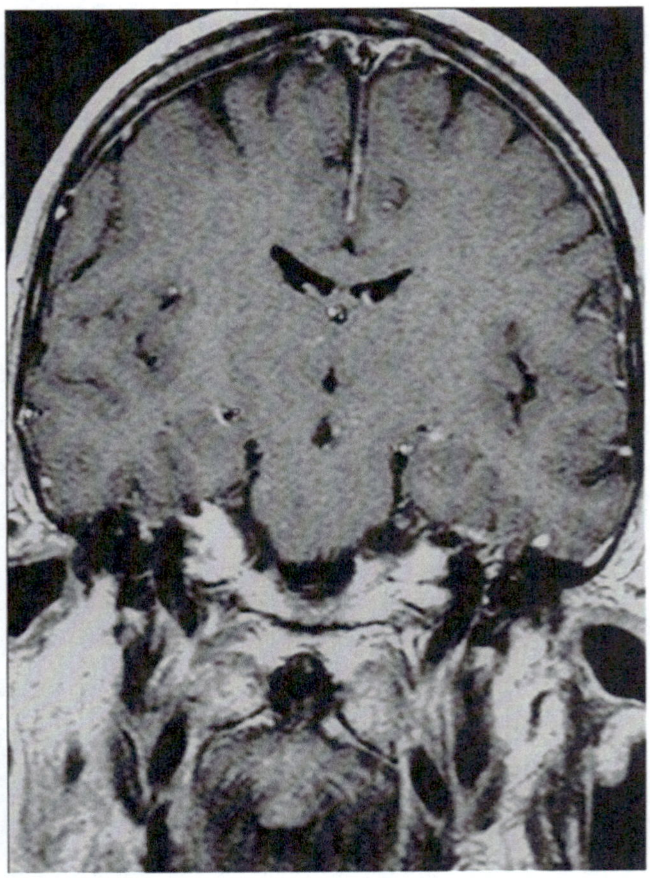

(T)

Fig. 37 (continued)

- Dizziness, balance, or coordination (ataxia) disturbances
- Severe postoperative headaches and pneumocephalus
- Mild or significant hydrocephalus

9. AVOIDING COMPLICATIONS IN AUTHOR'S EXPERIENCE

Major complications such as death, brainstem injury, quadriparesis, and hemiparesis are mostly avoided because dissection with the endoscopic approach is limited, and cerebellar retraction is not used. Bacterial or aseptic meningitis also occurs less frequently than with traditional surgery because the operative field is reduced, along with the duration of the surgery. In general, the two major and most feared complications are CSF leakage and cranial nerve injuries. Hearing loss and facial paresis or paralysis depend on the size of the tumor resected. In general, the smaller the tumor, the greater the chance for hearing preservation; with increasing size of the tumor within the CPA, the incidence of complications increases.

Acoustic tumors are typically in intimate contact with the facial nerve, which may be compressed, distorted, or, rarely, completely engulfed by the tumor; therefore, postoperative facial paralysis may result from nerve swelling or nerve damage. Despite the fact that facial nerve monitoring has greatly aided separation of the facial nerve from the tumor, anatomical and functional preservation of the facial nerve with complete tumor removal, especially in patients with large tumors, is still a challenge. Postoperative facial nerve paralysis is sometimes unavoidable. Fortunately, even when as little as 10% of the functioning facial motor neurons are left intact, normal facial nerve function can be preserved.

A high rate of functional cochlear nerve (hearing) preservation has been encountered in our vestibular schwannoma patient series, which reflects the improved outcome associated with the better visualization of the 0° and angled endoscopes. Resection of a macroscopically intact cochlear nerve in an attempt to seek complete tumor removal is not recommended; that nerve is almost never involved with tumor and can function well for decades. In these cases, total tumor removal should not result in unnecessary hearing loss.

Although vestibular nerve preservation is virtually impossible in the majority of cases as most vestibular schwannomas arise from the vestibular nerve, this may not constitute a problem. The vestibular function is usually considerably reduced or even totally lost before vestibular schwannoma surgery, and immediate postoperative vertigo is usually minimal and transient and seldom causes any disability. Postoperative vertigo, dizziness, balance, or coordination problems may result from vestibular or cerebellar dysfunction and may be severe for days or weeks following surgery before completely resolving; these complications tend to persist longer in older patients. In many cases, tinnitus remains the same as before surgery, but it may be more or less noticeable in the early postoperative period. Direct injuries of cranial nerves V or, rarely, VI or the lower cranial nerves, vascular injuries to the AICA/PICA or their branches, and venous injuries are extremely rare complications.

Traditional open approaches require a certain degree of cerebellar retraction; therefore, cerebellar edema or hematoma can occur. This does not occur with the endoscopic approach because it does not require the use of any retractors. Hemorrhage into the posterior fossa or subdural or extradural hemorrhage in the immediate postoperative period can produce brainstem compression and rapid death. The prevention of secondary bleeding relies on strict hemostasis, and it is essential to coagulate both ends of any minor surface vessels during tumor resection.

Early or delayed CSF leakage from the wound, rhinorrhea, or otorrhea (either directly through the wound or via the eustachian tube and middle ear) can occur even if all the precautions have been taken to avoid them. In some cases, the leakage may be iatrogenic; this emphasizes the importance of watertight dural closure. The path of CSF egress is most commonly through mastoid air cells that were opened during the craniotomy.

The keyhole craniotomy, even though limited, can still result in some postoperative headaches, but these resolve spontaneously in the majority of cases. Taking great care to avoid contaminating CSF with bone dust and replacement of the keyhole bone flap have significantly reduced the incidence of this complication in our experience. Mild transient postoperative hydrocephalus rarely occurs in the early postoperative period; even when present, it generally resolves without difficulty in the first few postoperative weeks, and CSF shunting is rarely, if ever, required.

10 The Fully Endoscopic Subtemporal Approach

This chapter discusses the surgical application of the fully endoscopic subtemporal approach. Performed through a small preauricular skin incision and a keyhole craniotomy, the endoscopic subtemporal approach provides a minimally invasive, short, and direct pathway to access the temporal base, the parasellar and retrochiasmatic regions, and the anterolateral petroclival region. In our practice, we have found that the great advantage of this approach is that it provides an excellent route for wide surgical exposure of the operative field from the ipsilateral greater wing of sphenoid anteriorly, including the suprasellar and parasellar regions, to the petroclival region posteriorly with virtually no temporal lobe retraction. The chapter provides a thorough description of the fully endoscopic subtemporal approach, including indications, operating room setup, patient positioning, operative technique, state-of-the-art illustrative cases (with clinical background on the most important pathologies in this area), potential complications, and ways to avoid these complications (in the authors' experience).

Keywords: Cavernous sinus; Endoscopic; Infratemporal; Keyhole; Middle fossa; Meningioma; Minimally invasive; Optic chiasm; Optic nerve; Parasellar; Skull base; Subtemporal; Suprasellar; Surgery; Transtemporal; Trigeminal schwannoma.

1. INTRODUCTION

The traditional subtemporal approach, originally adopted for trigeminal rhizotomy and later modified with anterior petrosectomy to access the internal auditory canal (IAC) and adjacent structures, represents a short and direct pathway to access the temporal base, the parasellar and retrochiasmatic regions, and the anterolateral petroclival region. Unfortunately, aggressive temporal lobe retraction to provide adequate visualization of the operative field; injury to the temporal veins, including the inferior anastomotic vein (of Labbé); and even the possibility of venous infarction of the temporal lobe have often outweighed the unique advantages of this approach.

From: *Endoscopic Skull Base Surgery: A Comprehensive Guide with Illustrative Cases.*
Edited by H. K. Shahinian © Humana Press, Totowa, NJ.

In our practice, we adopted the use of an endoscopic subtemporal keyhole approach; the great advantage of this approach is that it provides an excellent route for wide surgical exposure of the operative field from the ipsilateral greater wing of sphenoid anteriorly, including the suprasellar and parasellar regions, to the petroclival region posteriorly with virtually no temporal lobe retraction.

The ability to approach the middle cranial fossa with a variety of endoscopic approaches (supraorbital, subtemporal) is advantageous as it allows more options to be tailored according to each patient's individual needs. In this respect, the endoscopic subtemporal approach can be augmented by other endoscopic approaches when accessing complex lesions of the skull base. For instance, when the tumor involves Meckel's cave, the tentorium is opened to aid in dissection of the tumor. The addition of a zygomatic osteotomy, drilling along the floor of the middle cranial fossa to access the infratemporal region, or medial petrosectomy are all applied depending on the specifics of each case, providing both intradural and extradural exposure.

2. INDICATIONS

The fully endoscopic subtemporal approach provides minimally invasive surgical access to the ipsilateral petroclival, suprasellar and parasellar, cavernous sinus, and medial sphenoid wing regions. Pathologies in these areas may include hypothalamic gliomas; craniopharyngiomas, especially with a prefixedoptic chiasm; trigeminal schwannomas or neurofibromas; petroclival, sphenoid wing, and cavernous sinus meningiomas; arachnoid cysts of the middle cranial fossa; pituitary macroadenomas with major lateral extensions; chordomas of the middle and upper clivus; carcinomas; rhabdomyosarcomas; and other benign and malignant lesions extending to or through the middle skull base, with or without invasion of the cavernous sinus.

3. INSTRUMENTATION

The instruments needed to execute this procedure successfully include an endoscopic tower containing a high-definition digital camera, a xenon or halogen light source, 0° and 30° rigid

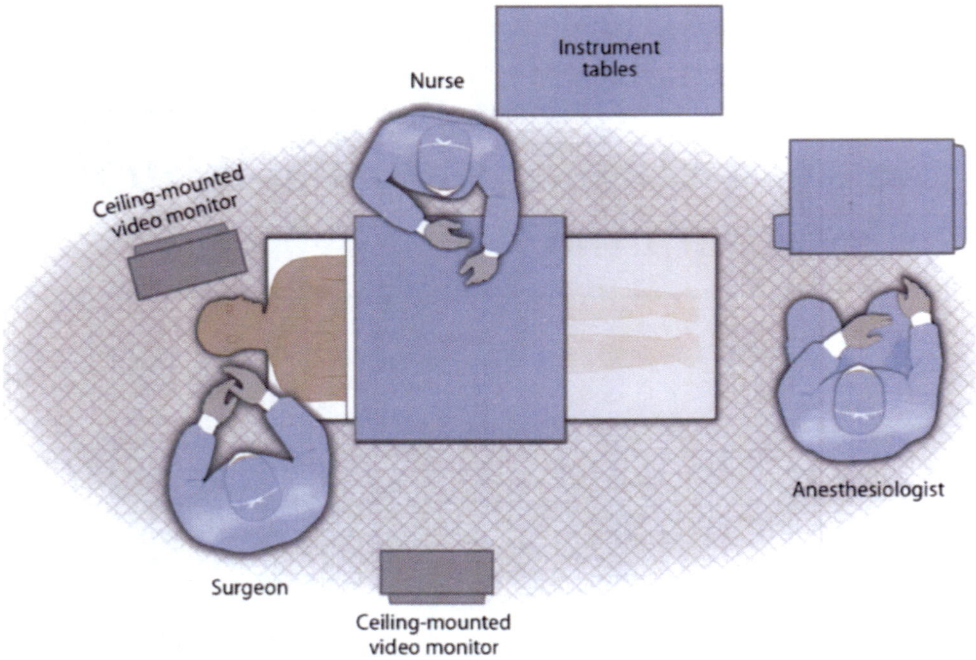

Fig. 1 Operating room setup.

endoscopes, two endoscope holding arms, endoscope irrigation sheaths and pumps, and precision microinstruments.

4. OPERATING ROOM SETUP (FIG. 1)

The patient is positioned supine on the operating room table. Following the induction of general anesthesia, the airway circuit is extended with corrugated tubing, and the head is rotated 180° away from the anesthesiologist, who stands at the foot of the operating room table. The surgeon stands at the head of the table on the side of the lesion, and the endoscopic tower is placed on the opposite side, directly facing the surgeon. Two separate pneumatically powered holding arms are affixed to the table, one on each side of the patient, and wrapped in sterile drapes. One holding arm is dedicated to holding the endoscope, and the other is used to hold other endoscopic instruments or soft silicone spatulas. A second monitor is placed on the ipsilateral side to allow the scrub nurse, who stands facing the surgeon, to monitor the operation.

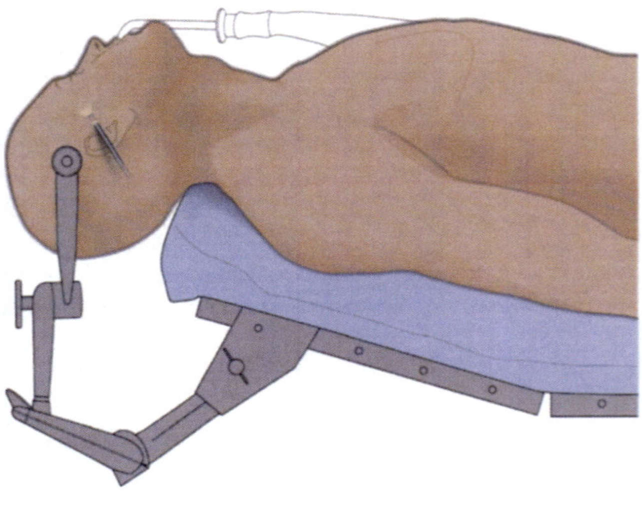

Fig. 2 Patient positioning.

5. PATIENT POSITIONING (FIG. 2)

The patient is positioned supine on the operating room table, and the head of the bed is slightly raised to improve venous drainage. The final position of the head is tailored according to the exact location of the lesion by rotating and tilting it up to 15° toward the contralateral side. This position facilitates gravitational temporal lobe retraction and provides wider access to the skull base anteriorly. The head is fixed in position using a three-pin Mayfield clamp.

6. OPERATIVE TECHNIQUE

Following general anesthesia, intraoperative monitoring leads are placed, and the preauricular temporal region is cleansed with an aqueous antiseptic solution and then draped. A standard 3-cm skin incision begins in the preauricular skin crease from the inferior rim of the zygomatic arch just anterior to the tragus and extends upward, curving first anteriorly then posteriorly within the natural hairline; curving the incision allows the surgeon to spread soft tissue widely to gain more access anteriorly. The deep temporalis fascia and muscle are then incised in line with the skin incision and dissected down to the squamous temporal bone in a subperiosteal plane. Small hooks are used for bilateral retraction of the skin and underlying muscle. The superficial and deep layers of the deep temporal fascia, attached to the lateral and medial surfaces of the zygomatic arch, respectively, are incised and dissected subperiosteally to expose the upper part of the temporal zygomatic root (Fig. 3A–D).

Using a microdrill, a 2-cm keyhole craniotomy is then performed in the squamous temporal bone just above the temporal zygomatic root with its base level with the zygomatic arch and extending anteriorly. The superior surface of the zygomatic arch is drilled flat, and any residual bone at the temporal base is removed or drilled extradurally to facilitate a more basal subtemporal view (Fig. 4A–D).

A semicircular incision is then made in the temporal dura, which is reflected basally (Fig. 5A-D). A combination of positioning, mild hyperventilation, mannitol, and slow cerebrospinal fluid (CSF) drainage relaxes the temporal lobe and enhances a subtemporal trajectory. Following adequate relaxation of the temporal lobe, a 0° endoscope is introduced and gradually advanced along the floor of the middle cranial fossa, displaying a panoramic view of the entire area from the sphenoid wing anteriorly to the petroclival region posteriorly. The procedure will vary from this point according to the pathological condition being addressed.

Once the intracranial portion is completed, the whole area is copiously irrigated, and hemostasis is secured. The dura is then

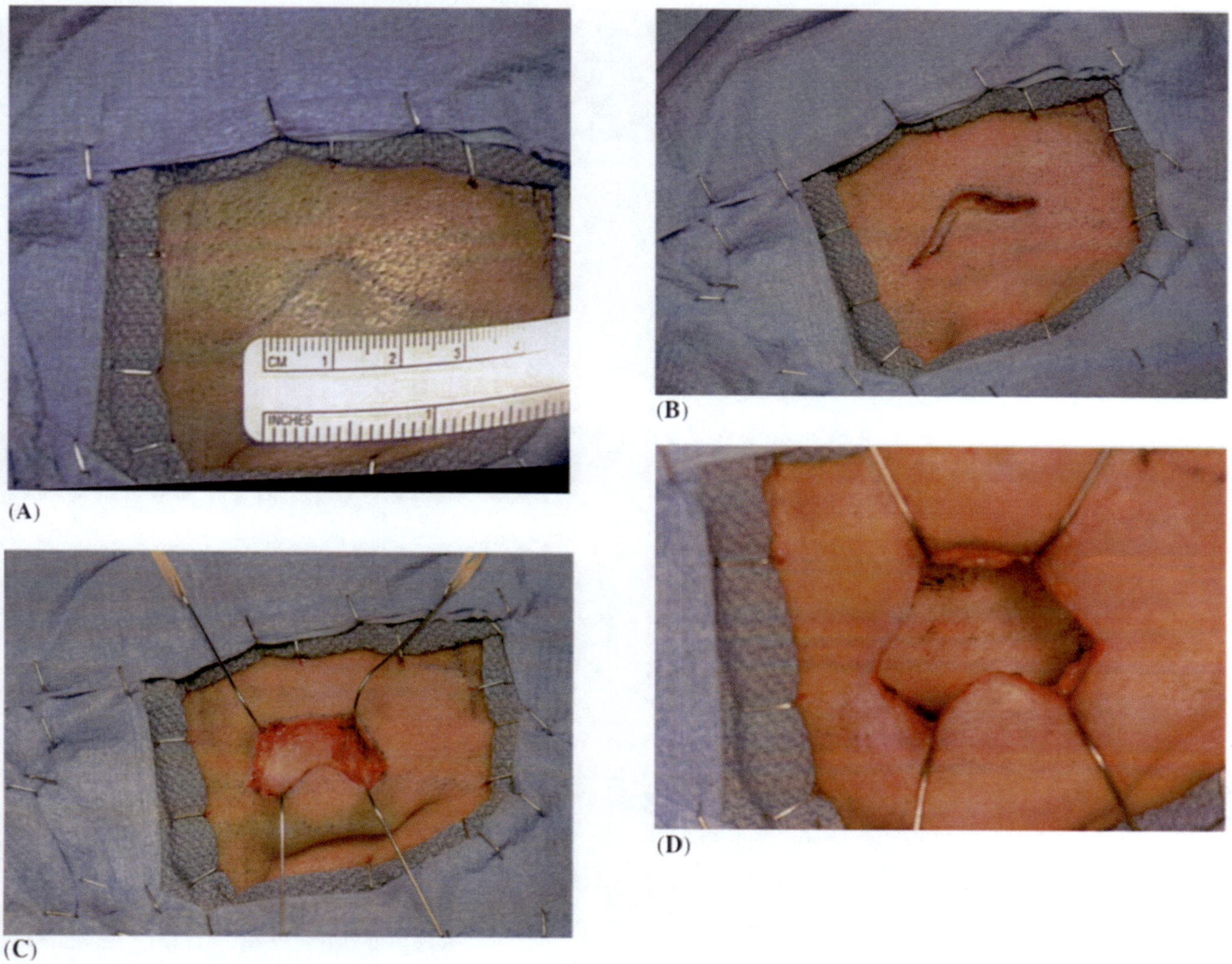

Fig. 3 (**A**)–(**D**) Marking, draping, and skin incision.

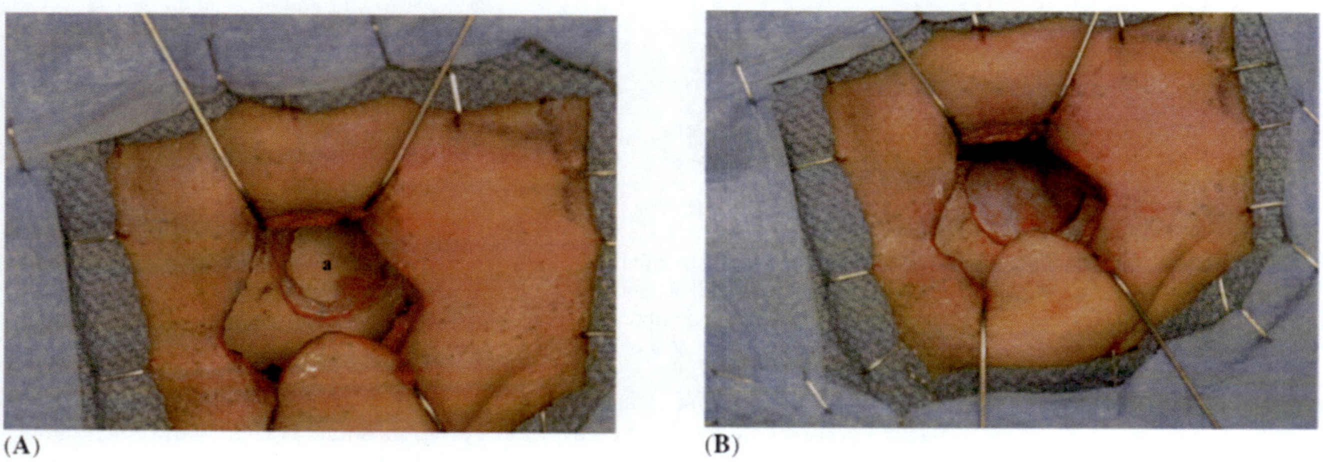

Fig. 4 (**A**)–(**C**) Keyhole craniotomy. (**A**) *a* Keyhole bone flap. (**C**) *a* Temporal dura. *b* Lateral skull base (middle cranial fossa floor).

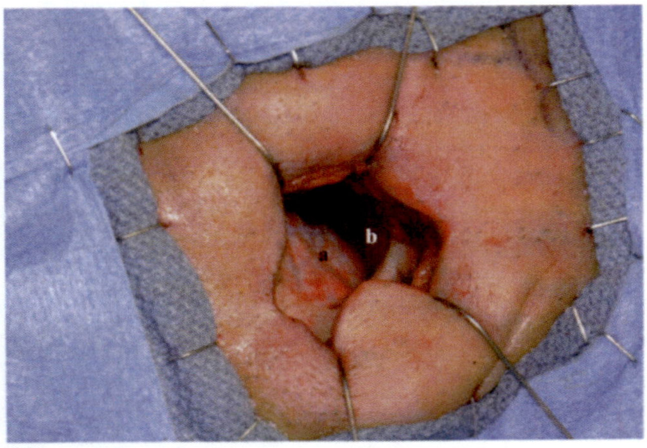

(C)

Fig. 4 (continued)

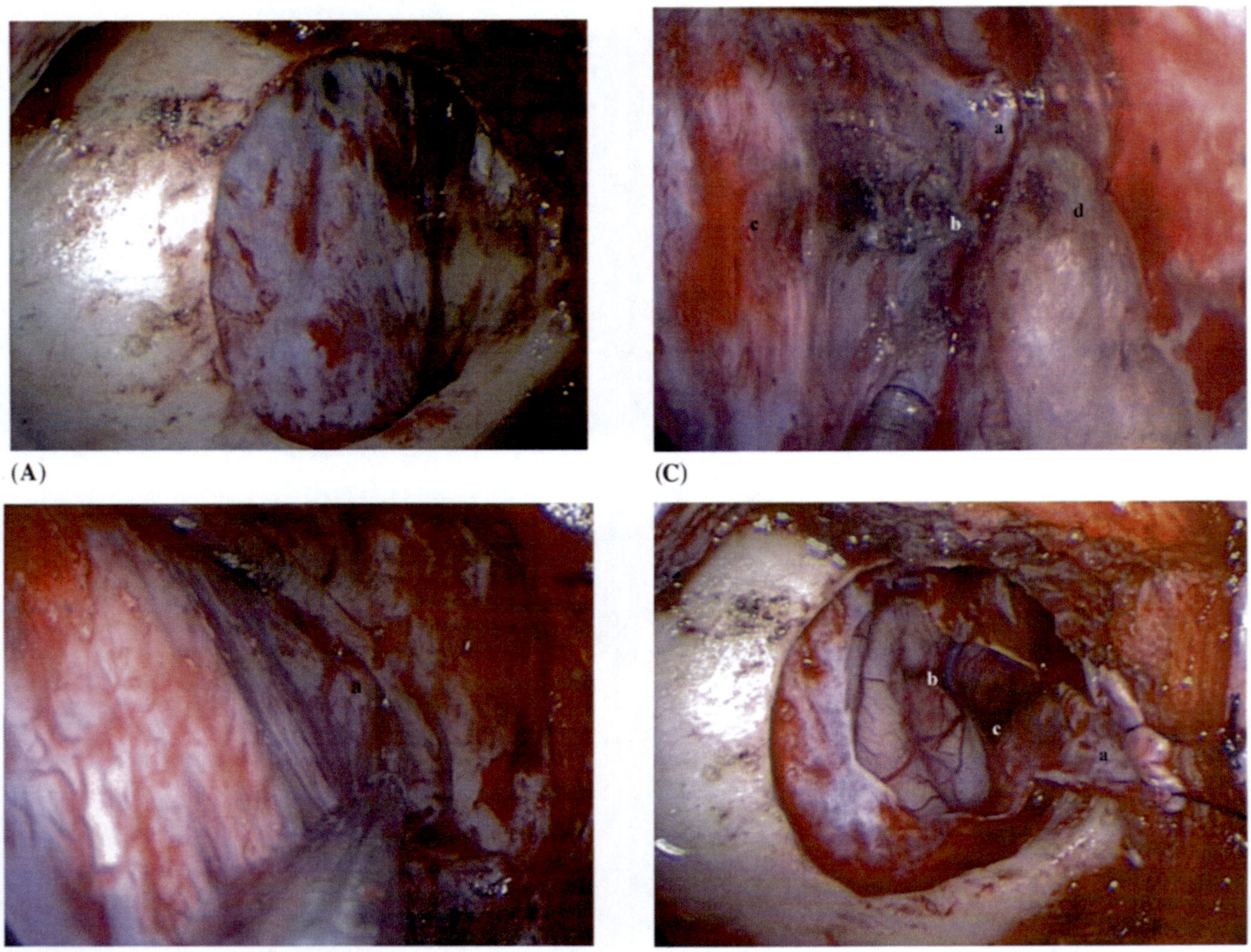

Fig. 5 (**A**)–(**D**) Extradural anatomy and dural opening. (**B**) *a* Mandibular (V3) division of trigeminal nerve (V). (**C**) *a* Mandibular (V3) division of trigeminal nerve (V) at foramen ovale. *b* Cauterized middle meningeal artery at foramen spinosum. *c* Temporal dura. *d* Lateral skull base. (**D**) *a*. Reflected dura. *b* Lower aspect of temporal lobe. *c* Endoscope trajectory.

closed watertight and covered with a layer of collagen dural substitute membrane and a dural sealant to prevent any CSF leak (Fig. 6A,B). The keyhole bone flap is then repositioned and fixed in place using resorbable microplates and screws; a hydroxyapatite bone substitute is applied to cement the defect around the keyhole bone flap, restoring integrity of the squamous temporal bone (Fig. 7A,B). The skin, subcutaneous tissues, and musculature are then sutured in layers without the use of any drains and with careful attention to the aesthetic repair. A small adhesive bandage is then applied to the preauricular suture line (Fig. 8A–D). The majority of patients undergoing this procedure are monitored in either the intensive care unit (ICU) or a step-down unit overnight and then transferred to the ward until discharged home, typically 48 h after the operation.

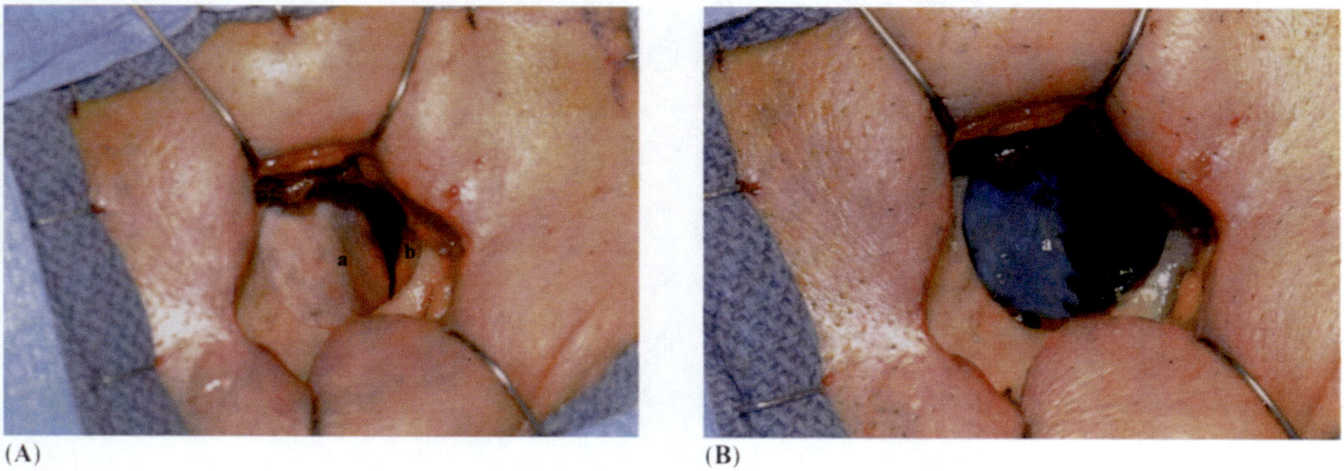

Fig. 6 (**A**) and (**B**) Dural closure. (**A**) *a* Collagen dural substitute (onlay graft). *b* Lateral skull base. (**B**) *a* Dural sealant.

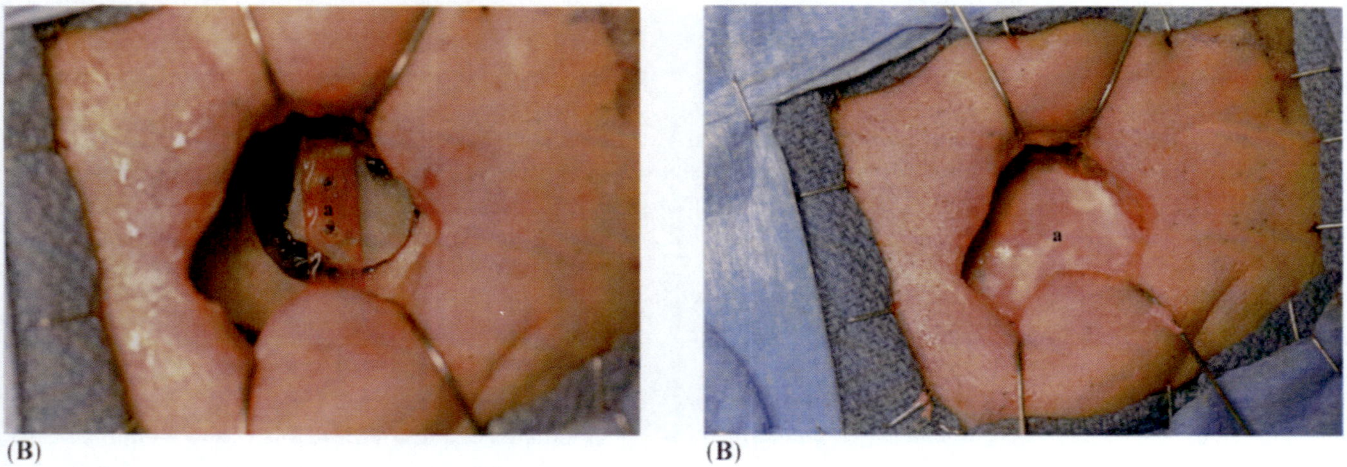

Fig. 7 (**A**) and (**B**) Cranioplasty. (**A**) *a* Microplate and screws. (**B**) *a* Hydroxyapatite bone substitute.

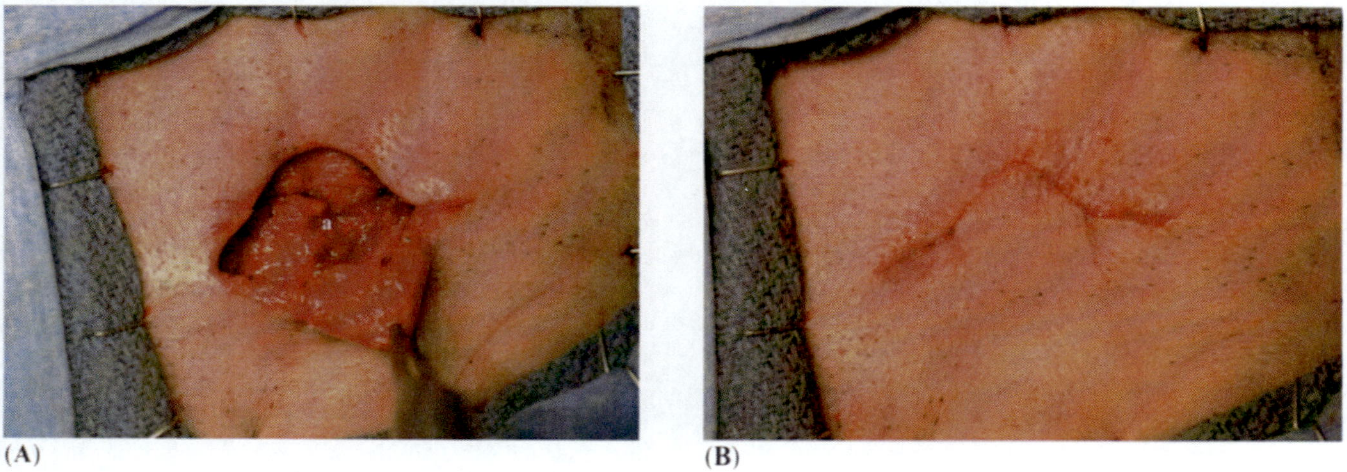

Fig. 8 (**A**)–(**D**) Skin closure and dressing. (**A**) *a* Temporal muscle and fascia closed.

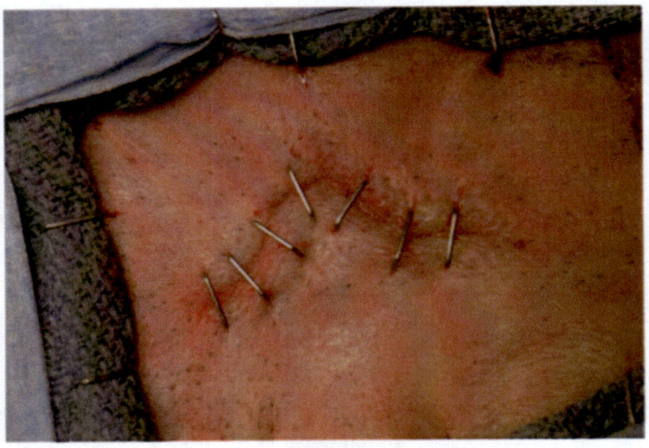

(C)

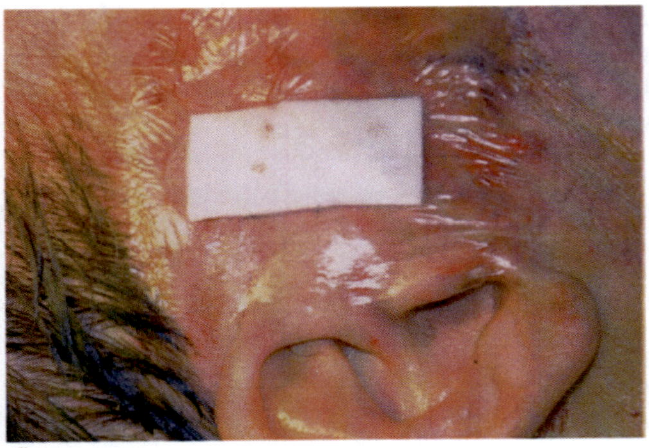

(D)

Fig. 8 (continued)

7. ILLUSTRATIVE CASES

7.1. Middle Cranial Fossa and Cavernous Sinus Region Tumors

7.1.1. Background Traditionally, surgical approaches to the cavernous sinus included the pterional, cranioorbitozygomatic, and extended middle cranial fossa approaches. Currently, advances in endoscopic skull base surgery, neuroanesthesia, neuroimaging, and nerve monitoring have helped tremendously in operating around the cavernous sinus, parasellar, infrachiasmatic, and posterior clinoid regions, and gross-total resection of previously unresectable tumors using endoscopic approaches has been possible in a wide range of patients with excellent functional and cosmetic outcomes.

Craniopharyngiomas, especially with a prefixed optic chiasm (because the endoscopic subtemporal approach provides excellent surgical access from above and beneath the optic chiasm and tracts); trigeminal schwannomas; cavernous sinus meningiomas (including those that arise from the dural reflection of the sinus or grow into it as part of a larger tumor involving the sellar/parasellar dural surfaces, medial sphenoid wing, orbit, clivus, petrous bone, or other areas of the skull base); arachnoid cysts; and others can be completely resected without the need for major exposures. Some tumors, however, might involve or even completely encase major neurovascular structures, such as the internal carotid artery (ICA) or the cavernous sinus, posing major impediments to such a complete removal. The extent of the tumor and the involvement of major vessels are defined by magnetic resonance imaging (MRI) and magnetic resonance angiography (MRA). The decision regarding the approach is dependent on the anatomical location of the lesion as well as the potential for some of these tumors, such as meningiomas and schwannomas, to extend into two cranial compartments, presenting further difficulties regarding the choice of approach. At the present time, we routinely use the endoscopic subtemporal or supraorbital approaches to access lesions of the cavernous sinus region according to their location, extent, and site of pathology.

7.1.2. Approach Under general anesthesia, after positioning, prepping, draping, and skin incision, a 2-cm temporal keyhole craniotomy is performed; the dura is then incised open, and CSF is slowly drained. After adequate relaxation of the temporal lobe, a 0° endoscope is introduced and gradually advanced medially along the floor of the middle cranial fossa.

For cavernous sinus region tumors, including meningiomas, schwannomas, and others, the tumor is exposed, and a small area of its lateral surface is electrocoagulated and biopsied for intraoperative frozen section confirmation of the pathology. The major lateral part of the tumor is then internally decompressed under direct endoscopic visualization using a combination of a micro-Cavitron ultrasonic surgical aspirator (microCUSA), bipolar electrocoagulation, microinstruments, and microdissecting techniques. Following internal debulking, the lateral portion of the tumor's capsule is gradually and circumferentially dissected and resected in a piecemeal fashion.

At this point, attention is shifted to the medial portion of the tumor, which is often attached to or extends within the cavernous sinus wall; straight and angled endoscopes are used to obtain different angles of view. Dissection within the cavernous sinus is continued only sharply using microdissectors and microscissors to prevent any traction on the ICA and cranial nerves. Once the cavernous sinus is entered, venous bleeding is controlled by applying gentle pressure to the sinus with hemostatic agents. Following tumor removal, the whole area is inspected with angled endoscopes to identify and remove any tumor remnants. Any bony hyperostoses, such as in meningiomas, are also removed.

The same principles apply to the resection of retrochiasmatic craniopharyngiomas and sellar tumors with significant lateral and retrochiasmatic extensions. These tumors are typically attached to the undersurface of the optic tracts and chiasm. After the tumor is identified, a biopsy is obtained, and the tumor is internally decompressed and gradually resected in the usual manner; the last portion of the tumor, adherent to the optic apparatus, is always sharply dissected.

After tumor resection is achieved, the 0° endoscope is slowly withdrawn, and a 30° or 70° endoscope is used to conduct a second survey of the entire region; any remaining tumor is further dissected and removed. Following that, hemostasis is secured, and the entire region is copiously irrigated, followed by dural closure, cranioplasty, and layered suturing of the subcutaneous tissues and skin.

7.1.3. Cases

7.1.3.1. Trigeminal Schwannoma (Right Sided) (Fig. 9A–S)

7.1.3.2. Middle Fossa Epidermoid Tumor (Left Sided) (Fig. 10A–U)

8. POTENTIAL COMPLICATIONS

Potential complications of the fully endoscopic subtemporal approach include the following:

- Bleeding, infection, meningitis, cerebrovascular accident, and death, as well as the potential risk for endocrinological morbidity, vascular complications, neuropsychological and behavioral disorders, and neurocognitive disorders (these are also potential complications associated with open approaches with more extensive dissection).
- Injuries during skin incision include transient or permanent injury to the frontotemporal branch of the facial nerve or, less commonly, the auriculotemporal branch of the mandibular nerve.
- Direct injuries can occur to cranial nerves, carotid artery, optic apparatus, or the pituitary gland/stalk.
- CSF leakage.

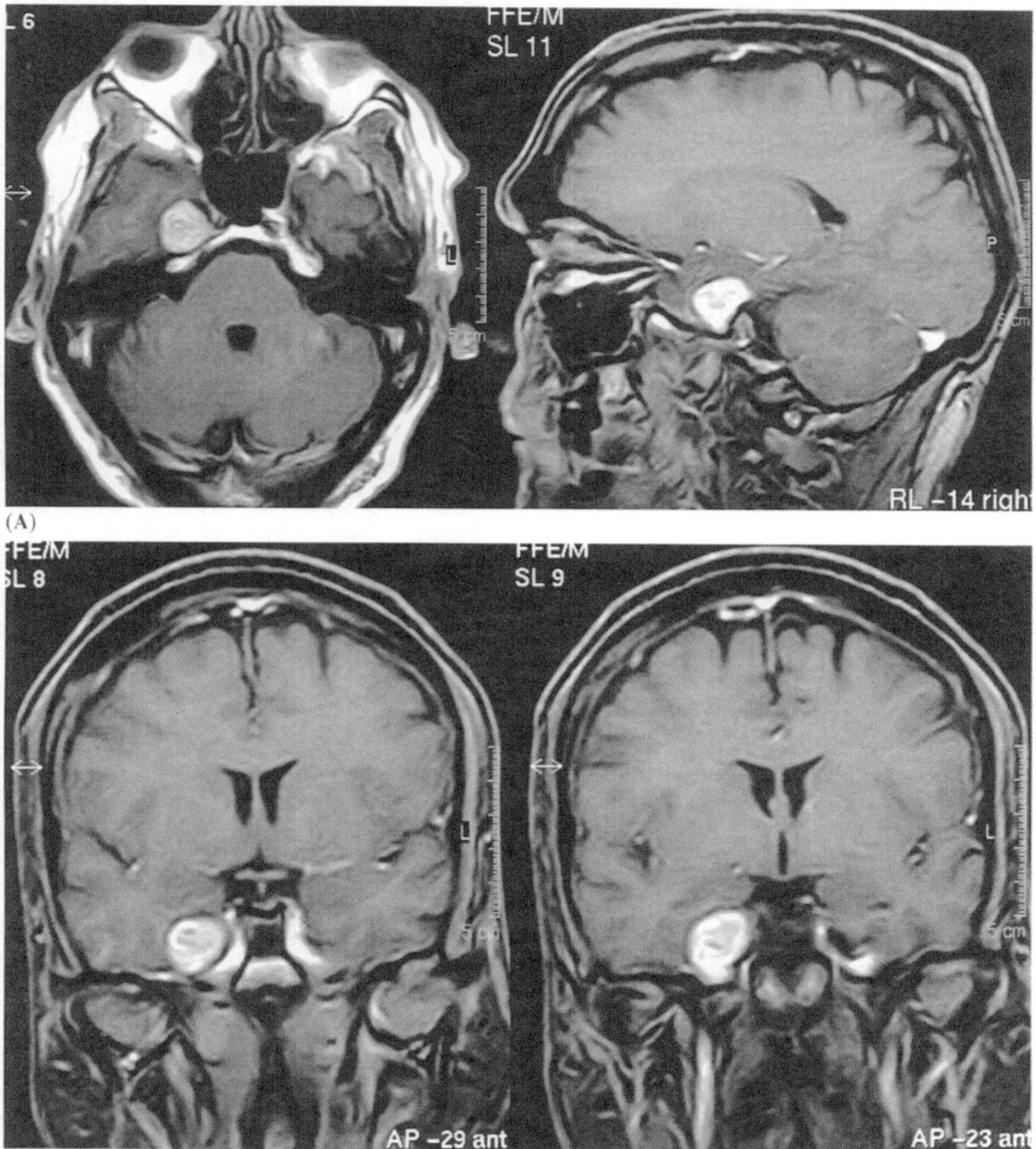

(B)

Fig. 9 (**A**) Contrast-enhanced axial and sagittal MRIs showing a trigeminal schwannoma. (**B**) Contrast-enhanced coronal MRIs showing a trigeminal schwannoma. (**C**)–(**E**) Intraoperative endoscopic view showing the initial exposure of trigeminal schwannoma. (**C**) *a* Trigeminal

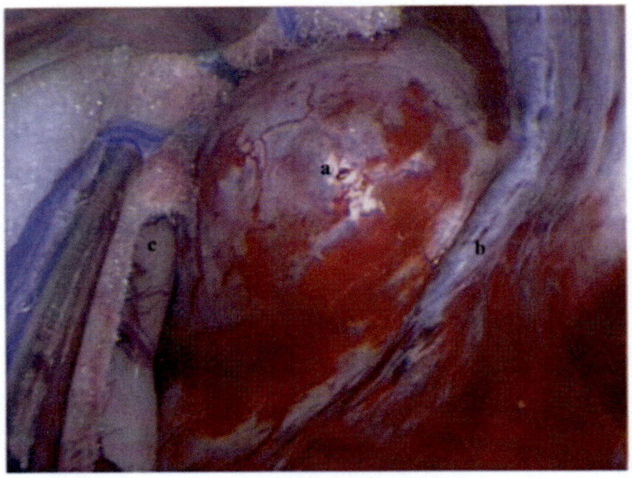

(C)

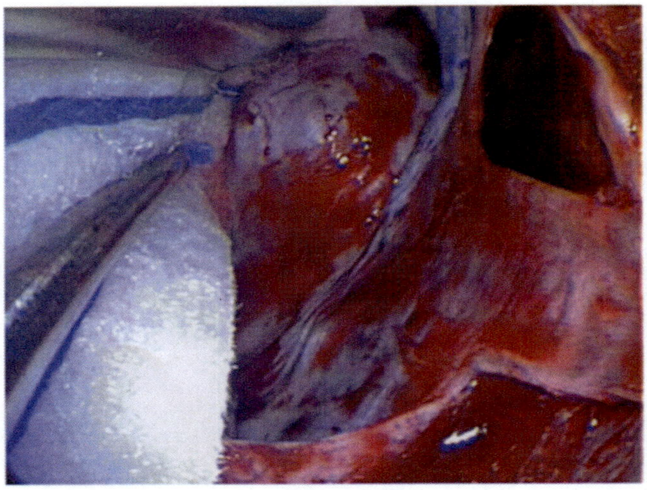

(D)

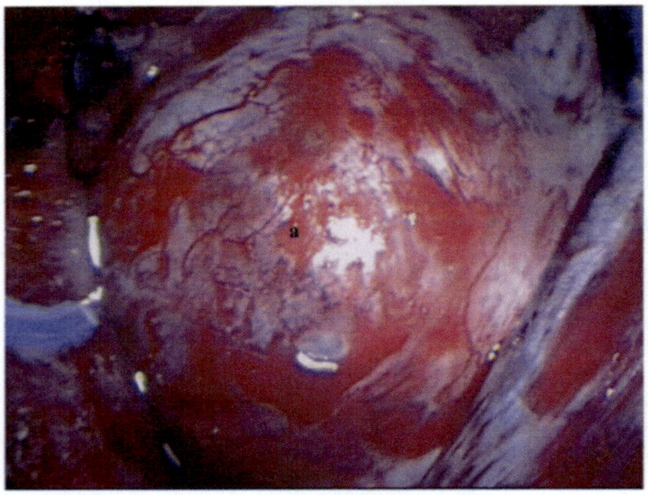

(E)

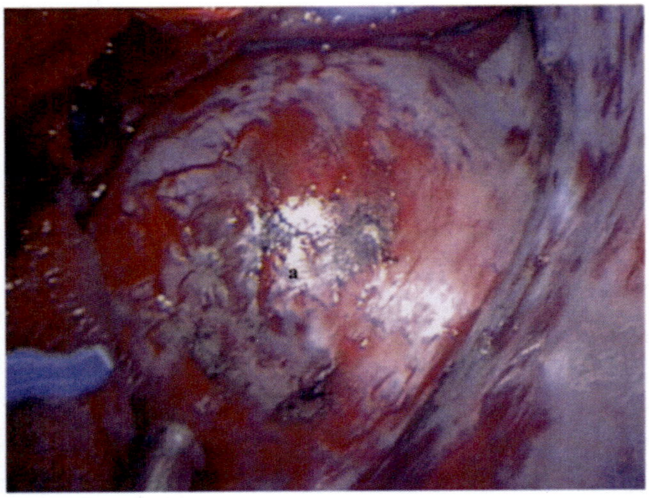

(F)

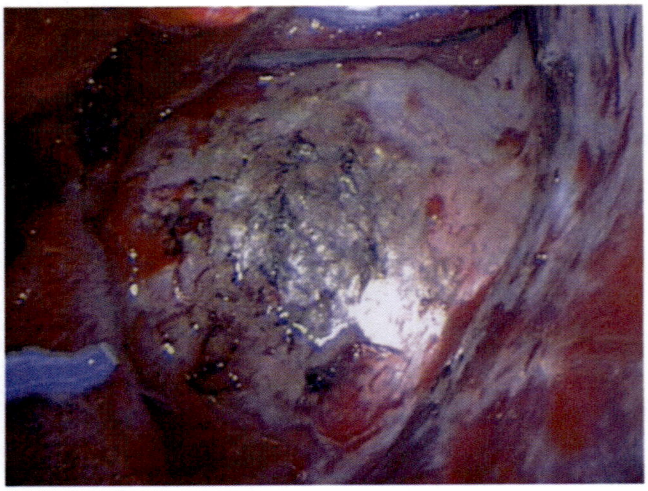

(G)

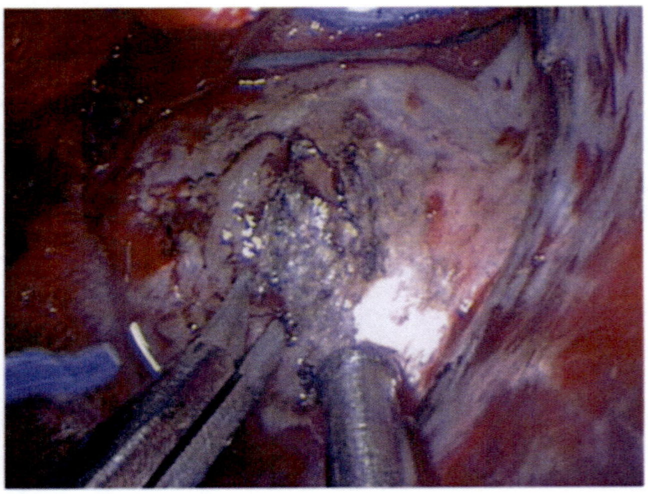

(H)

Fig. 9 (continued) schwannoma. *b* Lateral skull base. *c* Lower aspect of temporal lobe. **(E)** *a* Close-up view of trigeminal schwannoma. **(F)**–**(O)** Intraoperative endoscopic view showing gradual resection of trigeminal schwannoma. **(F)** *a* Tumor surface cauterized. **(I)** *a* Trigeminal schwannoma partly debulked. **(J)** *a* Capsule of trigeminal schwannoma. **(K)** *a* Sharp dissection of posterior capsule of trigeminal schwannoma. **(M)** *a* Maxillary (V2) division of trigeminal nerve (V). *b* Mandibular (V3) division of trigeminal nerve (V). **(N)** *a* Maxillary (V2) division of trigeminal nerve (V). *b* Mandibular (V3) division of trigeminal nerve (V). *c* Final portion of trigeminal schwannoma. **(O)** *a* Sharp dissection of final portion of trigeminal schwannoma. **(P)** and **(Q)** Intraoperative endoscopic view following complete tumor removal. **(P)** *a* Maxillary (V2) division of trigeminal nerve (V). *b* Mandibular (V3) division of trigeminal nerve (V). *c* Lower aspect of temporal lobe. **(Q)** *a* Gelfoam in tumor cavity. *b* Lower aspect of temporal lobe. *c* Basal temporal dura. **(R)** Postoperative contrast-enhanced axial and sagittal MRIs. **(S)** Postoperative contrast-enhanced coronal MRIs.

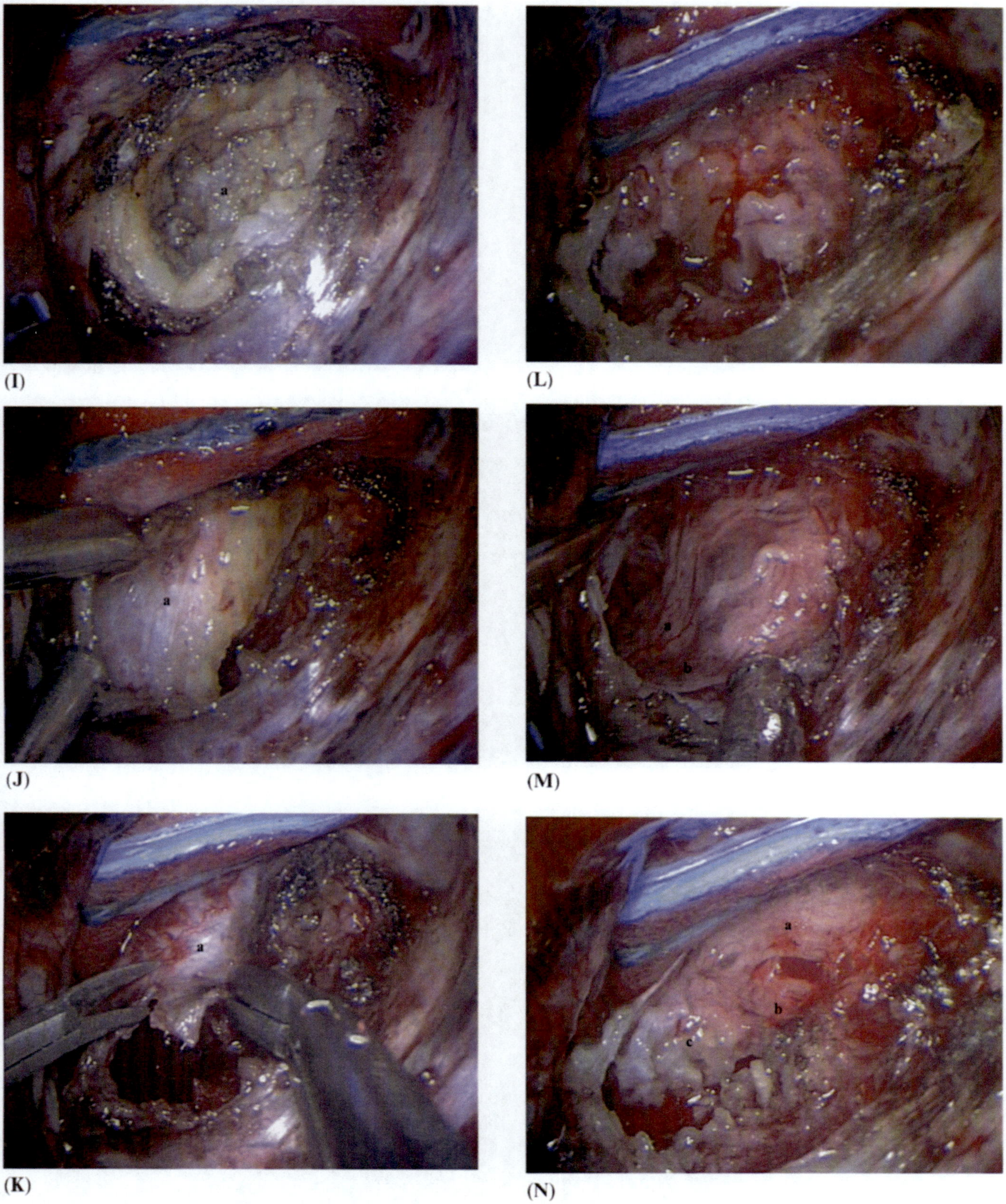

Fig. 9 (continued)

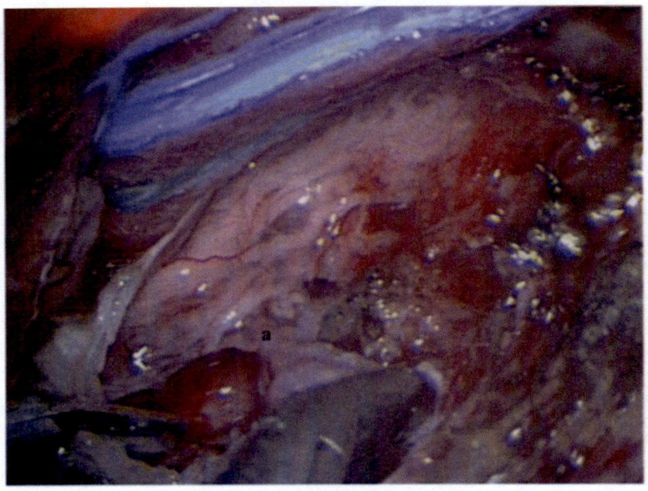

(O)

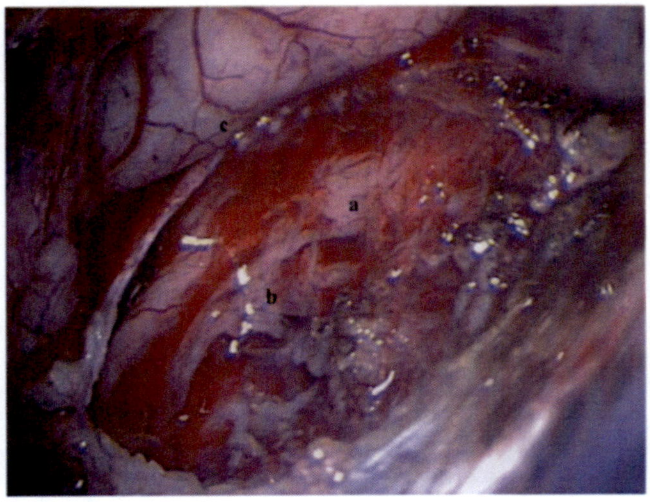

(P)

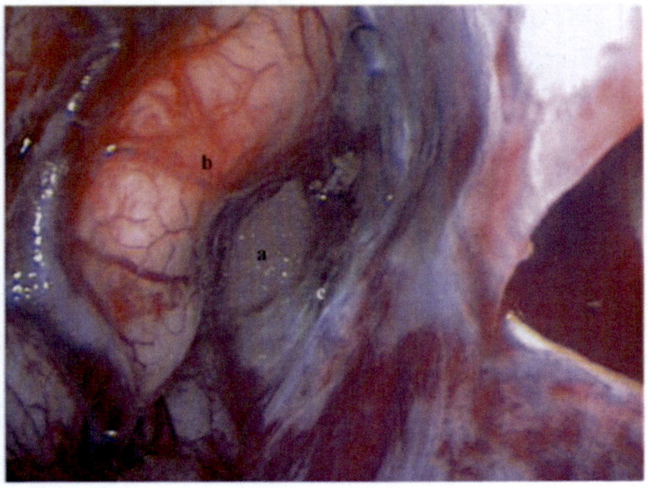

(Q)

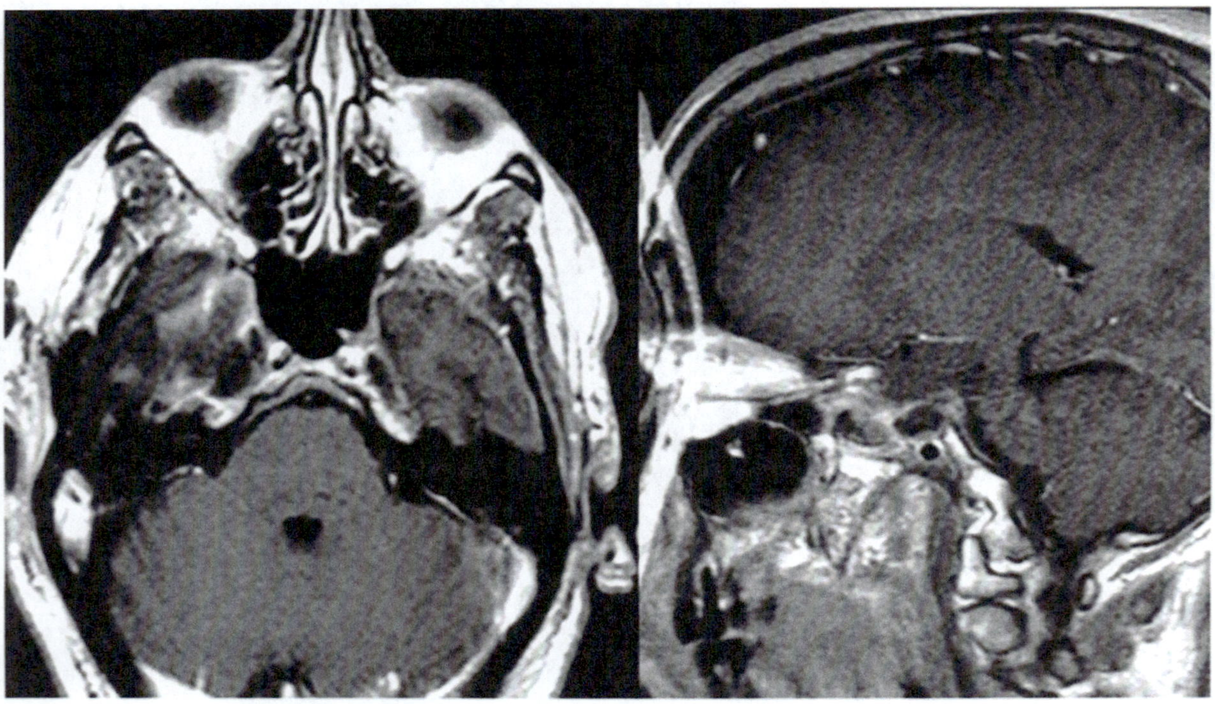

(R)

Fig. 9 (continued)

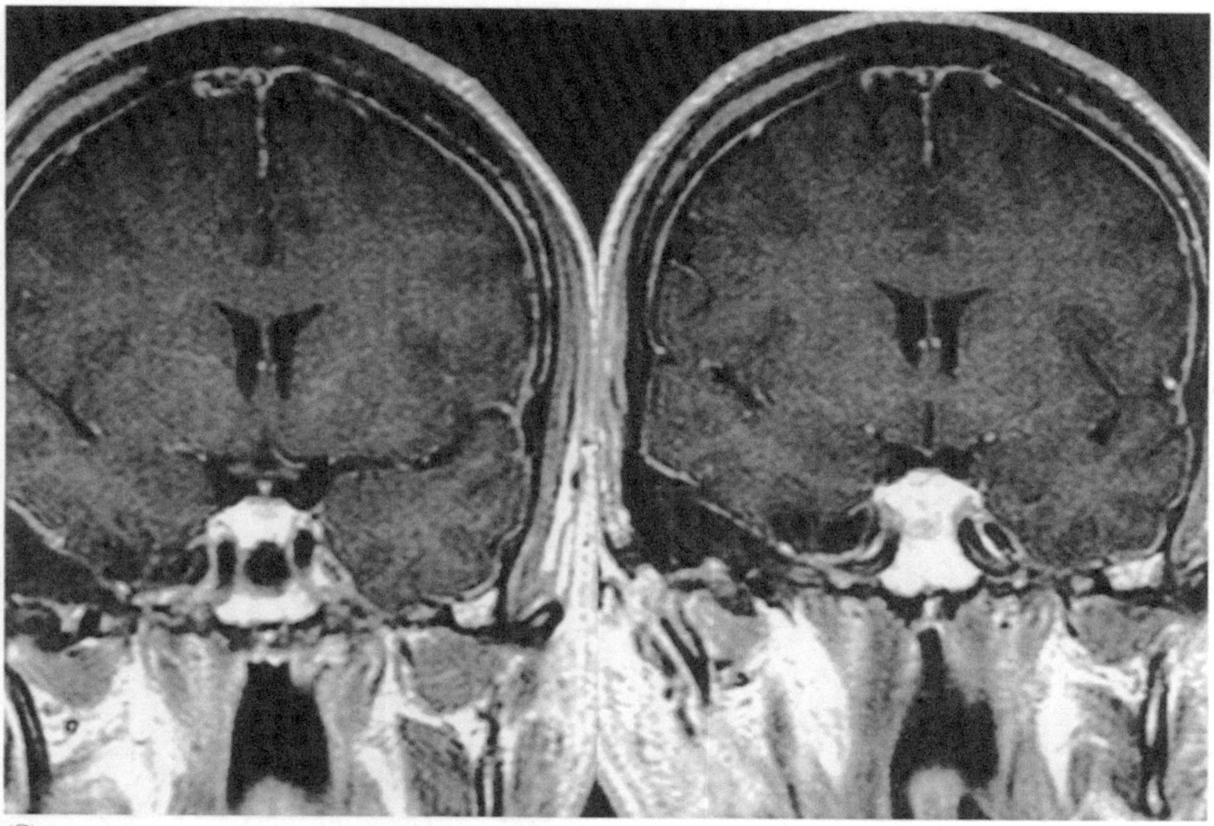

(S)

Fig. 9 (continued)

- Temporal lobe cortical injury can cause short term memory disturbance, aphasia, seizures, or hemiplegia.
- Hematoma (intracerebral/epidural/subdural), edema, or lateral herniation of the temporal lobe.
- Other complications with combined approaches (e.g., transtentorial, transpetrosal, subtemporal–infratemporal).

9. AVOIDING COMPLICATIONS IN AUTHOR'S EXPERIENCE

During the skin incision, the frontotemporal branch of the facial nerve is the most likely motor branch to be injured because it is vulnerable in its superficial path as it penetrates just below the zygomatic arch close to the temporomandibular joint and traverses an oblique course superiorly over and above the zygomatic arch. This is avoided by carefully elevating the lateral periosteum of the arch to protect the nerve and not extending the skin incision below the lower border of the zygomatic root. The course of the nerve over the zygomatic arch can be estimated by a line connecting a point 0.5 cm inferior to the tragus to a point 1.5 cm lateral to the superior brow.

The auriculotemporal nerve, a sensory branch of the mandibular division of the trigeminal nerve, lies posterior to the superficial temporal artery within the temporoparietal fascia (the surgeon may often encounter an anterior branch of the artery during the skin incision), and therefore elevation anterior to the frontal branch of the superficial temporal artery should proceed with caution to avoid injuring this nerve. Whenever possible, the anterior branches of the superficial temporal artery are preserved to maximize blood supply to the skin; if not, they can be ligated with nonabsorbable suture.

Cranial nerve morbidity caused by intimate involvement of the affected nerves with the lesion is a critical issue in the resection of tumors involving the cavernous sinus. This complication sometimes cannot be avoided regardless of the type of surgery; however, endoscopes with their superior visibility, precision microsurgical instruments, and intraoperative nerve monitoring allow many unnecessary injuries to be avoided. In general, existing preoperative cranial nerve deficits infrequently improve or resolve following resection, while the majority of new and often partial postoperative deficits resolve over time.

Closure after performing this approach requires meticulous attention to preventing CSF leakage; the dura may be thin, especially in old age. Also, the squamous temporal bone is thin and can often be easily fractured; therefore, it is important to avoid lacerating the dura during the bone flap removal. If watertight dural closure could not be obtained, a second layer (e.g., Duragen®, muscle) should be placed over the dura and secured in place with 2 cc fibrin glue.

Bleeding from small vessels at the operative bed usually subsides with copious irrigation. An epidural hematoma is an uncommon postoperative occurrence and is the result of inadequate hemostasis. Of note, bone bleeders, as well as bleeding on the dural surface from branches of the middle meningeal artery, may be encountered and controlled by bone wax application and bipolar electrocoagulation.

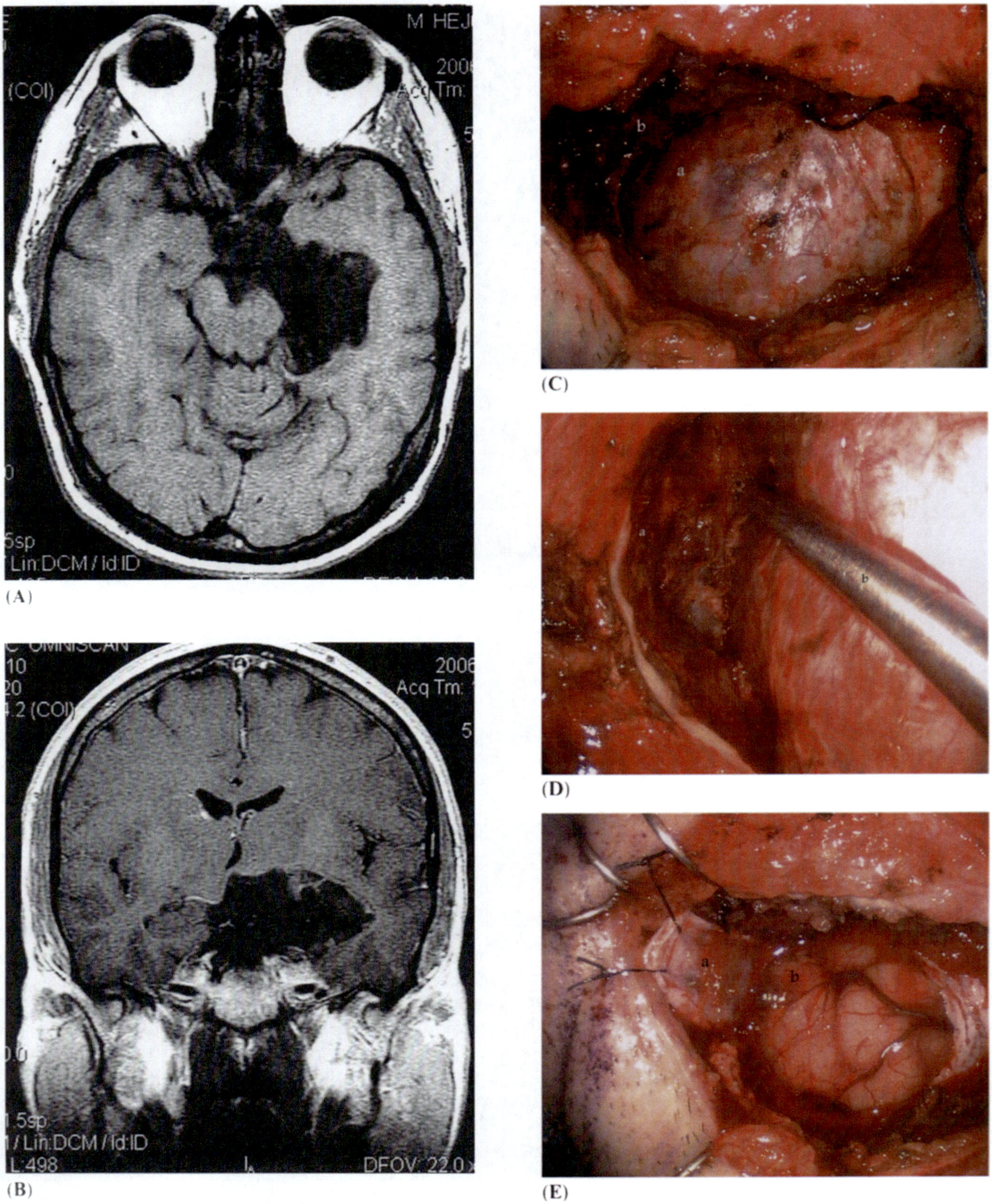

Fig. 10 (**A**) Contrast-enhanced T_1-weighted axial MRI showing a middle fossa epidermoid tumor. (**B**) Contrast-enhanced T_1-weighted coronal MRI showing a middle fossa epidermoid tumor. (**C**)–(**F**) Intraoperative endoscopic view showing initial exposure of middle fossa epidermoid tumor. (**C**) *a* Basal temporal dura. *b* Lateral skull base floor partially drilled. (**D**) *a* Drilled floor of lateral skull base. *b* Atraumatic suction. (**E**) *a* Temporal dura reflected. *b* Lower aspect of temporal lobe.

(continued)

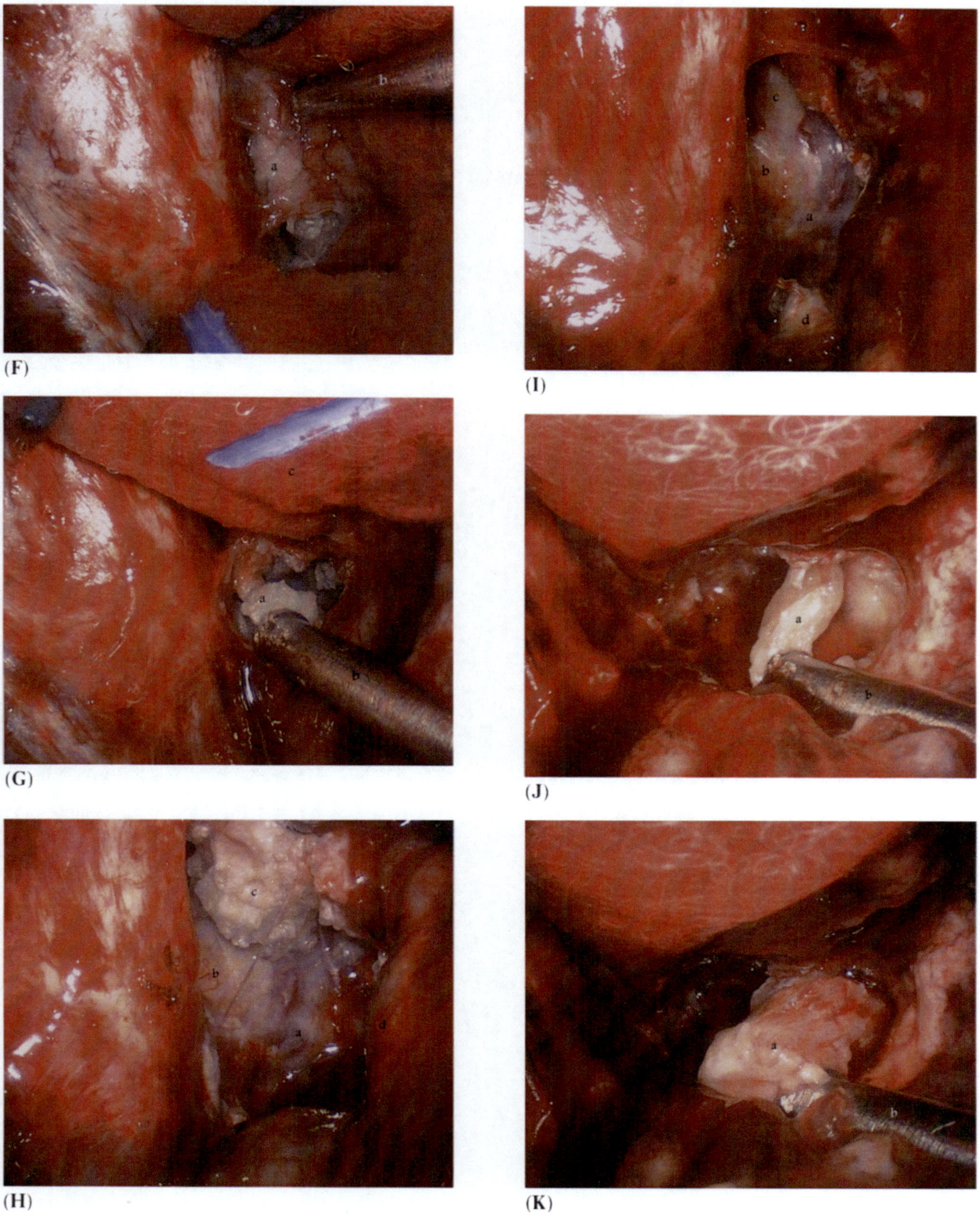

Fig. 10 (continued) (**F**) *a* Epidermoid tumor. *b* Atraumatic suction. (**G**)–(**O**) Intraoperative endoscopic view showing gradual resection of middle fossa epidermoid tumor. (**G**) *a* Epidermoid tumor. *b* Atraumatic suction. *c* Cottonoid over lower surface of temporal lobe. (**H**) *a* Trigeminal (gasserian) ganglion. *b* Mandibular (V3) division of trigeminal nerve (V). *c* Epidermoid tumor. *d* Lower aspect of temporal lobe. (**I**) *a* Trigeminal (gasserian) ganglion. *b* Mandibular (V3) division of trigeminal nerve (V). *c* Maxillary (V2) division of trigeminal nerve (V). *d* Epidermoid tumor. (**J**) *a* Epidermoid tumor. *b* Atraumatic suction. (**K**) *a* Epidermoid tumor. *b* Straight microforceps.

(continued)

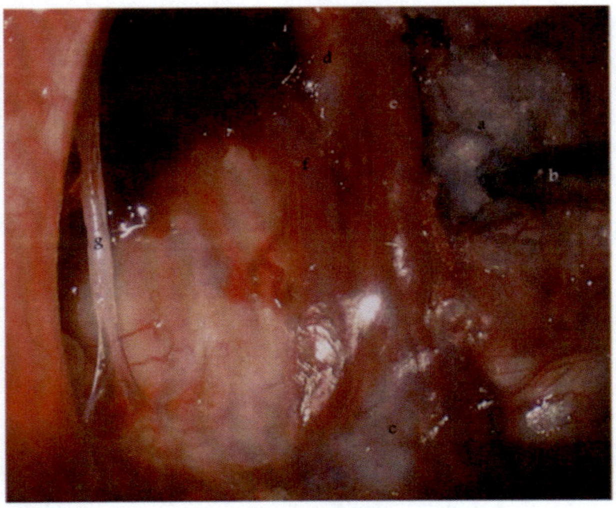

(L)

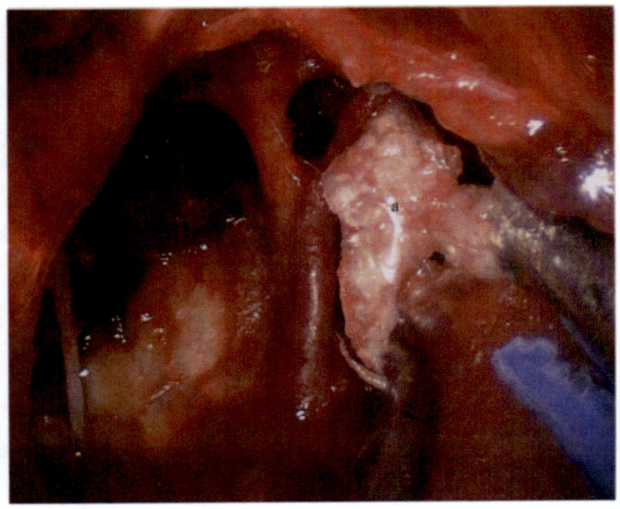

(O)

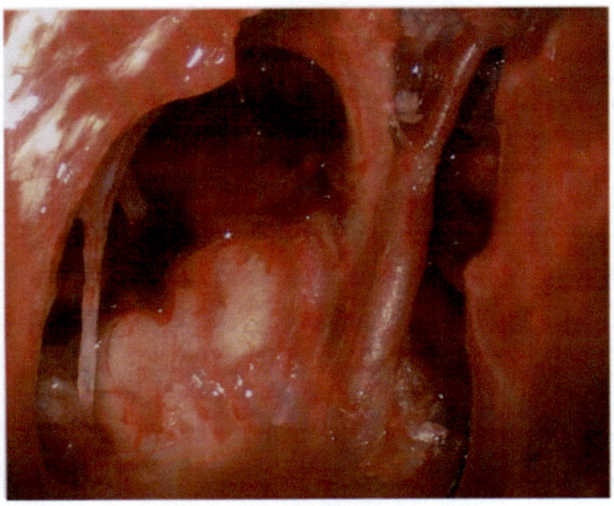

(M)

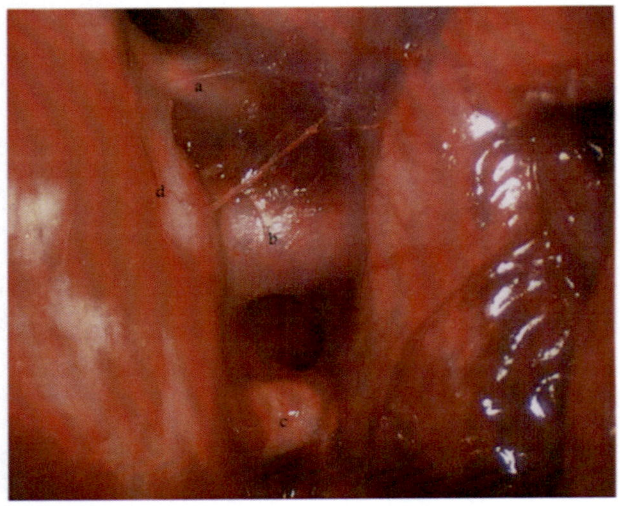

(P)

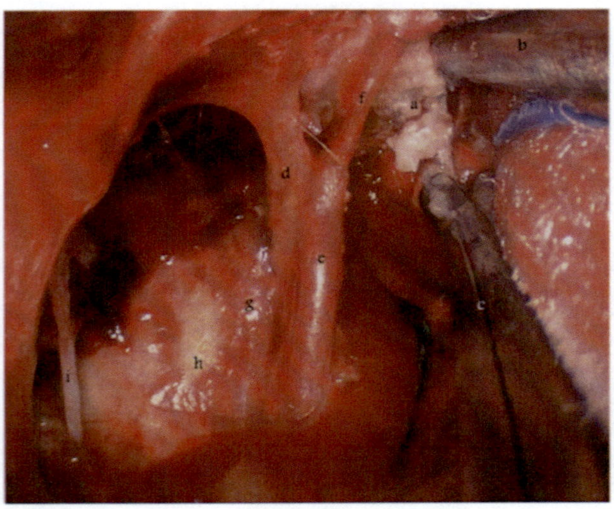

(N)

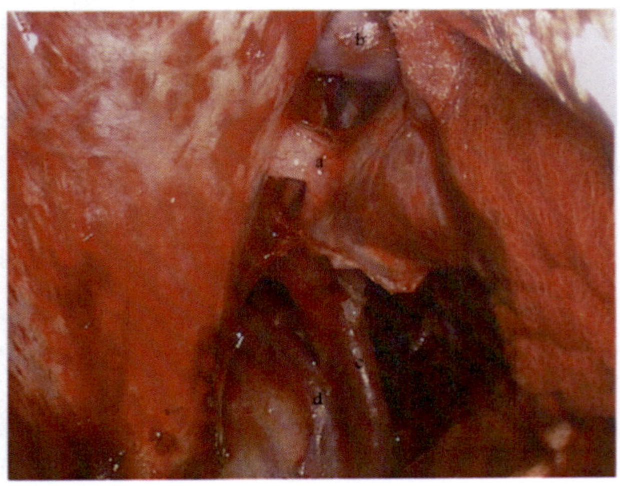

(Q)

Fig. 10 (continued) (**L**) *a* Epidermoid tumor. *b* Atraumatic suction. *c* Brainstem. *d* Occulomotor (III) nerve. *e* Posterior cerebral artery (PCA). *f* Superior cerebellar artery (SCA). *g* Trochlear (IV) nerve. (**N**) *a* Epidermoid tumor. *b* Atraumatic suction. *c* Left-curved tumor forceps. *d* Occulomotor (III) nerve. *e* Posterior cerebral artery (PCA). *f* Posterior communicating (PCOM) artery. *g* Superior cerebellar artery (SCA). *h* Brainstem. *i* Trochlear (IV) nerve. (**O**) *a* Close-up view showing resection of final portions of epidermoid tumor. (**P**)–(**S**) Intraoperative endoscopic view following complete tumor resection. (**P**) *a* Ipsilateral optic (II) nerve. *b* Internal carotid artery (ICA). *c* Occulomotor (III) nerve. *d* Dura overlying anterior clinoid process. (**Q**) *a* Occulomotor (III) nerve. *b* Internal carotid artery (ICA). *c* Posterior cerebral artery (PCA). *d* Superior cerebellar artery (SCA).

(continued)

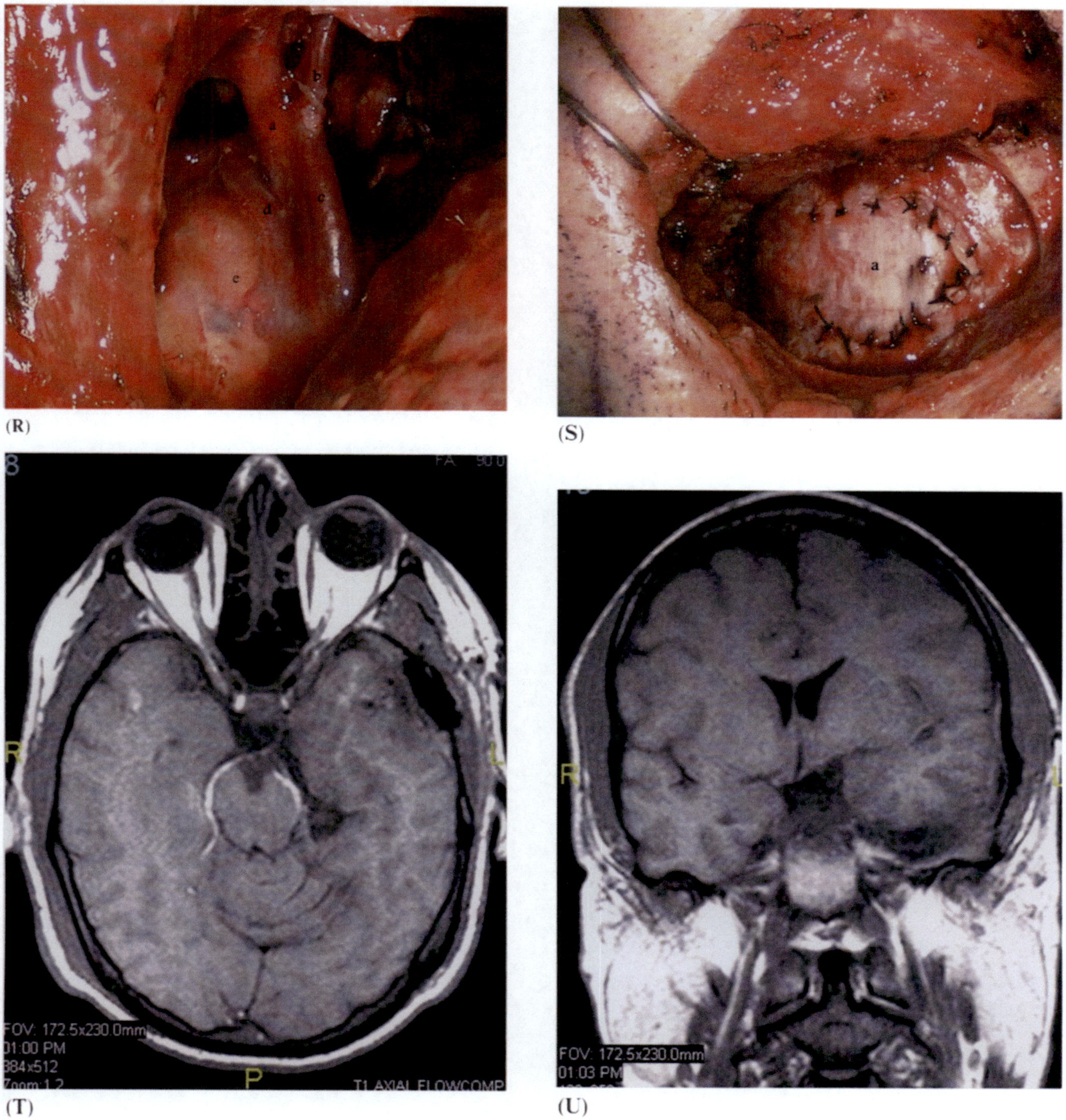

Fig. 10 (continued) (**R**) *a* Occulomotor (III) nerve. *b* Posterior communicating (PCOM) artery. *c* Posterior cerebral artery (PCA). *d* Superior cerebellar artery (SCA). *e* Brainstem. (**S**) *a* Temporal dura closed. (**T**) Postoperative contrast-enhanced T_1-weighted axial MRI. (**U**) Postoperative contrast-enhanced T_1-weighted coronal MRI.

The traditional middle fossa subtemporal approach requires long-standing placement of retractors on the temporal lobe; therefore, potential injury to the temporal lobe can occur (e.g., hematoma and edema resulting in aphasia, hemiparesis, or seizures). This concern should not be a problem with the described approach because temporal lobe retractors are not used. The floor of the middle cranial fossa is at the level of the upper edge of the zygomatic arch and the craniotomy should always be kept flush with the floor this, along with correct positioning and other measures, facilitates a subtemporal trajectory for the endoscope without requiring any temporal retraction.

Finally, it is necessary to replace the keyhole bone flap at the end of the operation as this improves both functional and cosmetic outcomes and avoids transmission of brain pulsations to the skin, which is cosmetically undesirable and may even cause lateral herniation of the temporal lobe.

Index

A

Acoustic tumors, 171
Acromegaly, 15–16, 49
ACTH-secreting tumors, 14. *See also* Pituitary tumors
AndroGel, testosterone cream, 17
Aneurysms, 114
Angiofibromas, 23
Anterior cerebral artery (ACA), 95
Anterior communicating artery (ACoA), 90
Anterior cranial fossa tumor, 93–95
  1.5- cm supraorbital keyhole craniotomy, 95
  cranioplasty, 95
  dissection of optic nerves, chiasm, and ACA complex, 95
  dissection with normal frontal lobes, 95
  0° endoscope, introduction, 95
  frozen section analysis, 95
  tumor decompression, 95
Anterior inferior cerebellar artery (AICA), 115
Antidiuretic hormone (ADH), 11, 17, 18
Arachnoid cysts, 77
Arginine vasopressin (AVP), 11, 17
Arterial pCO_2, 8
AVP analog DDAVP®, diabetes insipidus, 17

B

Bilateral inferior petrosal sinus sampling in cushing's disease (BIPSS), 15, 26
Bispectral index (BIS), 9
Brainstem auditory evoked potentials (BAEPs), 8, 31
Brainstem somatosensory-evoked responses, 8

C

Cabergoline (Dostinex), for prolactinomas, 13
Cavernous sinus, 173, 183
  and tumors of, 178
Cavitron ultrasonic aspirators (CUSAs), 29, 32
Cerebellar retraction, 171
Cerebellopontine angle (CPA), 2, 3, 109
  tumor and approach for, 120, 130
Chordomas, 12
Clival chordoma, 43, 60, 65
Corticotropin (ACTH), 11, 26, 48
Corticotropin-releasing hormone (CRH), 11, 27
Cosyntropin, $ACTH_{1-24}$, 17
Cranial nerves
  electromyograms, 8
  EMG monitor, 34
  stimulation, 8
Craniopharyngioma, 12, 43, 76, 78, 82–83, 173
  coronal contrasted T1-weighted MRI, 78
  with large cystic component, 78–81
  postoperative T1-weighted, contrast-enhanced coronal MRI, 81
  sagittal contrasted T1-weighted MRI, 78, 82
CSF rhinorrhea, 82, 129
Cushing's syndrome, 13–15, 26
Cystic craniopharyngiomas, 77

D

Deep inhalational anesthesia, 7
Dexamethasone suppression tests, 13–14. *See also* Cushing's syndrome
Diabetes insipidus (DI), 5, 107
Digital versatile disc (DVD), 31
Digital video camera (DVCAM), 31
Dopaminergic agents, hormonal abnormalities, 18

E

Electroencephalography (EEG), 31
Electromyograms (EMGs), 8
Electromyography (EMG), 31
Embolization, of skull base tumors. *See also* Neuroradiology, skull base surgery
  carotid bifurcation paraganglioma, 22
  foramen jugular paraganglioma, 22–23
  juvenile nasopharyngeal angiofibromas, 23
  nasal angiofibroma with intracranial extension, 24–25
  preoperative meningioma embolization, 25–26
  skull base meningiomas, 23, 25
Endocrine-inactive adenomas, 18
Endoscopic endonasal approach, 43
  anterior cerebrospinal fluid (CSF) fistulas, repair, 43
  anterior wall of sphenoid sinus, 47
  arachnoid membrane, prevention injury, 65
  CSF leak, avoidance, 65

Endoscopic endonasal approach (*Continued*)
for cysts, 78
double-layer closure technique, 71
dural sealant or fibrin glue, 47–48
70° endoscope and 30° lens, use of, 65
endoscopic anatomy of nose, 45
endoscopic supraorbital or transglabellar approach, 65
fat graft harvesting, 47–48
floor of sella, removing, 45–46
hidden tumor remnants removal, 47
instruments needed to, 43
intranasal dissection, 45
middle turbinate, 45
opening of sphenoid sinus, 46
operating room setup, 6, 43–44
posterior septoplasty, 46
potential complications of, 60, 65
sphenoid anatomy, MRI, 65
sphenoid sinus exposure, 45–46
supine placement, patient, 44
tumor remnants, 71
Valsalva maneuver, use of, 47
Endoscopic endonasal surgery, 6
Endoscopic pituitary surgery, 3
Endoscopic retrosigmoid approach, 109
cerebellar retraction and prevention of secondary bleeding, 171
cerebellopontine angle (CPA)
access to, petroclival, and foramen magnum regions, 109
endoscope advancement, 111, 112
endoscopic anatomy of, 111, 113
cranioplasty, 111, 114
dural opening, 110, 112
dural sealant, to prevent CSF leak, 111, 114
early or delayed CSF leakage, precautions, 171
hydrocephalus, to resolve, 171
instrumentation need, 109
keyhole craniotomy, 110, 112
marking and draping, 110–111
operating room setup, 109–110
postoperative facial nerve paralysis, to avoid, 171
potential complications of, 112, 115, 171
skin closure and dressing, 112, 115
skin incision, 110–111
three-pin Mayfield clamp and lateral oblique position, 110
Endoscopic retrosigmoid surgery, 8
Endoscopic skull base surgery, 2–3, 5
preoperative assessment, 5–6
unique operating room environment, 6
Endoscopic subtemporal approach, 173
auriculotemporal nerve, prevention in skin incision, 183
complications of, 179, 183
cranial nerve morbidity, to avoid, 183
cranioplasty, 177
CSF leakage, prevention, 183
draping, and skin incision, 174–175
Duragen®, use of, 183
dural closure, 176–177
epidural hematoma, prevention, 183, 187
extradural anatomy and dural opening, 176
hydroxyapatite bone substitute, 177
instruments need, 173–174
keyhole craniotomy, 175–176
minimally invasive surgical access areas, 173
operating room setup, 174
skin closure and dressing, 177–178
supine, patient position, 174
transmission of brain pulsations, to avoid, 187
trigeminal nerve, mandibular (V3) division, 176
zygomatic arch injury, prevention, 183
Endoscopic surgical anatomy, 3
Endoscopic transglabellar keyhole approach, 73
access for surgical resection of midline tumors, 73
burr hole and keyhole craniotomy, 74–75
complications of, 80, 82
craniopharyngiomas of suprasellar region with adhesions to optic chiasm, 82
cranioplasty, 77
dural opening and closure, 76
dural sealant, 76
general anesthesia, 74
hydroxyapatite bone substitute, 77
instruments needed, 73
marking, draping, and skin incision, 75
operating room setup, 73–74
pericranial graft, for sealing, 82
pericranium reflection, 75
postoperative visual deterioration, 82
preliminary endoscopic survey, 75–76
resection of tumor, 76
resection, suprasellar extensions of pituitary macroadenomas, 82
skin closure and dressing, 77
supine placement, patient, 74
Endoscopy-based specialty, 1
Epidermoid cysts, 12
Epidermoid tumors, 12
Esthesioneuroblastomas, 89, 95

F

Facial nerve, neurovascular anatomy, 123
Facial nerve paralysis, postoperative, 171
Fiber-optic technology, advancement, 1
Follicle-stimulating hormone (FSH), 11
Foramen magnum regions, 109
Foramen of Monro, 49

G

Glossopharyngeal neuralgia, 115, 118, 129
Gonadotropin-releasing hormone (GnRH), 11
Growth hormone (GH), 11
Growth hormone-releasing hormone (GHRH), 11

H

Hemifacial spasm, 115, 118, 120
left sided, 123–124, 127–128
right sided, 124–125, 126–127
Hemostasis, 111, 175
Hormone replacement therapy, 5
Hypercortisolism, 13
Hyperprolactinemia, 49
Hypogonadism, 17
Hypopituitarism, 49
Hypothalamic gliomas, 173

I
Iatrogenic injury, 1
Inferior petrosal sinus sampling, 26–27
Inflammatory, pituitary gland, 12
Insulin-like growth factor-1 (IGF-1), 11
Internal auditory canal (IAC), 29, 109, 173
Internal auditory meatus (IAM), 116
Internal carotid artery, test and permanent occlusion, 25
  clinical assessment, 26
  clinical tolerance, 26
  four-vessel cerebral angiography, 26
  hypotensive test, 26
  indications for test, 25
Intracanalicular acoustic neuroma, 130
Intracranial pressure (ICP), 11
Ipsilateral petroclival, 173

J
Juvenile nasopharyngeal angiofibromas, 23

K
Keyhole craniotomy, 2

L
Large acoustic neuroma, 130
  left sided, 136–139
  right sided, 131–132, 133–135, 139–143
Large-bore intravenous and arterial lines, 6
Lateral CPA meningioma, 130
  left sided, 165–167
LH- and FSH-secreting tumors, 16. *See also* Pituitary tumors
Liquid crystal display (LCD), 29, 31
Luteinizing hormone (LH), 11

M
Magnetic resonance imaging/magnetic resonance angiographic (MRI/MRA) scan, brain, 114
Medial CPA meningioma (left sided), 167–170
Medial sphenoid wing regions, 173
Medium acoustic neuroma, 130
  left sided, 146–149, 150–153
  right sided, 143–145
Meningiomas, 12, 95, 109
MicroCUSA handpieces and tips, 36–37
Microscopic transseptal pituitary surgery, 3
Microvascular decompression of cranial nerve, 8
Middle Cerebral Artery (MCA), 26
Middle cranial fossa tumors, 95, 97, 99, 178
Middle fossa epidermoid tumor
  atraumatic suction, 185, 186
  complete tumor resection, 186–187
  contrast-enhanced T1-weighted axial MRI, 184
  gradual resection, 185–186
  initial exposure of, 184–185
  mandibular (V3) division of trigeminal nerve, 185
  posterior cerebral artery (PCA), 186
  posterior communicating (PCOM) artery, 186
  postoperative contrast-enhanced T1-weighted axial and coronal MRI, 187
  temporal dura, closing, 187
  trigeminal (gasserian) ganglion, 186
Motor evoked potentials (MEPs), 31
Multiple endocrine neoplasia type 2 (MEN 2), 21

N
Neuroanesthesia
  for endoscopic technique
    endonasal approach, 6–7
    retrosigmoid approach, 7–9
    supraorbital approach, 7
Neuroanesthesiologist, role in endoscopy, 5–6
Neurofibromas, 173
Neurofibromatosis type 1 (NF-1), 21
Neuromuscular blockade, 8
Neuroradiology, skull base surgery
  embolization, skull base tumors, 21–25
  inferior petrosal sinus sampling, 26–27
  test and permanent occlusion, internal carotid artery, 25–26
Neurosurgical and microsurgical instruments, conventional
  cranial nerve monitors, 31–32
  digital monitors, 31
  DVD recorders, 31
  endoscopic microinstruments, 33–41
  high-definition digital cameras, 31
  irrigation sheaths and pumps, 29–30
  micro-cavitron ultrasonic surgical aspirator, 32–33
  microdrill handpieces, attachments, and burrs, 32
  pneumatic holding arms, 30–31
  polaroid digital printers, 31
  rigid endoscopes, 29
  xenon light sources, 31

O
Olfactory groove meningiomas (OGMs), 95, 96–97
  debulking of, 96
  postoperative contrast-enhanced, T1-weighted coronal MRI, 97
  resection of, 96
  T1-weighted coronal MRI, 96
Open craniotomy, 1
Optic nerve gliomas, 43
Osteomyelitis, 82
Otorrhea, 129

P
Panhypopituitarism, 49
Paragangliomas, 21–23
Periclival tumors, 53
  clivus or retroclival region, approach, 60
  dural defects, prevention, 60
  fibrin or dural sealant, 60
  frozen section analysis, 60
  operative techniques and approaches, 60
Perioperative antidiuretic hormone (ADH), 5
Phenylephrine, vasopressors, 9
Pituitary apoplexy, 49
Pituitary gland
  hormones secrete from, 11
  pathologies affecting, 12
  target organ hormone axis, 19
  tumors and disorders affecting, 12
Pituitary macroadenoma, 55–65, 77
  bone of sellar floor, removal, 49
  postoperative contrast-enhanced axial, saggital, and coronal MRIs, 65
  postoperative contrast-enhanced sagital MRI, 57
  T1-weighted axial, sagittal and coronal contrast-enhanced MRI, 61
  T1-weighted coronal contrast-enhanced MRIs, 58
  T1-weighted sagittal MRI, 55

Pituitary microadenoma
dura, electrocoagulation and opening, 48
hypophysectomy, 49
left one-third for pituitary microadenoma, 52–54
microadenoma, resection, 48
microadenomectomy, 49
left pituitary microadenoma, 49–51
pituitary microadenoma, 51–52
postoperative contrast-enhanced coronal MRI, 52
ring curette, 50
T1-weighted coronal contrasted MRIs, 49, 51–52
Pituitary tumors
acromegaly, 15–16
cushing's disease, 13–15
bilateral inferior petrosal sinus sampling, 15–16
hormonal deficiencies caused by, 16
ACTH, 17
central hypothyroidism, 17
diabetes insipidus, 17
gonadotropin, 17
growth hormone, 17
hypopituitarism, 18
LH- and FSH-secreting tumors, 16
nonfunctioning tumors, 16
patients, long-term follow-up, 18
prolactinomas, 12–13
TSH-secreting tumors, 16
Planum sphenoidale meningioma, 89, 97–101
Pneumocephalus, 82
Posterior cranial fossa, neurovascular anatomy, 109
Posterior fossa meningioma, 120
Prepontine epidermoid tumor, 60, 66–70
postoperative contrast-enhanced T1-weighted axial and sagittal MRIs, 70
T2-weighted axial and T1-weighted contrast-enhanced saggital MRIs, 66
Prolactinomas, 12–13, 18
clinical effects, 13
Prolactin (PRL), 11
Propofol, anesthetic management, 8
Pseudo-Cushing's syndrome, 13

R

Rathke's cleft cysts, 12, 18, 43, 77
Rigid lens scopes, parallel use, 2
Root entry zone (REZ), 114, 115

S

Schizophrenia, Haldol for, 12
Schwannomas, 109
Secretory tumors, 48
Selective serotonin reuptake inhibitors (SSRIs), 12
Sella turcica, 11, 45, 78
Skull base surgery
and endoscopic technique
anesthetic considerations, 5–9
evolution from traditional surgical approaches, 1–3
instrumentation in, 29–41
interventional neuroradiology aspects of, 21–27
neuroendocrine aspects of, 11–19
preoperative assessment patients, 5–6
adrenocorticoids, 5
airway abnormalities, 6
cartilaginous hypertrophy of arytenoids and tracheal rings, 5
childhood craniopharyngiomas, 5
Cushing's disease and acromegaly, 5
growth hormone-secreting pituitary adenomas, 5
mineralocorticoid-induced effects, 5
patients with pituitary neoplasms, 5
pituitary adenomas, 5
pituitary hyperfunction, 5
Rathke's cleft cysts, 5
Skull base tumors, 11
Small, intracanalicular acoustic neuroma
right sided, 158–161
Small, purely intracanalicular acoustic neuroma
left sided, 153–155
right sided, 156–157
Somatosensory evoked potentials (SSEPs), 31
Somatostatin (SMS), 11
Squamous temporal bone, 177
Superior cerebellar convexity meningioma, 130
extending to CPA (left sided), 162–164
Supraorbital endoscopic keyhole approach, 89
access to lesions of midline anterior skull base, 89–90
anterior cranial, regional endoscopic anatomy, 92
bone hyperostosis, removal, 107
burr hole and keyhole craniotomy, 91–92
collagen dural substitute membrane and dural sealant, use of, 93
CSF leak, prevention, 107
draping and skin incision, 91
dura closure, 93
dural opening, 92
enophthalmos and pulsatile exophthalmos, prevention, 107
instruments requirement, 90
keyhole bone flap, reposition, 93–94
operating room setup, 90
postoperative frontal edema or contusion, to avoid, 107
potential complications of, 101, 106–107
reflected dura, 92
Steri-Strips and adhesive bandage dressing, 93
supine placement, patient, 90
two-stage endoscopic approaches, for complete resection, 107
Suprasellar cystic lesions, 77
Suprasellar lesions, 76
Suprasellar meningioma, 84–88
coronal contrasted T1-weighted MRI, 84
olfactory and optic nerve, 84–85
postoperative T1-weighted, contrast-enhanced sagittal and coronal MRI, 87–88
resection of, 87
right and left anterior clinoid process, 85
sagittal contrasted T1-weighted MRI, 84

T

Temporal lobe retractors, 187
Thyroid-stimulating hormone (TSH), 11, 48
Thyrotropin-releasing hormone (TRH), 11
Thyroxine (T4), 11
Traditional middle fossa subtemporal approach, 187
Traditional pterional and bifrontal, 2
Traditional translabyrinthine, 2
Transseptal transsphenoidal microsurgical technique, 43
Transsphenoidal surgery, for cyst, 77
Trigeminal nerve irritation, 8

Trigeminal neuralgia, 113–115
  left sided, 116–118
  right sided, 119
  right sided, post-gamma knife twice, 115, 121–122
Trigeminal schwannoma
  gradual resection of, 181–182
  lower aspect of temporal lobe, 182
  maxillary (V2) division, of trigeminal nerve, 182
  postoperative contrast- enhanced coronal MRIs, 183
  sagittal and coronal MRIs, 179
  sharp dissection of posterior capsule of, 182
Triiodothyronine (T3), 11
TSH-secreting tumors, 16. *See also* Pituitary tumors

U

Urinary free cortisol (UFC), 13

V

Valsalva maneuver, 6, 8
Vestibular (acoustic) schwannoma, 120
Vestibular schwannoma surgery, 171
Vestibular schwannomas (VSs), 109
Videocassette recorders (VCRs), 31
Visual evoked potentials (VEPs), 31
von Hippel–Lindau (VHL), 21

FSC
www.fsc.org
MIX
Papier | Fördert gute Waldnutzung
FSC® C083411

Kolibri 360 GmbH
Ferdinand-Jühlke-Straße 7
99095 Erfurt, Deutschland
produktsicherheit@kolibri360.de